FUNCTIONAL ANATOMY

Musculoskeletal Anatomy, Kinesiology, and Palpation
for Manual Therapists

FUNCTIONAL ANATOMY

Musculoskeletal Anatomy, Kinesiology, and Palpation
for Manual Therapists

Christy Cael BS, ATC, CSS, LMP

Faculty member
Massage Connection School of Natural Healing
Tacoma, WA.

Wolters Kluwer | Lippincott Williams & Wilkins
Health
Philadelphia • Baltimore • New York • London
Buenos Aires • Hong Kong • Sydney • Tokyo

Acquisitions Editor: John Goucher
Marketing Manager: Christen Murphy
Manufacturing Manager: Margie Orzech
Development Editor: Jennifer P. Ajello
Design Coordinator: Doug Smock
Production Services: Absolute Service/MDC

Printed in the People's Republic of China

Library of Congress Cataloging-in-Publication Data

Cael, Christy.
  Functional anatomy : musculoskeletal anatomy, kinesiology, and palpation for manual therapists / Christy Cael.
    p. ; cm.
  Includes bibliographical references and index.
  ISBN 978-0-7817-7404-8
  1. Musculoskeletal system—Anatomy. 2. Kinesiology. 3. Manipulation (Therapeutics) I. Title.
  [DNLM: 1. Musculoskeletal System—anatomy & histology. 2. Movement—physiology. 3. Musculoskeletal Physiological Phenomena. 4. Palpation. WE 101 C127f 2010]
  QM100.C34 2010
  611'.7—dc22

2009010983

The publishers have made every effort to trace the copyright holders for borrowed material. If they have inadvertently overlooked any, they will be pleased to make the necessary arrangements at the first opportunity.

To purchase additional copies of this book, call our customer service department at **(800) 638-3030** or fax orders to **(301) 223-2320.** International customers should call **(301) 223-2300.**

Visit Lippincott Williams & Wilkins on the Internet: http://www.LWW.com. Lippincott Williams & Wilkins customer service representatives are available from 8:30 am to 6:00 pm, EST.

10 11 12 13 14
2 3 4 5 6 7 8 9 10

For Alla.

None of this would have been possible without your love, support, skill, knowledge, participation, insight, unwavering faith, and magical powers.

I am forever grateful.

Reviewers

Kate Anagnostis, ATC, LMT, CKTP
Sports Massage Instructor
Downeast School of Massage
Waldoboro, ME

Amy Appel
Program Director
Massage Therapy Department
P.H.D. Academy
Eau Claire, WI

William Burke, BA
Instructor
Department of Health, Human and Protective Services
Madison Area Technical College
Madison, WI

Patricia Coe, DC
Massage Therapy Clinic Supervisor
Department of Massage
National University of Health Sciences
Lombard, IL

Kirsten Grimm, BS, MS, LMT
Owner/Director/Therapist
Snug Harbor Natural Health Spa
North Muskegon, MI

Josh Herman, ATC, LMBT
Massage Therapy Program Director
Miller-Motte College
Cary, NC

William Raich, NCTMB
Massage Chair
Massage Therapy Department
Rasmussen College
Brooklyn Park, MN

Rachel Miller, BA, LMT
Massage Therapist
Private Practice
Harpswell, ME

Preface

Today's massage, bodywork, and fitness professionals are increasingly becoming members of the healthcare team. These professionals collaborate with physicians, physical therapists, occupational therapists, chiropractors, nurse care managers, attorneys, insurance companies, and other healthcare providers. Professionals must have a clear understanding of muscle and joint function beyond simple actions. This allows them to communicate clearly, maintain credibility, and obtain reimbursement for therapeutic work. The emerging requirement for "outcome-based" justification of treatments further supports the need for a thorough understanding of the body in motion.

Functional Anatomy was written to help students of human movement and bodywork understand how anatomical structures work together to create motion. Developing an understanding of the body in all of its complex synchronicity is critical for students of massage and bodywork. These careers require the therapist to create concise and effective treatment plans. Fitness and sports professionals are routinely called upon to analyze complex movement patterns in order to maximize the athlete's performance and prevent injury.

Beyond these pragmatic benefits, an understanding of functional anatomy develops heightened intellectual and artistic appreciation of the human body in motion. With a deep understanding of structure–function relationships, we begin to see the client's body as a living, breathing, *moving* marvel. *Functional Anatomy: Musculoskeletal Anatomy, Kinesiology, and Palpation for Manual Therapists* can assist you in exploring the structures and anatomical relationships responsible for movements such as walking, running, lifting, and throwing. You will be guided through activities that involve inspecting, touching, and moving these structures, enabling you to create a solid, three-dimensional image of the human body and its movement potential.

ORGANIZATION AND CONTENT

The chapters in *Functional Anatomy* are organized to build anatomical regions "from the ground up." This means deeper structures are identified first, and then structural layers are added. This organization helps readers understand the relationship between static structures such as bones, ligaments, and joint capsules and dynamic functions of muscles. Muscles are presented from superficial to deep to develop systematic palpation skills. *Functional Anatomy* also groups muscles together functionally. For example, the latissimus dorsi and teres major are located next to each other in the body, have a common insertion, and perform the same actions. Because of this, they are considered sequentially in Chapter 4.

The first three chapters in the book describe how the body is put together and how it achieves movement. In Chapter 1, the basic structures and systems of the body, the text's organization of the layers of the human body, and the language of anatomy and movement are discussed and explored. Chapter 2 provides an in-depth investigation of bones and joints, including their basic structure, various shapes and functions, classification, and location of the different types in the body. Chapter 3 delves into skeletal muscles, including their functions, properties, fiber directions and types, the different types of contractions they create, and how they are regulated. After studying these introductory chapters, you should understand the basic structures of the body and methods for creating movement. You will also have developed a language for discussing these concepts.

Each of the remaining six chapters explores a specific region of the body. These chapters follow a consistent template, with the same type of information occurring at the same place in each chapter. This predictability will help you locate any topic within a given chapter quickly and easily.

The recurring elements in the first half of each chapter include, in order:

- competency-based objectives
- overview of the region
- surface anatomy
- skeletal structures
- bony landmark palpation
- muscle attachment sites
- joints and ligaments
- superficial muscles of the region
- deep muscles of the region
- special structures located in the region (other than bones, ligaments, and muscles)
- movements allowed by the region's joints
- passive and resisted range of motion techniques

This opening section is followed by a set of one- or two-page profiles of each muscle pertinent to that region. Profiles include an illustration of the muscle showing its origin, insertion, and fiber arrangement and direction. Text descriptions of the muscle attachments, actions, and innervations are located next to this image. The profile also includes a description of the muscle's functional anatomy; that is, the relationships it has with other muscles, how it works in the body beyond its actions, and common imbalances or dysfunctions associated with it. Finally, the profile explains in simple, easy-to-follow steps how to palpate and fire the muscle against resistance. A photograph shows proper positioning of the practitioner and client, as well as the pertinent bony landmarks and muscle features. The simple, consistent design of each muscle profile ensures ease of use in the classroom or lab, as well as for studying and quick reference.

A section discussing the functional aspects of the body region follows the muscle profiles. This section includes information on synergist and antagonist relationships and a photo essay called *Putting It in Motion*, which explores the structure–function relationships involved during activities of daily living and sport.

Every chapter of the book closes with a concise summary, review questions, and study activities. The latter includes specific exercises aimed at kinesthetically engaging the covered material.

FEATURES

Functional Anatomy will guide you to a deeper understanding of the structure and function of the human body by engaging not only your mind, but also your other senses. Features include dynamic, colorful visuals, kinesthetic exercises to enhance your palpatory skills, and individual and group activities. Each region of the body is explored from the inside out to enhance understanding of structural relationships and movement possibilities. Simple, easy-to-follow instructions for palpation of bony landmarks and each muscle profiled are provided.

Functional Anatomy recognizes that you may be experiencing the challenges of learning a new language. To help you in acquiring this new language, we include within each muscle profile a guide to correct pronunciation of the muscle name. The companion Web site (thePoint.lww.com/cael) also includes an auditory guide to pronunciation, so you can hear proper pronunciation of each muscle profiled.

A *Synergist/Antagonist* table is included in each regional chapter. A photograph of a specific body motion, such as flexion or extension, is accompanied by a list of all muscles that contribute to that motion. Each motion is paired with its opposite in order to help you appreciate balanced muscle relationships.

Each regional chapter also discusses and illustrates passive and resisted range of motion procedures for assessing normal joint function. This is included to help you physically access the specific structures identified in this text.

As mentioned earlier, each regional chapter contains a section called *Putting It in Motion*, which identifies and explains specific actions that contribute to motions we use in daily activity or in sports. The photographs of these movements are enhanced to show the pertinent muscle groups driving the action. This feature is linked to the animations on the student resource site, which further explore some of these movements.

The *Try This* activity located at the end of each chapter includes a simple, kinesthetic activity that engages one or more key concepts identified in the chapter. Easy-to-follow steps are listed, as well as any special equipment that may be needed. For example, the *Try This* in Chapter 1 instructs readers to verbally position or move a partner in ways described on cards they create. This activity engages multiple senses and encourages correct use of anatomical terms and concepts.

The student resource site for this text has been developed alongside this manuscript in order to ensure strong connections between the special features of the book, student study materials, and teacher resources. Although the text is a stand-alone product, it can be greatly enhanced when used in conjunction with the companion student resource site at thePoint.lww.com/cael. Features of the resource site include animations that correspond with the *Putting It in Motion* segment in each regional chapter. These animations sequentially reveal muscle functions during common activities such as walking, jogging, standing, and throwing. Other features include video footage of palpation, study questions for self-assessment, a Stedman's audio glossary of the muscles profiled, and searchable full text online. The inside front cover of the text contains more details including the passcode you will need to gain access to the site. In addition to the student resources, instructors will also have access to lesson plans, PowerPoint presentations, and Brownstone Test Generator.

DESIGN

The design of *Functional Anatomy* creates a user-friendly, predictable, and interactive experience for readers. The text and art are arranged to allow quick-reference for study as well as maximum usability during classroom activities such as guided palpation exercises. Specific icons identify where these activities are located and when they are linked to the ancillary materials. All of these features will help you develop competency in the key skills identified in each of the chapter objectives.

FINAL NOTE

I hope that *Functional Anatomy* helps you discover new and exciting things about the human body. It is intended to enhance your personal and classroom experience and engage you in exploring how the body works. I encourage you to try as many of the activities as possible, utilize the learning tools provided, and embark upon your educational journey with wonder and curiosity.

Please contact me at functionalbook@hotmail.com with any comments or suggestions about this book. My students have always been both an inspiration and my toughest critics, and I wish for that to continue. Your perceptions, responses, and experiences with this text are valuable and I am interested in what you have to share. In the meantime, thank you and enjoy.

– Christy Cael

Acknowledgments

Producing *Functional Anatomy* has been a journey requiring the effort, enthusiasm, and patience of many. I would like to thank those who have believed in me and this project, contributed their vast knowledge and expertise, and tolerated my distraction, as well as my single-minded immersion.

First, the team at Lippincott, Williams, and Wilkins: Pete Darcy, thank you for the opportunity to begin the process. John Goucher, thank you for having a vision and giving me the chance to manifest my own. Your steady presence and joyful giggle are both greatly appreciated. Linda Francis, you helped me dive into uncharted waters with patience and grace and I am so happy to hear your calm and cheerful voice on the palpation video. Jennifer Ajello, you have talked me down so many times. I am so grateful to have you in my corner. I cannot express how much I appreciate your talent, dedication, and creativity. I have been lucky to have you. Rachelle Detweiler, a woman of so many talents. You have been willing to take on everything I've thrown your way without complaint. I appreciate your tireless commitment, no matter how many "do-overs" I have requested. Jennifer Clements, the "behind-the-scenes" art problem-solver. Your contributions have not gone unnoticed and I hope I have not proven as difficult as I think I have. And to all of the unsung heroes who made the pieces come together into something I feel very proud of, thank you.

Laura Bonozzoli, I am a better writer and researcher because you have challenged me and kept me honest. I have grown in so many ways because of your dogged determination to make this project great. I look back at early drafts and recognize the fruits of your steady mentorship. Photographer Bob Riedlinger, the images turned out so beautifully in great part to your steady hand, mindful approach, and gentle willingness. It has been a tremendous pleasure working with you personally and the images you have helped create. All of the artists, you have exceeded my expectations and I extend my deepest gratitude for all that you do. Specifically, I would like to acknowledge the tremendous efforts of Art Director Craig Durant and Artists Rob Duckwall, Mike Demaray, Rob Ferdirko, and Helen Wordham of Dragonfly Media Group. You have brought forth the vision that inspired this text.

Family, friends, and neighbors: Alla Kammers, you have contributed to the initiation and completion of this project on all levels. How lucky am I to have a partner who is also a massage therapist, kinesiologist, teacher, great listener, and contributor. Looking across my desk and asking, "Can you listen to this?" or "Does this make sense?" has been such a gift. Your willingness to problem-solve, demonstrate, critique, support, and take care of the mundane details of life has been a blessing. This success belongs to you equally. Cameron Buhl, Suzanne Wright, Dusty Hughes, and Eva Rasor, thank you for coming over at my whim to be poked, prodded, and photographed. Those informal "photo shoots" in the massage room were critical in realizing the visual components of this book. Thank you for being willing and available. Anne Williams, you have been my cheerleader from the very beginning. Your belief and willingness to hear me cry, rage, and celebrate has been invaluable. I am also tremendously grateful for your compassion and constructive criticism from one author to another. All my other friends and family, thank you for listening and tolerating my absence. Every one of you has been supportive in some way and I look forward to a collective celebration and return to normalcy.

My extended family at Ashmead/Everest College in Fife, Washington, please know that this accomplishment also belongs to you. You have incubated my career from wet-behind-the-ears instructor to what I am today. You are one of the most dynamic, creative, and supportive teams I have ever had the pleasure of working with. My students have been no less influential in my professional and personal development. Every class and every student has challenged me and forced me to grow and learn. I am also incredibly grateful for my family at Associated Bodywork & Massage Professionals. Everyone at ABMP has embraced me and created an environment where each of us can explore our talents and develop balanced, meaningful lives. Thank you.

Tony Holgado, Eva Rasor, Regina Logan, Mary Senecal, Sarah Formica, Nadia Flusche, Nicole Auble, Donnell House, Debbie Bates, Chris Woon, Brit-Simone Sutter, Marty Kneeland, Erin Murphy, Alla Kammers, and Suzanne Wright, thank you all for giving up so much time to model for the photos and video. You each went "above and beyond" in patience and willingness. Those were some long days and I cannot thank you enough for your contribution. I hope you are each as pleased as I am with the end result and can take pride in this accomplishment.

Finally, I want to extend a hearty thanks to all of the reviewers that provided insight and accountability to this text. Your experience and knowledge guided the process and helped me to always remember my audience. There were many times that I wondered if I was on the right track or if anyone would understand what I was trying to convey. Your thoughtful comments and suggestions reminded me why I took this on and rekindled my excitement for the project many times. Your enthusiasm helped keep me going. Thank you all.

Contents

Introduction to the
Human Body

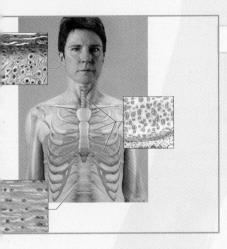

Imagine that a client is referred to you because he "can't use his arm." You might wonder what this means. Which joint is involved? What movements are affected? Or perhaps you've been further instructed to "look at his golf swing." How would you describe what you are seeing? Fortunately, a universal system of communication has been established to precisely describe the regions of the human body and their movements. This shared language, called *anatomical terminology*, allows for a common understanding and point of reference for professionals, scholars, and students. We begin by introducing you to this specialized language.

Human movement requires the coordinated efforts of several body structures. The bones and muscles provide a system of levers, which are held together by ligaments, tendons, joint capsules, and fascia. These are supported by special structures that provide nutrients, stimulation, or protection. We complete Chapter 1 by exploring these locomotive and special structures.

COMMUNICATING ABOUT THE BODY

When communicating about the human body, it is important to use the language that has been agreed upon by scientists, scholars, and health care providers.

Regional Terms

If a classmate were describing to you a tissue injury in a client's leg, you might assume that the injury was located in the thigh when your classmate actually meant the lower leg. To avoid such mix-ups, precise names are assigned to different regions of the body (FIG. 1-1). This is the first point of reference and the beginning of anatomical communication.

Anatomical Position

Even when using regional terminology, miscommunication can occur if both parties don't share the same point of reference. That's where the **anatomical position** comes in. In western medicine, anatomical position is described as body erect and facing forward, feet parallel, arms extended at the sides, and palms facing forward (FIG. 1-1A,B). This position of the body is used to describe the relative location of anatomical features as well as to describe movements of the various parts of the body. Most anatomical textbooks and charts utilize this position when depicting and describing the body's structures.

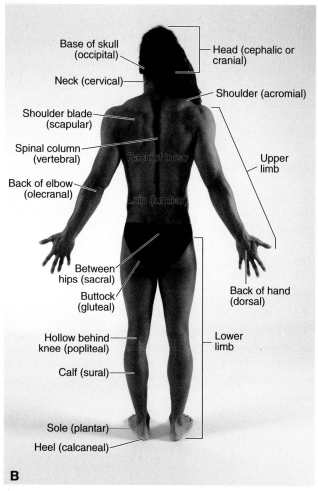

A

B

1-1. **Regions of the body in the anatomical position. A.** Anterior. **B.** Posterior.

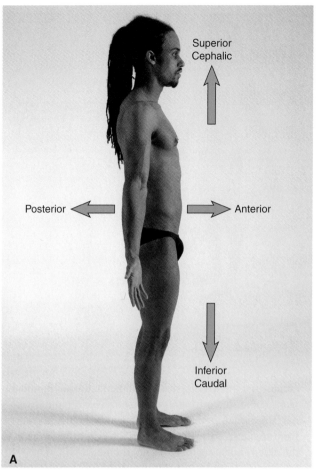

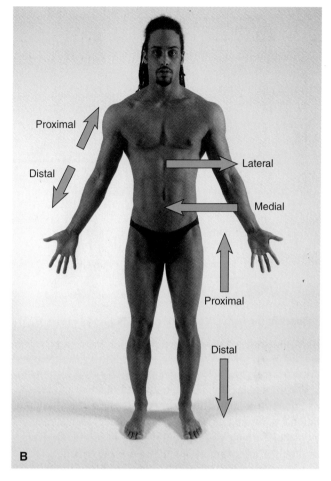

1-2. Directional terms. A. Lateral view. **B.** Anterior view.

Directional Terms

Starting from anatomical position, you can describe relative positions of different body structures (FIG. 1-2). For example:

- The chest is anterior to the spine.
- The hand is distal to the elbow; that is, the hand is farther from the point of attachment than the elbow, which is more proximal.
- The head is superior to the shoulders.
- The nose is medial to the ears; that is, the nose is closer to the body midline than the ears, which are more lateral.

Directional terms are useful for describing the location of injuries, as in, "The client is experiencing soreness about two inches proximal to the left patella." They are also useful when describing positions of the body, such as, "The athlete should finish the movement with the hands just lateral to the hips."

Relative terms not shown in Figure 1-2 describe how close to the surface of the body a structure lies. These include the terms **superficial** (closer to the surface) and **deep** (farther from the surface of the body). For example, the scalp is superficial to the skull, whereas the brain is deep to the skull.

Planes of Movement

Now that anatomical position and appropriate directional terminology have been established, we're ready to explore the language of human movement. The human body moves in complex ways, which can make description difficult. Scientists have categorized and simplified the terminology of human movement in an effort to heighten understanding and communication. This strategy encourages consistent description and analysis of complex human movements by breaking them down into simpler parts.

Motions occur at the joints of the body in one of three general directions: front to back, side to side, or rotationally. To describe these movements precisely, it helps to visualize the body transected by one of three large imaginary planes.

The first plane, which divides the body vertically into right and left halves, is called the **sagittal plane** (FIG. 1-3A). Front-to-back movements occur parallel to this imaginary plane. Swinging your arms and legs back and forth with walking are examples of sagittal movements.

The second plane divides the body into front and back halves. It is called the **frontal plane** (FIG. 1-3B). Side-to-side movements occur parallel to this imaginary plane. The arm and leg movements that occur when you do jumping jacks are examples of frontal movements.

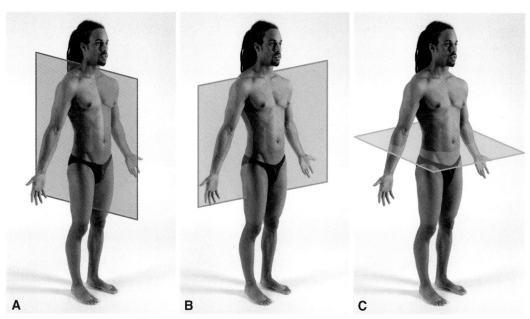

1-3. **Planes of the body. A.** Sagittal plane. **B.** Frontal plane. **C.** Transverse plane.

The third plane divides the body into superior and inferior regions. It is called the **transverse plane** (FIG. 1-3C). Rotational or turning movements occur parallel to this imaginary plane. Turning your leg out or your head to look over your shoulder are examples of transverse movements. The word *transverse* means "across," so a transverse view of the body is sometimes referred to as a *cross-section*.

Axes

Each of the three types of movement, sagittal (front-to-back), frontal (side-to-side), and transverse (rotational) must occur around an **axis** (a pivot point). Visualize a wheel turning on its axle. The axle is the axis that the wheel turns around. Each of the three planes of movements has a corresponding axis around which movement occurs. This axis is always perpendicular (at a right angle) to the corresponding plane.

Understanding these imaginary axes, along with their counterpart planes, helps us communicate precisely about movement. For example:

- The front-to-back movements that occur on the sagittal plane pivot around the **frontal axis** (FIG. 1-4A). This means that movements such as swinging your arms while walking (front to back) occur in the sagittal plane and pivot around an imaginary line that goes through the shoulder from right to left. This is also true when you bend forward at the waist. The body is moving in the sagittal plane (front to back) around a frontal axis (transecting at a right angle side to side) that goes through the pelvis.
- The side-to-side movements that occur in the frontal plane pivot around the **sagittal axis** (FIG. 1-4B). This

means that the leg and arm movements during jumping jacks occur in the frontal plane and pivot around imaginary lines that go through the hips and shoulders from front to back. This is also true when you tip your head to the side. This movement occurs on the frontal plane (side to side) around a sagittal axis (transecting at a right angle front to back) that goes through the cervical vertebrae of the neck.
- Finally, the rotational movements that occur on the transverse plane pivot around the **longitudinal axis** (FIG. 1-4C). For example, the movement of turning your head to look over your shoulder occurs in the transverse plane and pivots around an imaginary line that runs superiorly–inferiorly through the spine. Similarly, when you turn your shoulder to throw a Frisbee, your arm turns on the transverse plane (rotation) around a longitudinal axis through the shoulder (transecting at a right angle up and down).

Joint Movements

Movements that occur along each of the three planes and their corresponding axes have unique names. Motions that occur on the sagittal plane around the frontal axis are called **flexion** and **extension** (FIG. 1-5A). Flexion describes the bending of a joint on this plane so that the joint angle is made smaller. Extension describes the movement of a joint on this plane so that the joint angle is made larger.

Motions that occur on the frontal plane around a sagittal axis are called **abduction** and **adduction** (FIG. 1-5B). Abduction occurs when an extremity (arm or leg) or part of an extremity (hand, fingers, etc.) is moved away from the

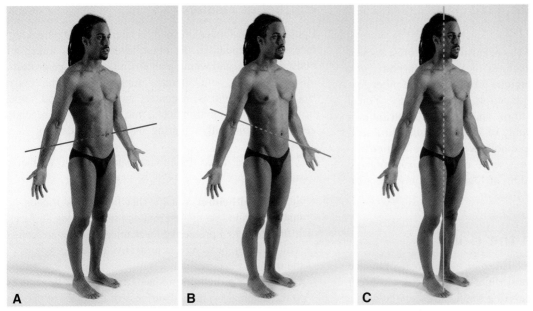

1-4. **Axes around which movement occurs.** **A.** Movements in the sagittal plane pivot around the frontal axis. **B.** Movements in the frontal plane pivot around the sagittal axis. **C.** Movements in the transverse plane pivot around the longitudinal axis.

center or **midline** of the body. Adduction occurs when an extremity or part of an extremity is moved toward the midline of the body. Remember, anatomical position is always the starting point when describing relative position or movement. Therefore, abducting the hand describes bending the wrist toward the thumb and adducting describes bending the wrist toward the pinky finger.

Finally, motions that occur on the transverse plane around the longitudinal axis are simply called **rotation** (FIG. 1-5C). Rotational movements in the trunk are differentiated as **right rotation** and **left rotation**, while these same move-ments in the extremities are termed **internal rotation** and **external rotation**. Internal rotation describes turning motions toward the midline and external rotation describes turning motions away from the midline of the body. These same motions are also called **medial** (internal) and **lateral** (external) rotation.

Specialty motions exist at several locations in the human body, including the scapula (shoulder blade), shoulder, forearm, wrist, hip, ankle, and foot. Each of these specialty motions will be discussed in appropriate chapters on these body regions.

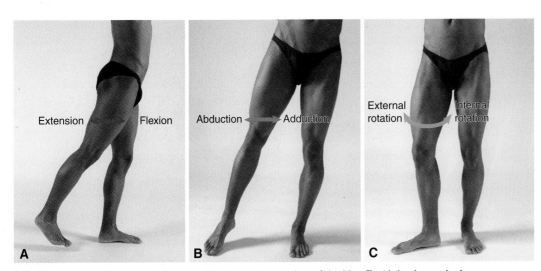

1-5. **Movements allowed by joints.** **A.** Flexion and extension of the hip. **B.** Abduction and ad-duction of the hip. **C.** Internal and external rotation of the hip.

STRUCTURES OF THE HUMAN BODY

Anatomy is the study of an organism's structures. As you begin to explore the structures of the human body, you will discover how their unique size, shape, and other features contribute to their function, or **physiology**. You'll also discover how both form and function contribute to human movement, the study of which is called **kinesiology**. Throughout this textbook, we will use written descriptions, images, and our sense of touch (palpation) to gain a deeper understanding of human anatomy, physiology, and kinesiology.

Tissue Types in the Body

A **tissue** is a group of cells that share a similar structure and function. The body is almost entirely composed of just four basic types of tissue: a covering tissue called *epithelium*, a supporting tissue called *connective tissue*, muscle tissue, and nervous tissue (FIG. 1-6).

Epithelial Tissue

Epithelial tissue covers the body's internal and external surfaces and is found in the outer layer of skin, lining the body's cavities, and within glands. Epithelial tissue protects, absorbs, filters, and secretes substances in the body. Because epithelium is in contact with external and sometimes destructive environments, this type of tissue regenerates easily, constantly repairing and replacing dead or damaged cells.

There are three functional categories of epithelial tissue:

- **Surface epithelium** contains sheetlike layers of cells that are located on the internal or external body surfaces. It functions as a protective mechanical barrier, as seen with the skin, or to secrete protective substances as in the urinary tract.
- **Glandular epithelium** produces and delivers substances to the external or internal surfaces of the body or directly into the bloodstream. Sweat glands, salivary glands, and tear glands are all comprised of glandular

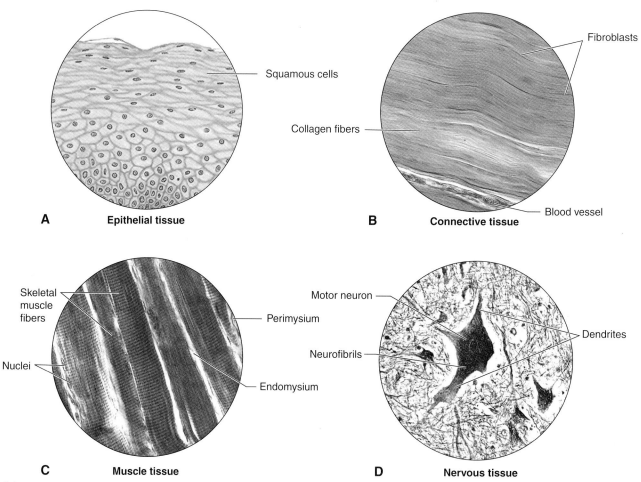

1-6. **The four tissue types in the body. A.** Epithelial tissue. **B.** Connective tissue. **C.** Muscle tissue. **D.** Nervous tissue.

epithelium, as are the pituitary, thyroid, and adrenal glands.
- **Sensory epithelium** contains specialized cells that are able to perceive and conduct specific stimuli. These cells are critical to the function of the special senses of hearing, sight, smell, and taste.

Connective Tissue

Of the four types of tissue, connective tissue is by far the most abundant: It is found in nearly all of the structures involved in human movement. Primary movement structures such as bone, tendons, ligaments, and fascia are considered connective tissues, as are support tissues such as cartilage, adipose (fat), and even blood.

Components of Connective Tissue

Connective tissue consists of individual cells scattered within an extracellular matrix (FIG. 1-7). The **extracellular matrix** is made up of various fibers suspended in a fluid known as **ground substance**. This fluid contains water, glycosaminoglycans, proteoglycans, and glycoproteins. Its unique chemistry allows the ground substance to exist as either watery liquid (sol) or firm solid (gel) depending upon chemical composition, amount of tension, and temperature. The term *thixotropy* describes the ability of the ground substance to become more liquid as movement and temperature of the tissue increases.

Suspended within the ground substance are three types of fibers:

- **Collagen fibers** are long, straight strands of protein wound together like rope. These fibers confer tensile strength and flexibility to connective tissue and are more abundant in tissues requiring strong resistance to force such as ligaments and tendons.

- **Reticular fibers** are thin proteins that resist force in multiple directions and help hold structures together. These fibers help hold supporting structures such as blood vessels and nerves in place.
- **Elastic fibers** contain the protein **elastin** and appear branched and wavy. Their presence confers resiliency to the connective tissue, allowing it to return to its original shape after being stretched.

Individual cells are scattered within the extracellular matrix. These cells vary according to the tissue's location and function, but typically include **fibroblasts**, cells that produce and secrete proteins that make up the fibers in the extracellular matrix. Specialized types of connective tissues have specific names for their fibroblasts; for example, in bone they are called **osteoblasts** and in cartilage they are called **chondroblasts**. Other examples of individual cells found in connective tissue include immune cells like **macrophages**, which respond to injury or infection, and **adipocytes** (fat cells) in which oil fills most of the internal space of the cell.

Types of Connective Tissue

Together the ground substance, specialized protein fibers, and individual cells within connective tissue make up a highly variable, dynamic structure. That is, connective tissue changes its appearance and function by varying the amounts and ratios of its component parts.

- **Loose connective tissue** has high levels of ground substance and fewer fibers. It includes adipose tissue (fat tissue) and the hypodermis, also called the superficial fascia, just below the skin.
- **Dense connective tissue** is thicker and stronger with more collagen fibers and less ground substance than loose connective tissue. Tendons, ligaments, joint capsules, and periosteum around bones are all examples of dense connective tissue.

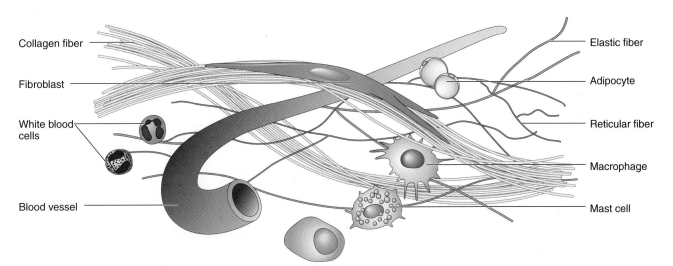

Collagen fiber

Fibroblast

White blood cells

Blood vessel

Elastic fiber

Adipocyte

Reticular fiber

Macrophage

Mast cell

1-7. **Cells and fibers of connective tissue.** Various cells within the ground substance allow connective tissue to support other tissues, transport nutrients and wastes, protect against invaders, and store energy. Collagen fibers, reticular fibers, and elastic fibers give connective tissue tensile strength, flexibility, and resiliency.

- **Fluid connective tissue** is watery because of the presence of plasma, which is 90% water, in the extracellular matrix. Blood and lymph are examples of fluid connective tissue.
- **Supporting connective tissue** is strong and solid because of the additional calcium salts deposited in its ground substance. Examples are cartilage and bone.

Since **connective tissue** is found throughout the body, it should not surprise you to learn that it has many functions; however, its main function is usually identified as supportive. Connective tissue forms a continuous network throughout the body, binding, supporting, and reinforcing other tissues. It also enables the body to transport nutrients and wastes, and houses immune cells that protect against harmful invaders. Finally, connective tissue stores energy in the form of fat cells.

Muscle Tissue

Muscle tissue is a network of muscle cells that contain contractile protein structures called myofibrils. The myofibrils are stimulated by the nervous system to contract or shorten, creating movement. The force generated by shortening of the myofibrils is transmitted into surrounding connective tissue called myofascia. This force is what drives internal and external human movement. Muscle tissue characteristics and types will be explored further in Chapter 3.

Nervous Tissue

Nervous tissue is a complex network of nerve cells, called *neurons*, and support cells. It has the unique ability to be stimulated, conduct a stimulus, and respond to stimulation. Electrical impulses travel from one neuron to another or between the neuron and other cells, such as muscle cells. These impulses serve as communication between the nervous system and other tissues, allowing the nervous system to monitor and regulate the body's internal and external environment. Nervous tissue and its role in movement will be explored further in "Special Structures" and later in Chapter 3.

BODY STRUCTURES INVOLVED IN HUMAN MOVEMENT

In this section we will explore the primary tissues of human movement, including bone, ligament, muscle, tendon, and fascia. It is important to understand the structure, function, location, and texture of each of these tissues. Important support structures are identified next, including skin, blood vessels, lymphatic vessels and nodes, nerves, cartilage, and bursae. Manual therapists must be aware of these structures to more clearly understand how the human body works and to avoid damaging these structures during palpation and engagement of other tissues.

| Box 1-1 | TIPS FOR PALPATION |

The following basic guidelines will help you learn to consciously explore anatomy through touch:

- **Visualize what you are about to feel.** It helps to have a picture or model of the structure nearby as you search and explore with your hands.
- **Go slowly and be patient.** Allow your brain time to register what is being felt with your hands.
- **Breathe and relax.** Consciously relax your hands and fingers by taking deep, calming breaths.
- **Close your eyes.** Removing sight heightens your other senses, including touch.
- **When in doubt, do less.** Don't force the structures you are palpating; rather, let them mold themselves into your waiting hands. Palpation should not be painful.
- **Allow for variation.** Expect differences from one person to another, as everyone has asymmetries and anatomical uniqueness.
- **Be curious.** You may find structures that differ from what you expect. This is because anatomy is influenced by genetic variation, habitual activities, and injury.
- **Practice.** Palpation is a skill that must be developed through repetition. Beginners are not expected to be perfect, just willing to try.

For each of the body structures discussed in this section, we will provide guidelines for palpation. In this way, you will learn to differentiate between different types of tissues by touch. General tips for palpation are provided in Box 1-1.

Bone

We are covering bone first because it is a fundamental structure of movement. It provides a complex architecture to the human body and a system of levers that muscles and tendons pull upon to create movement. It is also easy to palpate and provides crucial bony landmarks for finding muscles, tendons, and ligaments.

Also called *osseous tissue*, bone is a type of supporting connective tissue made up of collagen fibers and minerals that form the skeleton of the human body. The structure of this tissue resembles the rings of a tree on a microscopic level (FIG. 1-8). Individual bones are covered by a layer of dense connective tissue called *periosteum*.

Bone has many functions: It provides a framework that supports and allows movement of the body; it protects vulnerable structures such as the brain, spinal cord, and organs; it stores minerals such as potassium and calcium; and it is a site for hematopoiesis (formation of blood cells).

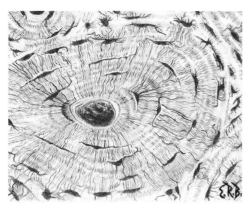

1-8. Microscopic view of bone. Osseous tissue is a mineralized supporting connective tissue that resembles the rings of a tree.

Shapes of Bones

Bones come in many shapes and sizes depending upon the person's age, gender, and activities, as well as the bone's function in the body (Fig. 1-9):

- **Long bones** have a distinct shaft in the middle with bumpy ends. Examples are the humerus (upper arm bone) and femur (thigh bone).

- Small, **short bones** are often cube-shaped and allow fine, gliding movements in the hand and foot.
- Some bones are **flat** and somewhat thin, like the sternum (breastbone) or ilium (one of the pelvic bones).
- **Irregular bones** are totally unique. These include the vertebrae of the spine and the facial bones.
- Finally, a unique type of bone called a **sesamoid bone** is encased in tendon and helps improve the leverage and strength of muscles that cross it. The patella (or kneecap) is a sesamoid bone.

The forces placed upon bones influence their shape. Gravity and compression determine the density of bones while tension from the pulling of tendons shapes their bumps and ridges. Familiarity with these topographical features can help you to understand the functions of bones and how they interact with other structures in the body. Types and functions of bones will be covered more thoroughly in Chapter 2.

Palpating Bone

We learn to palpate superficial bones next in our exploration because their firmness and constant shape make them easy to locate. Also, successful palpation of bone is necessary before we can find ligaments and tendons that hold bones

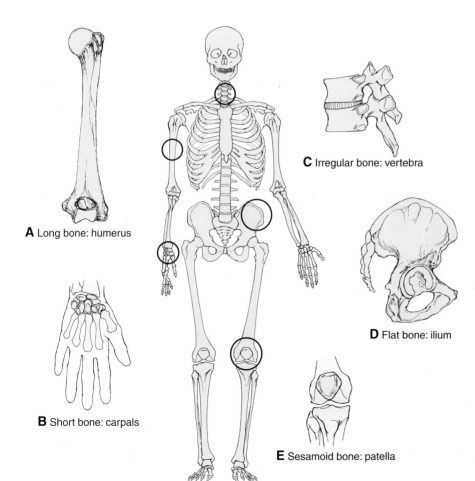

A Long bone: humerus

B Short bone: carpals

C Irregular bone: vertebra

D Flat bone: ilium

E Sesamoid bone: patella

1-9. Bone shapes. Bones come in many shapes and sizes depending upon the person's age, gender, and activities as well as the bone's function in the body. **A.** Long bones. **B.** Short bones. **C.** Irregular bones. **D.** Flat bones. **E.** Sesamoid bones.

together and connect muscles to them. Below are specific steps for palpating bone:

1. Hold your arm out in front of you with your elbow bent.

2. With the pads of your fingers and/or the palm of your hand, find the pointy end of your elbow (this is the olecranon process of the ulna) (FIG. 1-10).

3. Still palpating, bend and straighten your arm. The bone that you feel should retain its shape as you move your arm.

4. Keep the same position and move your fingertips and thumb toward the sides of your elbow. You should find two hard bumps, one on each side of your elbow (these are the epicondyles of the humerus).

5. Bend and straighten your elbow while gently holding these bumps with your fingers and thumb. They should also maintain their shape as you move your arm.

6. Gently feel for the edges and features of these structures. See how far you can follow the olecranon process of the ulna distally toward your hand. See how far you can follow the epicondyles of the humerus proximally toward your shoulder.

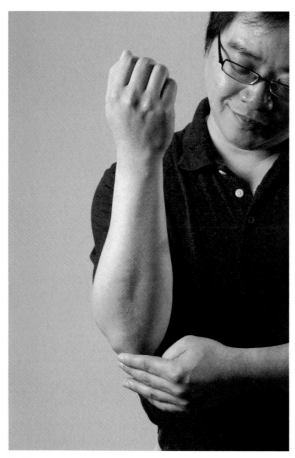

1-10. Palpating bone: finding the olecranon process.
The "point of the elbow" is the olecranon process of the ulna, a bone of the forearm. Joint movement at the elbow will not change the shape and feel of the olecranon process.

7. Practice this exercise on different parts of your body. Good places to practice are around the clavicle (collarbone), the patella (kneecap), and malleolus (ankle).

8. Practice this same exercise on different people. Compare yourself and these other people. What features and qualities are similar? What things are different?

Ligament

Ligaments are fibrous structures made of dense connective tissue that connect bones to each other. They prevent movements at joints and contribute to joint stability. Whereas muscles and tendons are considered **dynamic stabilizers** because of their ability to contract and stretch, thereby contributing to movement, ligaments are considered **static stabilizers** because they do not move.

Structure of Ligaments

Ligaments are composed of a complex network of collagen fibers that resist stress in multiple directions (FIG. 1-11). This tissue complexity also contributes to the gristly feel of ligaments as compared to the smooth feel of parallel-oriented tendons.

Ligaments are present at the ends of bones where they help form joints. Sometimes a network of ligaments will wrap around an entire joint, creating a **joint capsule**. We will explore the structure and function of joint capsules more thoroughly in Chapter 2.

Another structure related to ligaments is the **interosseous membrane**. This is a broad sheet of dense connective tissue that is thinner than ligaments and connects bones along the length of their shafts. Interosseous membranes are found in the forearm and lower leg and are too deep in the body to palpate.

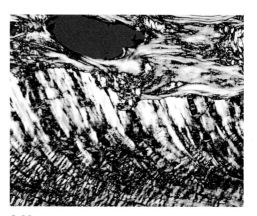

1-11. Microscopic view of ligament.
Ligaments connect the bones of the body to each other, providing static stability and preventing unwanted motion. The varying angles of collagen fibers allow ligaments to stabilize in multiple directions and contribute to their "gristly" feel when palpated.

Palpating Ligaments

Because ligaments and tendons often reside in similar locations in the body, they can be difficult to differentiate. One strategy for finding ligaments is to palpate the ends of two adjacent bones and then search for the fibrous connections between them. Movement will also help you differentiate these two types of tissue. Tendons will change shape and become more taught during muscle contractions, while ligaments remain relatively constant.

1. To palpate ligaments, let's move to our feet. Remove your shoes and socks and cross your legs with one foot resting on the opposite knee.

2. Find the medial malleolus (inside ankle bone) with the pad of your thumb (FIG. 1-12).

3. Move your thumb to the bottom edge of the anklebone and slightly anterior.

4. Actively move your foot around in circles as you press down with your thumb, locating the space between the ankle and foot bones. You should notice the gap between the bones opening and allowing the deltoid ligament to become closer to the surface and more easily palpated.

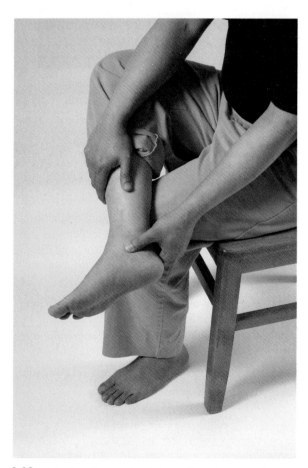

1-12. Palpating ligaments of the ankle. Cross one foot over the opposite knee and find the bottom edge of the anklebone. The deltoid ligament is gristly and connects the tibia to the calcaneous, navicular, and talus on the inside of the foot.

5. Several ligaments in addition to the deltoid ligament stabilize the ankle joint. Practice feeling the difference between the bones, the ligaments, and the tendons that reside around the ankle and foot.

6. Practice this exercise with different people and compare your results.

Muscle

Muscle is one of the four main types of body tissue. Although it is not connective tissue itself, it produces movement by pulling on the dense connective tissue that forms tendons and attaches to the periosteum of bones. Specific characteristics and functions of muscles will be discussed further in Chapter 3.

Types of Muscle

There are three types of muscle in the human body:

- **Smooth muscle** is present in the walls of hollow organs, vessels, and respiratory passageways, where it functions in digestion, urinary excretion, reproduction, circulation, and breathing. We cannot consciously control smooth muscle; thus, it is referred to as **involuntary**.
- **Cardiac muscle** makes up the wall of the heart. It creates the pulsing action necessary to circulate blood through the body. This muscle type is also involuntary.
- **Skeletal muscles** are connected to bones and create movements at joints. This type of muscle tissue is **voluntary**; that is, it is under our conscious control. Of the three types of muscle tissue, skeletal muscle is most pertinent to our study of human movement.

Skeletal muscles have several unique features that help differentiate them from other tissues such as bones. First, they are made up of distinct bundles of parallel fibers, giving them a corrugated feel compared with bones and tendons, which are smoother (FIG. 1-13). These "corrugations"

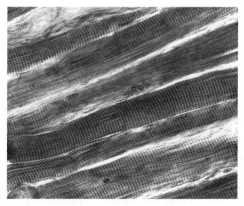

1-13. Skeletal muscle fibers. The parallel bundles of skeletal muscle fibers help distinguish them from other structures such as bones, tendons, and ligaments when palpated.

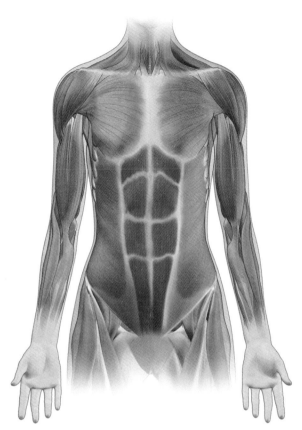

1-14. Fiber directions. Skeletal muscles have distinct fiber directions and arrangements, which reflect their function. Knowing these directions will help you identify the muscles during palpation.

also have distinct alignments, referred to as their **fiber direction**. As you palpate muscles, knowing a given muscle's fiber direction can help you identify it and distinguish it from other muscles nearby (FIG. 1-14). The properties of muscle tissue and functions of muscles will be explored further in Chapter 3 of this text.

Skeletal muscles change shape as the body moves. When a muscle is stretched, it becomes longer and the fibers feel taught, like a tightened rope. In contrast, when a muscle contracts it becomes thicker in the center and firmer throughout. You can see this on your own body by viewing your arm fully relaxed, and then with your hand clenched in a tight fist.

Palpating Muscle

Deep muscles are difficult for beginners to palpate. So let's begin our exploration of muscle palpation with some superficial muscles:

1. Wrap your hand around your opposite forearm, just distal to the elbow. With your forearm relaxed, the flesh should feel soft and pliable (FIG. 1-15).

2. Slowly bend your wrist back and forth. Notice how the flesh under your palm changes as you move your other wrist back and forth.

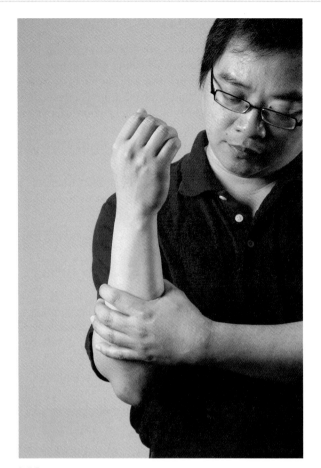

1-15. Palpating muscle tissue. Find the forearm muscles by grasping with your opposite hand. The muscles will change shape as they alternately contract and stretch.

3. Pay attention to which movement makes the muscles feel stretched and taught and which makes the muscles feel contracted and thick.

4. Wrap your hand around different locations on the forearm and continue this exercise. Are there locations that move more than others? Can you visualize what the muscles look like under your hand? How does muscle feel compared to bone?

5. Try this exercise on different parts of your body. Good places to practice are around the shoulder and knee. Use movement to stretch and contract muscles in order to more clearly visualize them.

6. Try this same exercise with different people. Compare your findings.

Tendon

The dense connective tissue that surrounds muscles converges to form a **tendon** (FIG. 1-16), which thereby connects the muscle to a bone. Tendons contain abundant collagen fibers, a basic component of connective tissue. These give tendons strength and elasticity as they transmit the forces produced by muscles into joint movement.

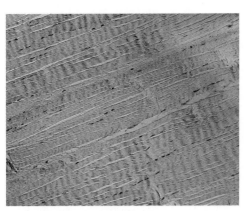

1-16. Microscopic view of tendon. Connective tissue surrounding bundles of muscle fibers converge to form tendons. This structure attaches muscles to the bones they move. The transition point between muscle and tendon is felt as tissue becomes smoother and firmer.

Shapes of Tendons

Like bones and muscles, tendons come in a variety of shapes and sizes depending on their function and location. They can be broad and flat like those in the small of the back, or long and cablelike such as those in the arm and wrist.

Tendons, like muscles, change shape as they stretch and contract. This feature helps us differentiate tendons from bones and ligaments. They also tend to be denser and smoother than muscles, another distinguishing characteristic.

Palpating Tendons

When palpating tendons, it helps to find a muscle and then follow the fibers until they become smoother prior to attaching to bone. This transition to smoother tissue is that convergence from the muscle's connective tissue wrapping to its tendon.

1. To explore palpation of tendons, let's use a group whose location and movement we can find easily: lay the pad of your thumb across the inside of your opposite wrist (FIG. 1-17).

2. Gently strum your thumb back and forth, feeling the tendons just under the skin.

3. Hold your thumb still as you open and close your hand. Do the tendons move and change? How?

4. Continue to hold your thumb still as you wiggle your fingers. Do the tendons move and change? How?

5. Follow the tendons with the pad of your thumb proximally toward the elbow. Can you feel when the tendons transition to muscle?

6. Follow the tendons distally toward the hand. Can you feel where the tendons insert on the bone? This is more easily felt when following tendons on the back of the hand.

7. Repeat this process at different locations in your body. Good places to practice are around the patella (kneecap) and the dorsal surface of the foot.

8. Try this exercise with different people and compare your findings.

Fascia

Fascia (pronounced fash´ē•ǎ) is a thin membrane of loose or dense connective tissue that covers the structures of the body, protecting them and binding them into a structural unit. Different configurations of fascia surround bones, muscles, and joints. Fascia also separates skin, layers of muscle, body compartments, and cavities. In addition, it forms sheaths for nerves and vessels that anchor them near the structures they regulate or nourish. It also forms or thickens ligaments and joint capsules. In short, fascia creates a continuous matrix that interconnects all structures of the body.

Structure of Fascia

Fascia comes in many forms and is separated into layers. Multiple layers with individual collagen fiber directions give fascia its unique appearance and feel (FIG. 1-18).

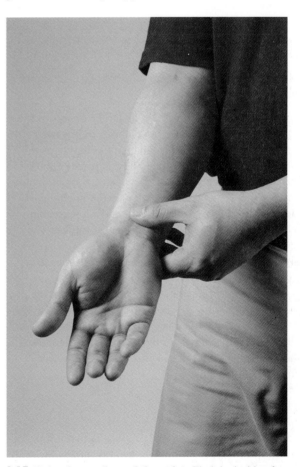

1-17. Palpating tendons of the wrist. Find the inside of the wrist with the pad of your opposite thumb. Joint movement at the wrist and hand will change the tension of underlying tendons.

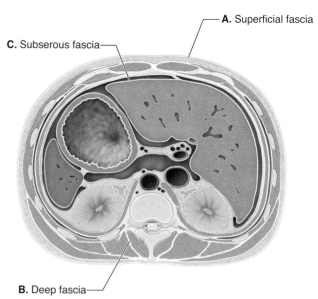

1-19. **Layers of fascia.** The different layers of fascia help organize and compartmentalize the structures of the body. **A.** *Superficial fascia* separates the skin from the hypodermis. **B.** *Deep fascia* separates individual muscles and muscle groups. **C.** *Subserous fascia* separates organs from the abdominal cavity.

1-18. **Microscopic structure of fascia.** Collagen fibers are arranged in fascia according to lines of tension and stress. This connective tissue creates overlapping sheets that resist tension and bind and separate structures, yet remain flexible.

Fascia Layers

As shown in FIGURE 1-19, there are three distinct layers of fascia:

* **Superficial fascia** lies directly under the dermis of the skin. It stores fat and water and creates passageways for nerves and vessels. We encountered this earlier as the *hypodermis*. The fascia located here is made of loose connective tissue.
* **Deep fascia** forms a convoluted network around muscles and their internal structures. It aids in muscle movements, provides passageways for nerves and vessels, provides muscle attachment sites, and cushions muscle layers. This fascial layer is made of dense connective tissue.
* **Subserous fascia** separates the deep fascia from the membranes that line the thoracic and abdominal cavities of the body. The loose connection between these layers allows for flexibility and movement of the internal organs. Like the deep fascia, subserous fascia is dense connective tissue.

Palpating Fascia

Fascia is unique from other body tissues in that it links different structures together, binding and organizing the body. The complexity of the fascial network is hinted at on the surface of the body with *Langer's lines*: normal, permanent skin creases that reflect the fiber orientation of the fascia and muscles that lie below (FIG. 1-20). Fascia can feel wavy,

dense, or smooth upon palpation, depending on location and the health of the tissue.

Like all connective tissue, fascia has the ability to be solid and firm or liquid and fluid in nature. Which form it takes depends upon temperature, pressure, and tension applied to the tissue. This, in combination with its presence in multiple layers and nearly everywhere in the body, can make palpation of fascia more challenging than palpation of the other structures of human movement. Let's start by trying to palpate the fascia of your elbow and forearm:

1. Slightly flex one arm and grasp the loose skin at the point of your elbow with the thumb and fingers of your opposite hand (FIG. 1-21).
2. Grasp firmly and see if you can roll the flesh between your fingers. This is the superficial fascia.
3. Bend and straighten your elbow as you keep hold of the flesh between your fingers. Feel the alternating tension and slack.
4. Grasp in the same way at different locations on your forearm. Find a mark on your skin, such as a freckle, mole, or scar, or make a pen mark somewhere on your arm. Keeping your eyes on the mark, see if you can cause it to move by pulling the flesh on different parts of your arm.
5. Practice this exercise at different locations on your body such as your patella (kneecap) or abdomen (belly). Compare the "movement" of the flesh at different locations. See if the amount of movement changes the more you palpate the area.

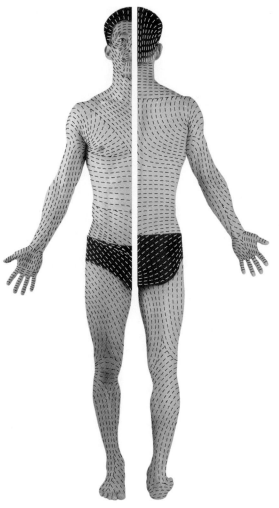

Anterior view   Posterior view

1-20. Langer's lines. These are normal, permanent skin creases that reflect the fiber orientation of the superficial fascia and the muscles that lie below.

6. Practice this exercise on different people. Compare "movement" as well as sensitivity in different areas and people.

SPECIAL STRUCTURES

As we explore the structures responsible for human movement, we must be aware of complementary structures existing within the body. Bones, muscles, tendons, ligaments, and fascia are mechanically responsible for movement, but other body systems and structures protect, nourish, regulate, and support their function. These special structures include skin, blood vessels, lymphatic vessels and lymph nodes, nerves, cartilage, and bursae. Each contributes to healthy and efficient movement.

Skin

One continuous structure, the **skin** covers the entire body. It protects against outside invaders and radiation, helps regu-

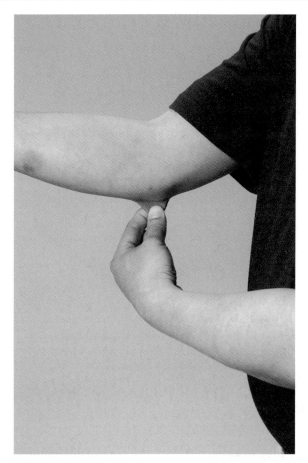

1-21. Palpating fascia at the elbow. Using your thumb and forefinger, grasp the loose superficial fascia around the olecranon process of the elbow. Roll it between your fingers and gently pull it in different directions to see how fascia feels and is moved.

late internal temperature, and excretes certain waste products. Through its complex system of sensory receptors, skin helps us interact with the outside environment.

Structure of the Skin

The skin is composed of three tissue layers (Fig. 1-22): the epidermis, dermis, and hypodermis:

- The covering *epidermis* is epithelial tissue, one of the four main types we introduced earlier. It contains several thin layers of cells, which produce a protective protein called *keratin* and a pigment protein called *melanin*. The epidermis also contains defensive cells that protect against foreign substances.
- Beneath the epidermis is an underlying *dermis*, which is mostly dense connective tissue. It contains hair follicles, glands, nerves, blood vessels, and tiny muscles.
- The *hypodermis* lies beneath the dermis (*hypo-* means beneath). This loose connective tissue layer contains adipose cells that cushion and protect underlying structures. Another name for the hypodermis is the *superficial fascia*.

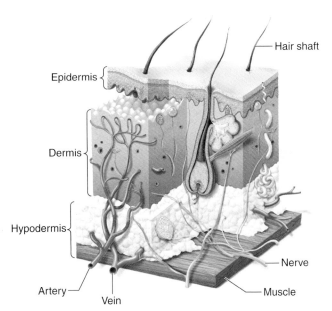

1-22. **Layers of the skin.** The skin is composed of three layers: a covering *epidermis*; a thicker *dermis* containing hair follicles, glands, nerves, blood vessels, and muscles; and an underlying layer containing fat cells, called the *hypodermis.*

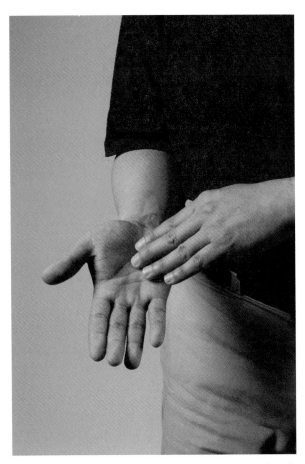

1-23. **Palpating skin.** Palpation of the skin on the palm of the hand.

Like all anatomical structures, the skin adapts to its location, function, and environment. For example, the epidermis is thickened where it encounters friction on the fingertips, palms of the hand, and the soles of the feet. The dermis contains more nerve cells on the fingertips, which give us tactile sensitivity, than on the soles of the feet, which have to endure constant pressure.

Palpating Skin

Skin is the most superficial tissue and therefore very easy to palpate. Pay attention to the temperature, pliability, and texture of skin as you palpate. Below are specific steps for palpating skin:

1. Place the pads of your index finger on the palm of your opposite hand (FIG. 1-23).

2. Brush your fingertips lightly over the skin without moving it. Is the skin smooth or rough? Are there ridges, bumps, or calluses? Is the skin oily, sweaty, or dry? What color is the skin? Repeat on the back of the hand.

3. Bring your fingertips again to the palm of your hand.

4. Keep both hands relaxed and make small, deep circles with your fingertips on your palm. Try and make the skin move.

5. Open your hand wider and observe if the skin changes.

6. Repeat this exercise on the back of your hand. What qualities are different about the skin on the palm of your hand compared to the back? What qualities are the same? Do any of these qualities change with your touch?

7. Try this exercise on different parts of your body and compare your findings.

8. Try this exercise on different people and compare your findings.

Blood Vessels

Blood vessels are part of the circulatory system, the pathway by which blood flows throughout the body (FIG. 1-24). The circulation of blood is necessary to deliver oxygen and nutrients to the body's tissues, and remove wastes. Blood vessels vary in size from large arteries and veins to smaller arterioles and venules to the smallest capillaries where gases, nutrients, and waste products are exchanged between the blood and individual cells (FIG. 1-25).

This network of blood vessels is woven throughout the body, existing side by side with lymphatic structures, nerves, and the structures of movement. Use caution when palpating near these structures to avoid damaging these vessels. Palpating a pulse under your fingers is an indication that you have compressed a blood vessel, particularly an artery.

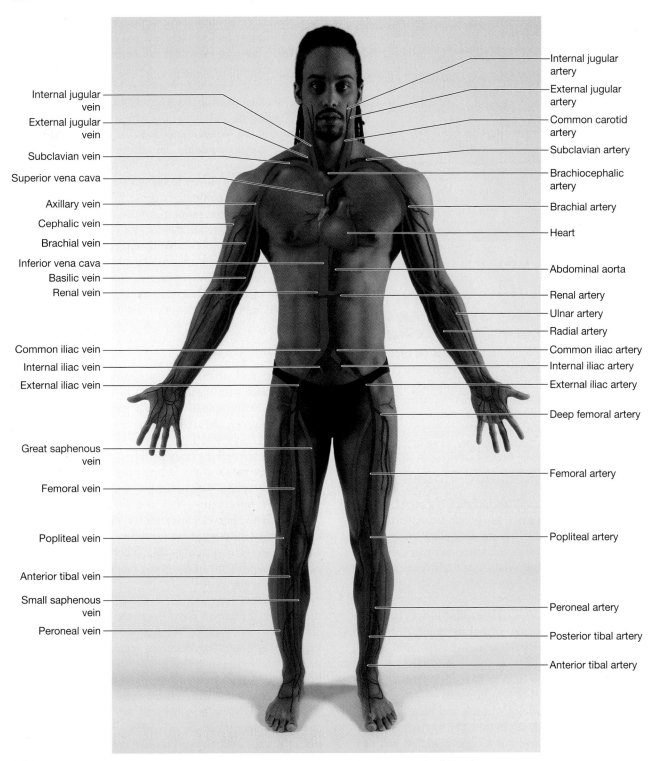

Internal jugular artery

External jugular artery

Common carotid artery

Subclavian artery

Brachiocephalic artery

Brachial artery

Heart

Abdominal aorta

Renal artery

Ulnar artery

Radial artery

Common iliac artery

Internal iliac artery

External iliac artery

Deep femoral artery

Femoral artery

Popliteal artery

Peroneal artery

Posterior tibial artery

Anterior tibial artery

Internal jugular vein

External jugular vein

Subclavian vein

Superior vena cava

Axillary vein

Cephalic vein

Brachial vein

Inferior vena cava

Basilic vein

Renal vein

Common iliac vein

Internal iliac vein

External iliac vein

Great saphenous vein

Femoral vein

Popliteal vein

Anterior tibal vein

Small saphenous vein

Peroneal vein

1-24. Circulatory system. The circulatory system includes the heart and a vast network of blood vessels that ensure the transport of blood to and from all body tissues.

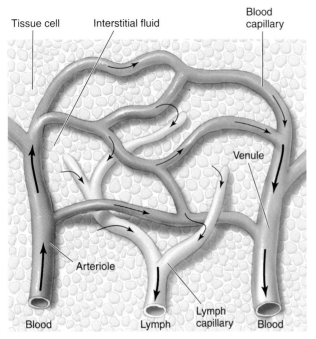

1-25. Capillary bed. This is the smallest unit of the circulatory system, where the exchange of nutrients and waste products occurs. Lymph vessels lie near these circulatory structures collecting fluid from surrounding tissue.

Lymphatic Vessels and Nodes

The complex lymphatic system includes lymphoid organs, lymph nodes, lymphatic ducts, and lymphatic vessels (FIG. 1-26). Its two primary functions are to collect excess fluid, called **lymph**, from the body's tissues and return it to the circulatory system, and to produce and distribute *lymphocytes*, which are special cells that help the body fight infection and disease.

Lymph circulates in a manner that is very different from the circulation of blood. Lymphatic capillaries collect the lymph from the blood capillaries and *insterstitial space*, or space between tissue cells, as shown in Figure 1-24. They then transport the lymph fluid to larger lymphatic vessels, along which lie hundreds of **lymph nodes**, tiny organs that cleanse it of foreign particles, viruses, and bacteria (FIG. 1-27). Lymph enters the node via the *afferent lymphatic vessels*, is filtered and cleansed of foreign particles, and then exits the node via the *efferent lymphatic vessel*, continuing its journey through progressively larger vessels of the lymphatic system. From the larger vessels, cleansed lymph drains into either of two lymphatic ducts in the chest, the *right lymphatic duct* or the *thoracic duct*, which then release the lymph into large veins of the chest.

Lymphoid organs include the lymph nodes, as well as larger organs such as the spleen, thymus gland, tonsils, and Peyer's patches of the intestine. All of these organs are critical to the body's immune system, a complex group of organs, tissues, cells, and chemicals that protect the body from harmful external invaders and internal events.

The lymphatic system is not pressurized in the same way as the circulatory system, as it has no pump comparable to the heart. Thus, the circulation of lymph relies heavily on skeletal muscle contraction and body movement. Breathing and the pulsation of nearby arteries also help propel lymph along. When lymph does not circulate efficiently, the tissue develops **edema**, an abnormal accumulation of fluid.

Lymph nodes cluster in certain areas of the body. For example, they are particularly dense in the cervical region (neck), axillary region (armpit), and inguinal region (groin). Lymph nodes clustered in these regions tend to be anchored in the surrounding connective tissue, close to the surface. They are usually small, shaped like a kidney bean, and pliable when healthy. Diseases such as viral or bacterial infections can prompt enlargement of the associated lymph nodes, making them feel swollen and full.

Nerves

Nerves are part of the nervous system that controls and communicates with the rest of the body. This system includes the brain, spinal cord, and peripheral nerves that monitor, interpret, and affect changes in the body (FIG. 1-28).

Nerves carry electrical signals to and from the brain and spinal cord and the body periphery. For example, **sensory nerves** monitor the internal and external environment and relay this data to the brain. Once the brain integrates this information and decides upon a reaction, action-oriented nerves called **motor nerves** carry out the response. By utilizing these reception and response pathways, the nervous system is able to control and communicate with all systems of the body, including those responsible for movement.

Recall that nervous tissue is one of the four primary tissue types in the human body. Under the microscope, nerves are revealed as cablelike bundles of excitable cells called *neurons* (FIG. 1-29). The functional center of a neuron, where the nucleus resides, is called the *cell body*. As you can see in FIGURE 1-30, it looks something like a many-legged spider. When a nerve impulse stimulates these short "legs," which are called *dendrites*, they transmit the impulse to the cell body. Branching from the cell body is one lengthy extension, the *axon*, which receives the impulse from the cell body and sends it down its length to a neighboring cell.

As with muscle fibers, each individual neuron is wrapped in connective tissue, as is each bundle of neurons and each whole nerve. Notice in Figure 1-29 that nerves are nourished by tiny blood vessels.

Nerves traverse the body in much the same way as blood vessels, beginning as large roots near the spinal cord and then branching into smaller and smaller segments throughout the body periphery. Large nerve branches feel taught and ropey upon palpation and do not change shape

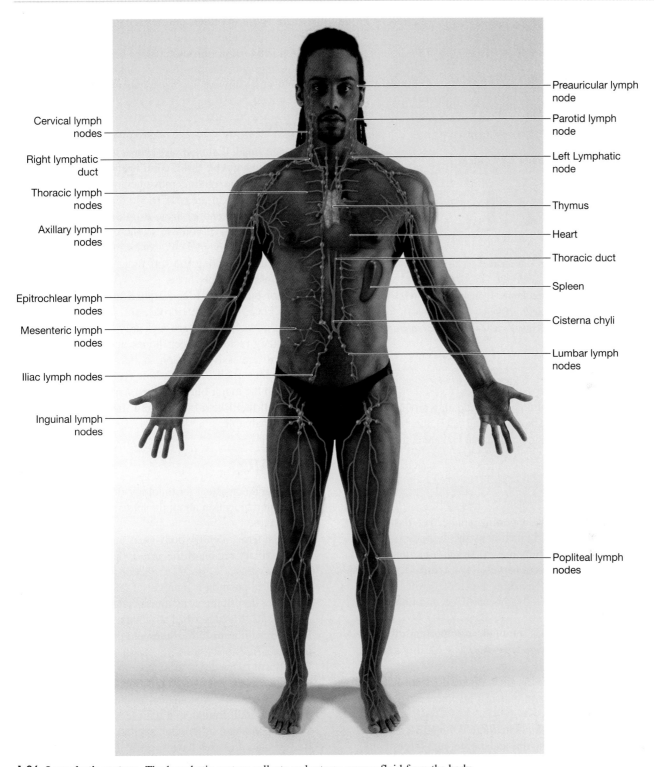

Cervical lymph nodes

Right lymphatic duct

Thoracic lymph nodes

Axillary lymph nodes

Epitrochlear lymph nodes

Mesenteric lymph nodes

Iliac lymph nodes

Inguinal lymph nodes

Preauricular lymph node

Parotid lymph node

Left Lymphatic node

Thymus

Heart

Thoracic duct

Spleen

Cisterna chyli

Lumbar lymph nodes

Popliteal lymph nodes

1-26. Lymphatic system. The lymphatic system collects and returns excess fluid from the body tissues to the circulatory system and helps the body resist infection and disease. It includes lymphoid organs such as the tonsils, thymus, and spleen, as well as lymph nodes and lymphatic vessels.

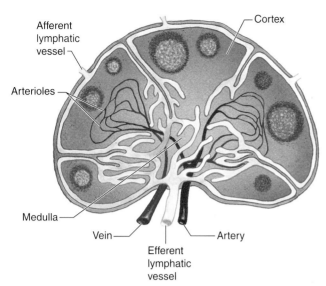

1-27. Structure of a lymph node. Lymph flows into the node via *afferent lymphatic vessels*, is filtered and cleansed of foreign particles, and then exits the node via the *efferent lymphatic vessel.*

with movement. Use caution when palpating around superficial nerves. Provoking hot, shooting pain, numbness, tingling, or weakness is an indication that you are compressing a nerve.

Cartilage

Cartilage is a type of supporting connective tissue that varies in consistency and function by the proportion of proteins distributed through its matrix. Because cartilage does not contain blood vessels or nerves, it has a limited ability to heal following injury. The three types of cartilage in the body are elastic cartilage, hyaline cartilage, and fibrous cartilage (FIG. 1-31).

Elastic cartilage has the highest proportion of elastic fibers of the three cartilage types (FIG. 1-31A). It is found in the nose and ears, where it creates a structure that is self-supporting, but flexible. Elastic cartilage does not have the same direct application to human movement as the other types of cartilage.

Hyaline (or *articular*) **cartilage** is found in the voice box (larynx), between the ribs and the sternum (breastbone), and on the surfaces of bones where they form joints. Hyaline cartilage is smooth and rubbery and helps reduce friction during movement (FIG.1-31B). It responds to increased activity by increasing the number and size of cartilage cells, which thickens the tissue and increases its ability to cushion and lubricate joint surfaces. Damage to the hyaline cartilage can result in chronic inflammation of the joint, commonly termed **osteoarthritis**.

Fibrous cartilage has a dense network of collagen fibers (FIG. 1-31C). It makes up part of the disks between the vertebrae and the meniscus between the femur and tibia at

the knee. These structures cushion the joint surfaces and enhance joint continuity, or the way the bones fit together. The collagen network in fibrous cartilage helps it resist pulling, compressing, and shearing forces, making it an ideal cushion while still allowing slight movement.

Bursae

Bursae are small, flattened sacs (*bursa* is Latin for "purse"). They contain **synovial fluid**, a lubricant that helps decrease friction and create gliding movement between structures. Bursae are located in areas of friction in the body, such as where muscles or tendons have to glide over bony prominences. In FIGURE 1-32, you can see how the bursa serves as a cushion between the gluteal tendons and greater trochanter of the femur, protecting the soft tissue from damage as it moves across the harder bone.

Major bursae are found around the shoulder, elbow, hip, and knee. They are fibrous, soft, and pillowy when palpated; however, they are normally difficult to palpate because they reside between bones and large tendons. If exposed to excessive friction, a bursa can become enlarged and swollen. This pathology, called **bursitis**, is common in the major bursae. When irritated and inflamed, a bursa will feel like a bag of fluid. It may be observable as well as palpable.

SUMMARY

* Precise and consistent terminology is necessary for clear communication about the human body and its movements.
* Regional terms identify body areas and structures, such as the axillary region of the arm or the pectoral region of the chest.
* Anatomical position is a universal reference position useful for describing structural locations and human movements. It is described as standing upright, facing forward, with arms to the sides and palms facing forward.
* Directional terms describe relative locations of body structures in the anatomical position.
* The body can be envisioned as divided by imaginary planes (sagittal, frontal, and transverse). Each plane has a corresponding axis (frontal, sagittal, and longitudinal).
* Body planes and axes have specific motions associated with them. These include flexion, extension, abduction, adduction, internal rotation, and external rotation.
* Several structures in the human body work together to make movement possible. These include bones, muscles, tendons, ligaments, and fascia, as well as nerves and other special structures. These structures can be identified through observation and palpation.
* Various special structures nourish, regulate, or otherwise support the structures of human movement. These include blood vessels, nerves, lymphatic vessels and nodes, cartilage, and bursae.

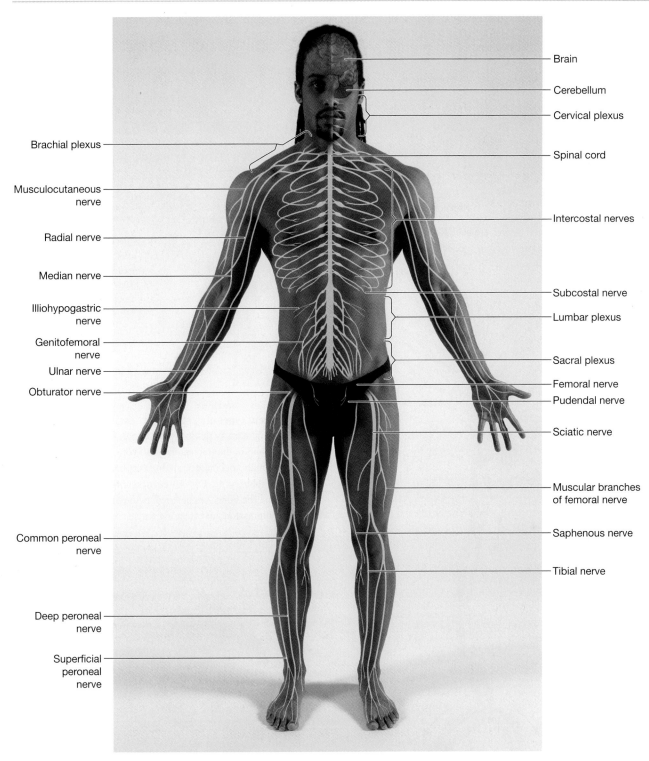

Brain

Cerebellum

Cervical plexus

Spinal cord

Brachial plexus

Musculocutaneous nerve

Radial nerve

Median nerve

Illiohypogastric nerve

Genitofemoral nerve

Ulnar nerve

Obturator nerve

Intercostal nerves

Subcostal nerve

Lumbar plexus

Sacral plexus

Femoral nerve

Pudendal nerve

Sciatic nerve

Muscular branches of femoral nerve

Saphenous nerve

Tibial nerve

Common peroneal nerve

Deep peroneal nerve

Superficial peroneal nerve

1-28. Nervous system. The nervous system controls and communicates with the rest of the body. This system includes the brain, spinal cord, and peripheral nerves that monitor, interpret, and affect changes in the body.

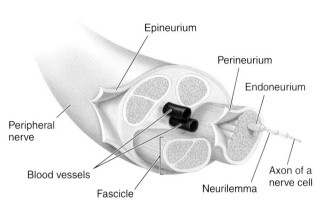

1-29. **Structure of a nerve.** Nerves are cablelike bundles of nerve cells (called *neurons*) enclosed in connective tissue wrappings.

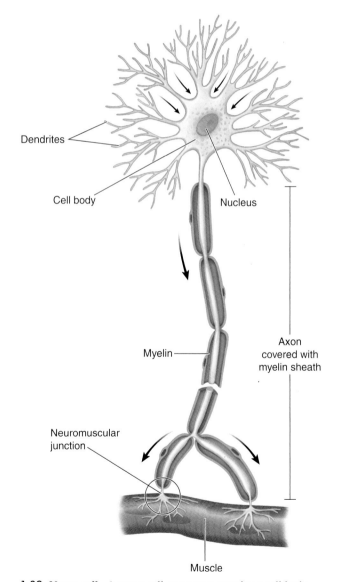

1-30. **Nerve cell.** A nerve cell or *neuron* contains a cell body, which contains the nucleus and is the functional center of the cell; dendrites, which transmit impulses to the cell body; and an axon, which transmits impulses away from the cell body and toward adjacent cells.

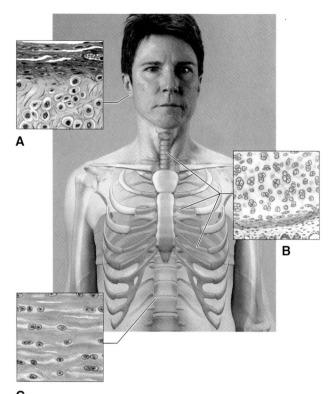

1-31. **Different types of cartilage. A.** *Elastic cartilage,* found in the nose and ears, is flexible and supple. **B.** *Hyaline cartilage,* found in the trachea, larynx (voice box), between the ribs and sternum, and on articulating surfaces of bones, is smooth and rubbery. **C.** *Fibrous cartilage,* found between the vertebrae and the bones of the knee, is tough and resistant to tension, compression, and shearing forces.

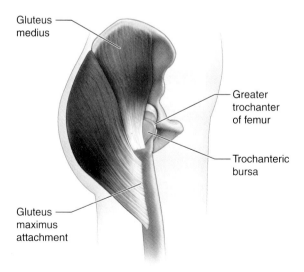

1-32. **Bursa of the hip: lateral view.** Bursae are located in areas of friction in the body, such as where muscles or tendons have to glide over bony prominences. This function is apparent in the hip, where several gluteal tendons are protected from the bony trochanter of the femur.

FOR REVIEW

Multiple Choice

1. When describing relative position, the wrist is _____ to the elbow.
   A. superior
   B. caudal
   C. anterior
   D. distal

2. When describing relative position, the head is _____ to the chest.
   A. proximal
   B. anterior
   C. superior
   D. lateral

3. When describing relative position, the nose is _____ to the ears.
   A. lateral
   B. anterior
   C. cephalic
   D. distal

4. When describing relative position, the spine is _____ to the abdomen.
   A. caudal
   B. posterior
   C. proximal
   D. medial

5. When describing relative position, the shoulder is _____ to the wrist.
   A. anterior
   B. cephalic
   C. proximal
   D. lateral

6. Bending the elbow to bring the hand toward the shoulder describes:
   A. abduction
   B. extension
   C. flexion
   D. rotation

7. Raising the entire arm up to the side until overhead describes:
   A. abduction
   B. extension
   C. flexion
   D. rotation

8. Straightening the knee to stand up from a sitting position describes:
   A. adduction
   B. rotation
   C. abduction
   D. extension

9. Swinging your arms back and forth while walking describes:
   A. abduction
   B. flexion
   C. extension
   D. both B and C

10. Looking over your shoulder while driving describes:
    A. adduction
    B. rotation
    C. abduction
    D. extension

Matching

Different anatomical structures are listed below. Match the correct function with its structure.

11. _____ Bursa
12. _____ Cartilage
13. _____ Muscle
14. _____ Capillary
15. _____ Nerve
16. _____ Tendon
17. _____ Fascia
18. _____ Bone
19. _____ Skin
20. _____ Lymph node

A. Facilitates smooth movement, cushions, and reduces friction on the surfaces of bones.

B. Carries signals to and from the brain and spinal cord.

C. Cleanses excess tissue fluid of foreign particles, viruses, and bacteria.

D. Provides location for blood cell formation and storage of inorganic salts.

E. Decreases friction and creates gliding movement between body structures such as tendons and bony landmarks.

F. Connects muscles to bones.

G. Protects against outside invaders and interacts with external environment through sensory receptors.

H. Generates force, which produces movements at joints.

I. Covers or binds the structures of the body.

J. Location where gases, nutrients, and waste products are exchanged between the blood and individual cells.

Different motions are listed below. Match the correct plane and axis with its motion. Answers may be used more than once.

21. _____ Internal rotation   A. Frontal axis

22. _____ Flexion   B. Longitudinal axis

23. _____ Abduction   C. Sagittal axis

24. _____ Lateral rotation   D. Sagittal plane

25. _____ External rotation   E. Transverse plane

26. _____ Adduction   F. Frontal plane

27. _____ Medial rotation

28. _____ Extension

Short Answer

29. Briefly describe the anatomical position.

30. Identify what qualities about bones make them distinguishable from other structures during palpation.

31. Identify what qualities about muscles make them distinguishable from other structures during palpation.

32. Identify each region of the body in the picture below.

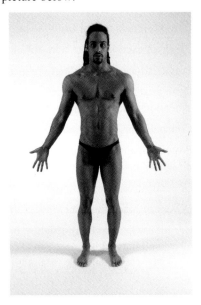

Try This!

Activity: Describe and/or draw specific body movements on a set of 3 × 5 cards; for example, doing jumping jacks, bowling, making snow angels, etc. Find a partner and have them get into anatomical position. Draw a card and do not let your partner see what it says/depicts. Using proper directional and movement terms only, have them move their body in the way described on the card. If in a group setting, this can be a contest. The first pair to correctly describe and perform a movement wins!

Switch partners and draw another card. Repeat the steps above. Practice with several different movements and partners. Challenge yourself by selecting increasingly difficult movements.

SUGGESTED READINGS

Hendrickson T. *Massage for Orthopedic Conditions*. Baltimore: Lippincott, Williams & Wilkins, 2003.

Juhan D. *Job's Body*. 3rd Ed. Barrytown, NY: Station Hill, 2003.

Kendall FP, McCreary EK, Provance PG, et al. *Muscles: Testing and Function with Posture and Pain*. 5th Ed. Baltimore: Lippincott, Williams & Wilkins, 2005.

Mage DJ. *Orthopedic Physical Assessment*. 2nd Ed. Philadelphia: Saunders, 1992.

Myers TW. *Anatomy Trains: Myofascial Meridians for Manual and Movement Therapists*. Edinburgh, London, New York: Churchill Livingstone, 2001.

Premkumar K. *The Massage Connection Anatomy & Physiology*. 2nd Ed. Baltimore: Lippincott, Williams & Wilkins, 2004.

Scheumann DW. *The Balanced Body: A Guide to Deep Tissue and Neuromuscular Therapy*. 3rd Ed. Baltimore: Lippincott, Williams & Wilkins, 2007.

WEBSITES

1. Anatomy & Histology Center: (http://www.martindalecenter.com/MedicalAnatomy.html) Part of Martindale's Health Science Guide, this metasite provides links to a comprehensive list of anatomy resources. It includes links to atlases, courses, images, databases, teaching files, and exams.

2. Visible Human Project: (http://www.nlm.nih.gov/research/visible/visible_human.html) The Visible Human Project provides transverse CT, MRI, and cryosection images of a representative male and female cadaver at an average of 1 millimeter intervals. This site provides a description of the project and information on how to access the images.

3. American Association of Anatomists: (http://www.anatomy.org/) AAA is the professional association for biomedical researchers and educators interested in anatomical form and function. The site provides professional information and links to a variety of anatomy-related resources for researchers, educators, and students.

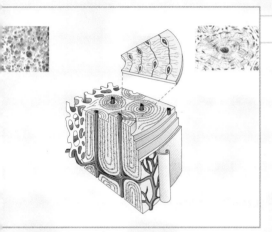

Osteology and Arthrology

Learning Objectives

After working through the material in this chapter, you should be able to:

- Identify the functions of bones in the human body.

- Compare and contrast spongy bone and compact bone.

- Describe how tendons and ligaments attach to bones.

- Identify the bones of the human skeleton and distinguish between the axial and appendicular divisions.

- Describe the different types and shapes of bones and relate them to function.

- Identify categories and functions of bony landmarks on the human skeleton.

- Describe how joints in the human body are named and identify all joints in the axial and appendicular divisions of the skeleton.

- Classify the different types of joints in the human body by structure and function and give an example of each.

- Label the basic structures of a synovial joint and summarize the function of each structure in the body.

- Identify the six types of synovial joints and provide an example of each.

- Describe the three types of accessory motion and give an example of each.

Chapter Outline

The bones of the human skeleton are living, changing structures that reflect their function in the body and the daily demands placed upon them. For example, bones develop specific landmarks—depressions, ridges, bumps, and other features—according to forces that act upon them. These forces include the compression of gravity and the tension of muscles and tendons.

Most bones connect with other bones to form joints, complex structures that vary in their ability to move according to their shape and composition. Some joints have little or no movement, while others move considerably and in multiple directions. In this chapter, we explore the structure and functions of bones and joints. Understanding the functional anatomy of these structures is essential to our understanding of human movement. The type and direction of movement available at a joint will influence the configuration and function of associated structures such as ligaments and muscles.

BONES OF THE HUMAN SKELETON

Learning the basic function, structure, and classification of bones helps us understand human movement. The prefix *osteo-* means bone. **Osteology,** the study of bones, examines how bones develop and respond to our environment.

Functions of Bone

Bones serve four primary functions in the body, including support and protection, levers for movement, hematopoiesis, and storage of minerals and fats.

Support and Protection

The human skeleton is a framework that supports all the soft tissues of the body and protects many critical organs. For example, the bony skull protects the brain from trauma, and the vertebrae of the spine protect the spinal cord. The protective function of bones is also apparent in the architecture of the ribcage, which protects the heart and lungs.

Movement

Bones also act as rigid levers upon which muscles pull to produce movement. As the body sits or stands in a stationary position, an orchestrated interaction between muscles, bones, and outside forces such as gravity work to maintain its position in space. More complex interactions are required to create and control movement.

Hematopoiesis

Certain types of bones have an interior cavity that contains **red bone marrow**, a loose connective tissue where blood cells are made. This process of blood cell production, called **hematopoiesis**, occurs primarily in the skull, the pelvis, the ribs, the sternum, and the ends of the femur and humerus in adults. During infancy red marrow also resides within the shafts of long bones. Later in life, this red marrow is converted to yellow marrow, mainly comprised of fatty tissue. Yellow marrow serves as a reserve for hematopoiesis and can be converted back to red marrow if the need arises for massive blood cell formation.

Storage of Minerals and Fats

The storage of minerals within bones is part of what makes them rigid. Minerals such as **calcium** and **phosphate** form the "cement" of bones, forming crystals that deposit along the bone's collagen fibers. These minerals not only give bones their hardness, but can be withdrawn from bone to serve critical chemical functions in the body. For example, calcium is alkaline (a base) and the body uses it to help maintain the acid–base balance of the blood. If the blood becomes too acidic, the calcium deposited in the bones is withdrawn to stabilize blood pH. Calcium is also used for transmitting nerve impulses, assisting with muscle contraction, maintaining blood pressure, and initiating blood clotting following injury. We need to consume adequate amounts of calcium, phosphate, and other bone minerals or the "storage bank" in our bones can become depleted and our bone density reduced. This can result in a condition called *osteoporosis* (literally meaning *porous bone*) and an increased risk of fracture.

While it is tempting to think of the human skeleton as a rigid, static structure, in reality it is dynamic and responsive, adjusting itself to the forces it encounters. This phenomenon is described by **Wolff's Law**, which states "bone forms in areas of stress and reabsorb(s) in areas of nonstress." In other words, bones, like muscles, change throughout our lives according to how we use them. This adaptive ability will be clarified further as we explore bone tissue.

Bone Tissue

Recall from Chapter 1 that bone tissue is an example of supporting connective tissue. Almost all bones of the body contain two types of bone tissue: **spongy** and **compact**. Both are created and maintained by two types of bone cells, or **osteocytes** (*osteo-* means bone and *–cyte* means cell). **Osteoblasts** are bone-forming osteocytes. They lay down calcium-containing crystals along the collagen fiber "struts" in the extracellular matrix. As new and different stresses are placed on bone throughout life, **osteoclasts** break down old bone, freeing chemicals that degrade the mineral crystals, and releasing their stored calcium into the bloodstream. This action prepares the way for osteoblasts to lay down new bone. This constant work of osteoclasts and osteoblasts breaking down and building up bone ensures maximal strength with minimal bulk and weight.

Spongy Bone

Spongy bone is a three-dimensional latticework of porous bony tissue filled with red bone marrow (Fig. 2-1). It is less dense than compact bone and resembles a household sponge. The osseous "struts," or **trabeculae,** of spongy bone

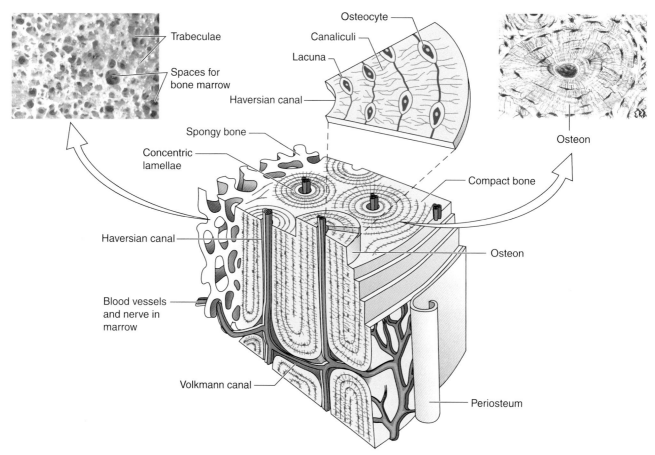

2-1. Bone tissue. Both inner spongy and outer compact bone can be seen in this view. Notice the system of transport canals, including the *Haversian canal, Volkmann canal,* and tiny *canaliculi.* The concentric rings of *llamelae* are visible from the top and side views. A single *osteon* is raised at the top, highlighting the system of bone cells (*osteocytes*), the cavities that house them (*lacunae*), the central Haversian canal, and its corresponding canaliculi. The protective *periosteum* forms the outermost layer of bone. The micrograph (left) of spongy bone clearly shows its porous nature. The small, dark spots on the micrograph (right) of compact bone are osteocytes within their lacunae. The larger dark areas indicate the central Haversian canals.

form and reform according to lines of stress. This provides maximal strength, like the braces used to support a building. Spongy bone is usually found in the bone core, deep to compact bone. Nourishment reaches the central spongy bone via a system of blood vessels that emerge from canals within the denser outer compact bone.

Compact Bone

As you look at Figure 2-1, the first thing you notice about compact bone is how much more dense it is than spongy bone. Several features are present. Tiny cavities within the bone matrix house osteocytes. These cavities are called **lacunae** and are wrapped in concentric circles (called **lamellae**) around central **Haversian canals**. Notice that blood vessels and nerves run within these Haversian canals, bringing nourishment to the tissue. Together, the lamellae and Haversian canals form the functional unit of bone, called an **osteon** (or *Haversian system*). These units resemble the rings of a tree.

Several canals radiate from the central Haversian canals. **Canaliculi**, literally "tiny canals," penetrate the compact bone matrix, bringing microscopic blood vessels and nerve branches to the outlying osteocytes. **Volkmann's canals** (also called *perforating canals*) run perpendicular to the Haversian canals. They complete the pathway from the surface of the bone to its interior.

As you can see in Figure 2-1, this entire complex is covered in a dense connective tissue called **periosteum**. Periosteum surrounds the bone, nourishing and protecting it. This covering is well supplied with blood vessels, which bring nourishment to the bone, and nerves, which enable communication, such as a warning of mechanical impact. Periosteum also participates in the regeneration of bony tissue and the formation of new bone following an injury, such as a fracture.

The Human Skeleton

The 206 bones of the human skeleton can be divided into two parts (Fig. 2-2). The **axial skeleton** forms the body's

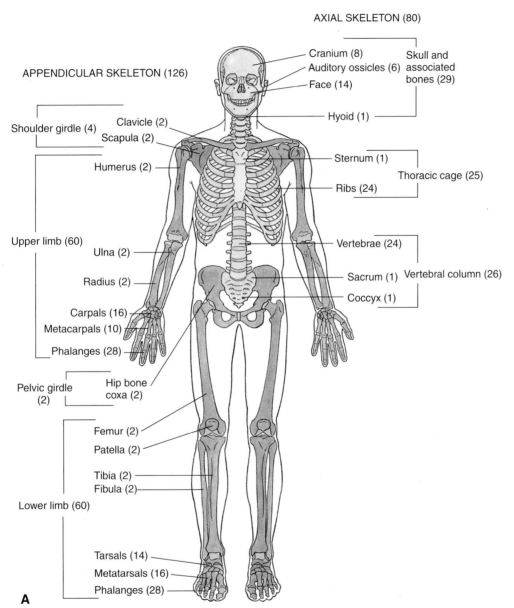

AXIAL SKELETON (80)

APPENDICULAR SKELETON (126)

Cranium (8)
Auditory ossicles (6)
Face (14)
Skull and associated bones (29)

Shoulder girdle (4)
Clavicle (2)
Scapula (2)

Humerus (2)

Hyoid (1)

Sternum (1)
Ribs (24)
Thoracic cage (25)

Upper limb (60)
Ulna (2)

Radius (2)

Carpals (16)
Metacarpals (10)
Phalanges (28)

Vertebrae (24)

Sacrum (1)
Coccyx (1)
Vertebral column (26)

Pelvic girdle (2)
Hip bone coxa (2)

Femur (2)
Patella (2)

Tibia (2)
Fibula (2)

Lower limb (60)

Tarsals (14)
Metatarsals (16)
Phalanges (28)

A

2-2. The human skeleton. There are 206 bones in the typical human skeleton, 80 in the *axial* skeleton (in yellow) and 126 in the *appendicular* skeleton (in pink) **A.** Anterior view. *(continued)*

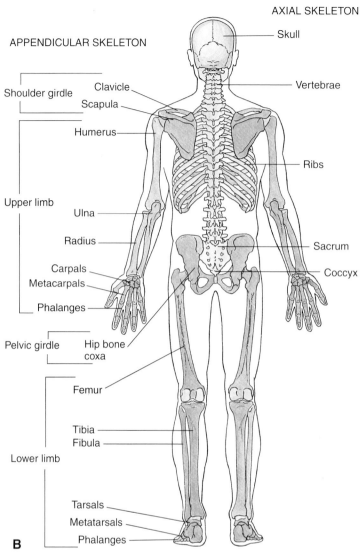

AXIAL SKELETON

APPENDICULAR SKELETON

Shoulder girdle
Clavicle
Scapula
Humerus

Skull

Vertebrae

Upper limb

Ulna

Radius

Ribs

Carpals
Metacarpals

Sacrum

Coccyx

Phalanges

Pelvic girdle   Hip bone
coxa

Femur

Tibia
Fibula

Lower limb

Tarsals
Metatarsals
Phalanges

B

2-2. **The human skeleton. B.** Posterior view.

"axis": that is, it makes up the center of the body. It is composed of bones of the head and trunk, including the skull and associated bones, hyoid, sternum, ribs, vertebrae, sacrum, and coccyx. A typical adult skeleton contains 80 bones in the axial division.

The **appendicular skeleton** is "appended" to the axial skeleton. In a typical adult, it contains 126 bones arranged in the following structures:

- The *shoulder girdle* includes the clavicle and scapula.
- The *upper limb* includes the humerus, radius, ulna, carpals, metacarpals, and phalanges.
- The *pelvic girdle* includes the coxal bone (*coxa* means hip), which is actually three fused bones (the ilium, ischium, and pubis).
- The *lower limb* includes the femur, tibia, fibula, tarsals, metatarsals, and phalanges.

The upper and lower limbs, or *appendages,* are essential to independent movement and full interaction with the environment, but wheelchairs, artificial limbs, and other devices have made it possible to live a rewarding life without them.

SHAPES OF BONES

Bones come in various shapes and sizes depending on their function in the body (Fig. 2-3). Some are long and slender, others are small and square, and some are totally unique in their configuration.

Long Bones

Long bones are longer than they are wide (Fig. 2-3A). These bones are divided into a **diaphysis** (shaft) and two **epiphyses** (the bumpy ends). The diaphysis is made up of compact bone with **yellow marrow** filling the center. Yellow marrow stores fat within the bone. After infancy, it replaces red marrow in the central cavity, called the **medullary cavity**.

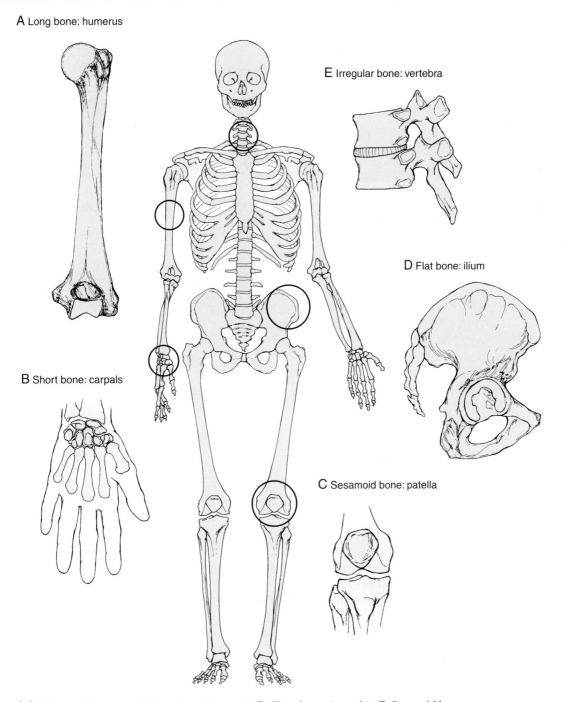

A Long bone: humerus

E Irregular bone: vertebra

D Flat bone: ilium

B Short bone: carpals

C Sesamoid bone: patella

2-3. **Shapes of bones.** **A.** Long bone (humerus). **B.** Short bones (carpals). **C.** Sesamoid bone (patella), a specialized short bone. **D.** Flat bone (ilium). **E.** Irregular bones (vertebrae). Wormian bones are not shown.

Each epiphysis is composed of spongy bone surrounded by a thin layer of compact bone. The region where the epiphysis meets the diaphysis is called the **epiphyseal plate**, or *growth plate*. Long bones grow in length via the development and **ossification** of hyaline cartilage at this plate. In the process of ossification, osteoblasts lay down bone tissue, which eventually replaces the cartilage. Ossification ends after puberty when the epiphyseal plates are entirely replaced by bone and *close*.

The external surfaces of the epiphyses are usually covered with hyaline cartilage where they articulate with other bones. This provides a smooth surface that reduces friction at the joints between bones. Examples of long bones in the human body include the humerus, radius, ulna, femur, tibia, and fibula.

Short Bones

Short bones, which tend to be cube-shaped, are composed mainly of spongy bone (Fig. 2-3B). A thin layer of compact bone surrounds the spongy bone. The carpals of the wrist and tarsals of the foot are short bones. The networks formed by multiple short bones in these locations allow fine, complex hand and foot movements.

A specialized short bone called a **sesamoid bone** is of particular importance to human movement (Fig. 2-3C). These bones resemble sesame seeds and are formed within tendons. Sesamoid bones strengthen the tendon and improve the traction mechanics of the corresponding muscle(s). The largest sesamoid bone in the human body is the patella, but there are smaller ones in the hand and foot.

Flat Bones

Flat bones are thin and flattened and tend to be curved (Fig. 2-3D). These bones are not developed by hyaline cartilage, but rather by the ossification of a fibrous network. Once mature, they consist of a thin layer of spongy bone surrounded by compact bone. The spongy bone at the center of these flat bones is a location for hematopoiesis. Most of the cranial bones, the sternum, scapula, clavicle, ribs, and ilium are examples of flat bones.

Irregular Bones

Irregular bones are those that have unique shapes and therefore do not fit into the previous categories (Fig. 2-3E). The vertebrae, with their unique shape and function, and the ischium and pubis of the pelvis are considered irregular.

Wormian Bones

Wormian bones are small, irregular bones found along the sutures of the cranium. They are areas of ossification outside of the usual cranial bones. Wormian bones tend to be symmetrical on the two sides of the skull and vary in size. These bones are not present in all human skulls and their number is generally limited to two or three.

BONY LANDMARKS

Bones have or develop over time specific landmarks that serve a variety of functions. Each bony landmark has a unique name that helps indicate its purpose and location. Table 2-1 lists some of the more common terms for these landmarks.

Depressions and Openings

Depressions are basins and channels that house muscles, tendons, nerves, and vessels. Clinicians distinguish two types of depressions. A *fossa* is a shallow depression. There is a fossa at the distal end of the humerus of the upper arm and a fossa in the ilium of the pelvis. A *sulcus* or a *groove* is a narrow depression, such as that found at the head of the humerus.

Openings are holes and channels that allow passage of nerves, vessels, muscles, and tendons. They also create air-filled cavities called *sinuses*. Terms used to describe openings are *fissure, foramen,* and *meatus*. A *fissure* is a cleft somewhat like an enlarged crack or slit in a bone. An example is the superior orbital fissure of the skull behind the eye. A *foramen* is a small to large, usually circular opening, such as the foramen magnum, which allows for the passage of the spinal cord to connect with the brain stem. A *meatus* is a tiny passageway. An example is the external auditory meatus of the temporal bone.

Projections That Form Joints

Several bumps, or **projections,** can be found on bones that help form joints. These tend to be at the ends of bones and include rounded *condyles*, flat *facets*, and the large *heads* of long bones, and *rami* (plural for *ramus*), which form bony bridges.

Attachment Sites

Bumps and ridges indicate tendon and ligament **attachment sites**. Their size and shape varies according to the type and amount of force that creates them. Some are long and narrow like a *crest, line,* or *ridge*. Others are rounded like a *tubercle, tuberosity,* or *trochanter*. *Epicondyles*, *processes,* and *spines* are other prominences where soft tissues connect to bone.

Some of these bony features are present at birth, whereas others develop in response to forces placed upon the skeleton. For example, the external auditory meatus of the temporal bone is present at birth. In contrast, the mastoid process (large bump directly behind the ear) develops over several years as the neck muscles pull on this bony attachment. Thus, bone has the ability to develop bony prominences where ligaments and tendons attach. This ability, in

▶ TABLE 2-1. BONE MARKINGS

Type of Bone Marking	Description	Example	Illustration
Fissure	Deep furrow, cleft, or slit	Orbital fissures of skull	
Foramen	Round opening through bone	Foramen magnum of skull	
Fossa	Long, basinlike depression	Glenoid fossa of scapula	
Groove	Narrow, elongated depression	Bicipital groove of humerus	

(continues)

▶ TABLE 2-1. BONE MARKINGS *(continued)*

Type of Bone Marking	Description	Example	Illustration
Meatus	Passage or channel	Auditory meatus of temporal bone	
Sinus	Cavity or hollow space in bone	Ethmoid sinus	

Projections that form joints:

Condyle	Rounded articular projection	Condyles of the femur	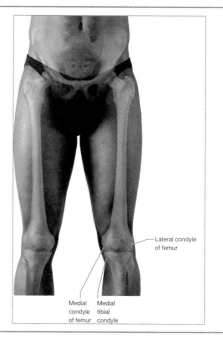

▌ TABLE 2-1. BONE MARKINGS *(continued)*

Type of Bone Marking	Description	Example	Illustration
Facet	Small, smooth area	Costal facet of thoracic vertebrae	The **costal facet** of the **transverse process** is a point of articulation with the ribs. The **superior costal facet** of each vertebra articulates with a rib. The **inferior costal facet** of one vertebra, and the superior costal facet of the vertebra beneath, together articulate with each true rib.
Head	Rounded extremity, protruding from narrow neck	Head of the fibula	Head of fibula
Ramus	Projecting part, elongated process, or branch	Ramus of the mandible	Ramus of the mandible

(continues)

▶ **TABLE 2-1. BONE MARKINGS** *(continued)*

Type of Bone Marking	Description	Example	Illustration
Projections that are attachment sites:			
Crest	Narrow prominence or ridge	Iliac crest	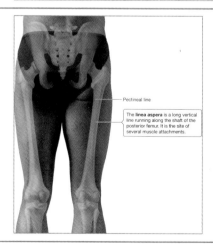
Epicondyle	Prominence on or above a condyle	Epicondyles of the humerus	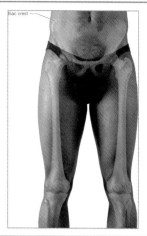
Line	Ridge, less prominent than a crest	Linea aspera of the femur	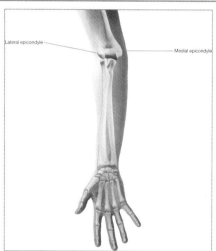

▶ TABLE 2-1. BONE MARKINGS *(continued)*

Type of Bone Marking	Description	Example	Illustration
Process	Any bony prominence	Coracoid process of the scapula	The **Coracoid process** of the scapula protrudes anteriorly and inferior to the clavicle, to form a strong bony attachment for several muscles of the shoulder.
Ridge	Linear elevation	Supracondylar ridge of the humerus	Supracondylar ridge of the humerus
Spine	Sharp, slender prominence	Spine of the scapula	Spine of the scapula

(continues)

▶ TABLE 2-1. BONE MARKINGS *(continued)*

Type of Bone Marking	Description	Example	Illustration
Tubercle	Small, rounded prominence	Adductor tubercle of the femur	
Tuberosity	Large, round, roughened prominence	Tibial tuberosity	
Trochanter	Large, blunt prominence found only on the femur	Greater trochanter	

addition to changing trabecular configurations of spongy bone and increasing thickness of compact bone, makes the skeleton a highly adaptive structure.

JOINTS OF THE HUMAN SKELETON

Bones come together in the body to form **joints**. The prefix *arthr-* indicates joints. **Arthrology** is the study of joints and how and why joints move the way they do.

Naming Joints

Joints are named according to the bones that form them. For example, the humerus bone of the upper arm articulates with the ulna of the forearm. To name this joint, we simply modify the two bone names and place an "o" between them. Thus, these bones form the *humeroulnar* joint (humer + o + ulna + r). Typically, the larger or more stable bone is named first, followed by the smaller or more mobile bone(s).

Sometimes a bone will participate in more than one joint. This is true of the scapula, which forms two joints. In such cases, we name the joint according to the bony landmark that forms it. Since the scapula articulates with the humerus at the glenoid fossa, the joint they form is called the *glenohumeral* joint (glen + o + humer + al). The scapula also articulates with the clavicle at the acromion process to form the *acromioclavicular* joint (acromi + o + clavicul + ar).

There are a few exceptions to these rules. For example, the hip joint is called the *coxal* joint. Here, the femur articulates with the coxa or hipbone, formed by the ilium, ischium, and pubis. Using the bone + o + bone rule, this would be the ilioischiopubofemoral joint. That's quite a mouthful! Using the term "coxal joint" is much simpler. As another example, the clinical name for the ankle joint is the *talocrural* joint. Three bones, the tibia, the fibula, and the talus, form this joint, but the name is derived from *talus* plus the region of the body (crural = lower leg) it connects with.

Joint Structure

Three major structural categories are used when describing joints: fibrous, cartilaginous, and synovial.

Fibrous Joints

Fibrous joints have firm connections between bones. There is minimal joint cavity (or space between the articulating surfaces), and a collagen-dense connective tissue holds the bones tightly together. Little or no movement is possible at these joints; thus, they are the most stable type. There are three types of fibrous joints:

- **Sutures** (Fig. 2-4A) are continuous periosteal connections between bones, such as between the cranial bones.
- **Syndesmoses** (Fig. 2-4B) are fibrous joints held together with a cord (ligament) or sheet (interosseous membrane)

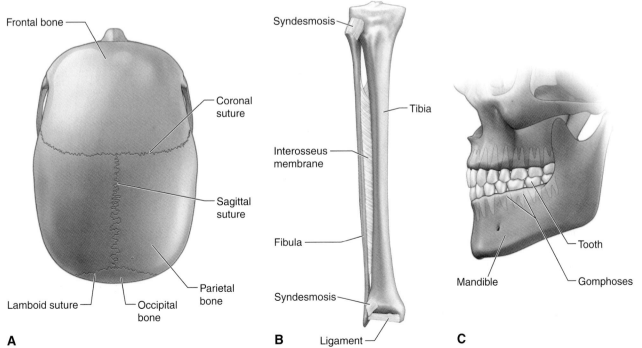

Frontal bone — Coronal suture — Sagittal suture — Parietal bone — Occipital bone — Lamboid suture

Syndesmosis — Tibia — Interosseus membrane — Fibula — Syndesmosis — Ligament

Tooth — Gomphoses — Mandible

A   **B**   **C**

2-4. **Fibrous joints.** Strong fibrous connections between bones prevent movement at these joints. **A.** Sutures of the skull. **B.** Syndesmosis formed by the ligaments and interosseous membrane of the lower leg. **C.** Gomphoses between the teeth and their sockets in the mandible.

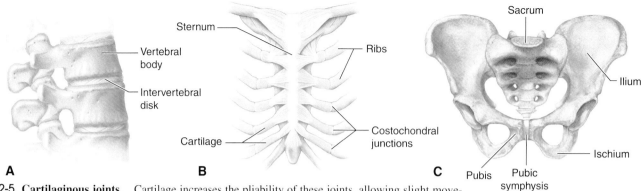

A   **B**   **C**   Pubis   Pubic symphysis

2-5. Cartilaginous joints.   Cartilage increases the pliability of these joints, allowing slight movement. **A.** Intervertebral disks of the spine. **B.** Costochondral junctions of the ribcage. **C.** Pubic symphysis of the pelvis.

of connective tissue. The connection between the tibia and fibula in the lower leg is a syndesmosis.
- **Gomphoses** (Fig. 2-4C) are the specific fibrous joints at which teeth fit into sockets in the jaw (*gomphos-* means bolt or nail).

Cartilaginous Joints

Cartilaginous joints have slightly more movement than fibrous joints. Here cartilage separates the articulating surfaces of adjacent bones (Fig. 2-5). The cartilage increases the pliability of the joint, allowing slight movement. This type of joint is present between the bodies of the vertebrae (Fig. 2-5A), allowing the vertebral column to absorb loads from walking, running, jumping, and lifting. At the costochondral junctions (where the ribs meet the sternum) (Fig. 2-5B), cartilaginous joints allow the ribcage to expand and contract for breathing. Cartilaginous joints are also found at the pubic symphysis (where the two pubic bones meet at the front of the pelvic girdle) (Fig. 2-5C). When we are walking and running, particularly on uneven surfaces, this slight capacity for movement allows the pelvic girdle to serve as a suspension system.

Synovial Joints

Synovial joints are the most mobile of all the joints. They are named for their distinctive structure (Fig. 2-6), which resembles an egg (*syn-* means together and *ovi-* means egg). Their specialized anatomy, as well as their types, will be discussed in more depth shortly.

Joint Function

Now that we have identified different types of joints, it is time to explore their unique functions. There are three categories that describe a joint's function:

- **Synarthrotic joints** have little or no movement.
- **Amphiarthrotic joints** are slightly movable.
- **Diarthrotic joints** are the most mobile of all joints.

Synarthrotic Joints

Synarthrotic joints have articulating surfaces that are very close together, (*syn-* means together, with, or joined and *arthrosis* means joint articulation). This limits their mobility. Some fibrous joints are synarthrotic, as is another type of joint called a **synostosis** (osseous connection between bones). An example of a synostosis is the connection between the ilium, ischium, and pubis of the pelvic girdle.

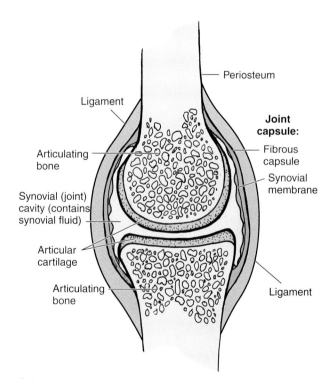

2-6. Synovial joint anatomy.   Several unique features are present in this type of joint, including a thick *joint capsule*, divided into an outer *fibrous capsule* and inner *synovial membrane*. The synovial membrane produces *synovial fluid*, reducing friction in the *joint cavity*. Smooth *articular cartilage* covers the articulating bone ends to further reduce friction during movement. *Ligaments* support the fibrous capsule, providing stability to the joint.

Amphiarthrotic Joints

Amphiarthrotic joints have articulating surfaces that are farther apart, with a pliable structure between or around them (*amphi-* means surrounding). This allows greater mobility at amphiarthrotic joints. The pliable structure can be in the form of ligaments *(syndesmosis)* or fibrocartilage *(symphysis)*. Amphiarthrotic joints are found between the tibia and fibula of the lower leg and the anterior pelvic girdle.

Diarthrotic Joints

Diarthrotic joints are freely movable because their joint surfaces are furthest apart (*di-* means separate or apart). This separation allows the greatest mobility of all joint types. Synovial joints tend to be diarthrotic. Their joint cavity, in conjunction with other anatomical features discussed shortly, creates a highly mobile joint.

When structures and functions of joints are examined together, we develop a clearer understanding of how a joint's anatomical structure influences how it moves. Some examples of joint structure and function are listed in Table 2-2.

STRUCTURE AND FUNCTION OF SYNOVIAL JOINTS

Synovial joints will be discussed in depth because they are responsible for most of the movement allowed in the human body.

Synovial Joint Anatomy

We have already learned that synovial joints are freely movable diarthrotic joints. They contain several unique features (see Fig. 2-6).

The articulating ends of the bones are encased in a thick **joint capsule**. This capsule is divided into two parts: the **fibrous capsule** and the **synovial membrane**. The outer fibrous capsule provides stability and protection for the joint. Additional ligaments often aid this function by limiting specific motions. The inner synovial membrane lines the joint cavity and produces **synovial fluid**, a lubricant that decreases friction and nourishes the articular cartilage. Synovial fluid fills the **joint cavity**, a slight space unique to diarthrotic joints and essential to free movement.

Incidentally, synovial fluid is also found in areas of friction aside from joints. Sacs of synovial fluid are called *bursae* and can be found throughout the body (see Chapter 1). *Synovial sheaths* surround long tendons in the hands and feet.

Synovial Joint Types

All synovial joints consist of the basic structures just identified, but their shape varies, allowing different movement possibilities (Table 2-3).

- **Ball and socket joints** have a spherical head on one bone that fits into a rounded cavity on another. These joints have the greatest movement possibility and are considered **triaxial** because they can move in all three planes: sagittal, frontal, and transverse (see Chapter 1). Examples of ball and socket joints in the body include the glenohumeral joint of the shoulder and the coxal joint.
- **Hinge joints** have a cylindrical prominence on one bone that fits into a corresponding depression on another. These joints are **uniaxial** in that they move in a single plane. An example of a hinge joint in the body is the humeroulnar joint of the elbow. The temporomandibular joint of the jaw and the tibiofemoral joint of the knee are *modified* hinge joints: both of them allow additional movements besides their primary hinging motion.
- **Pivot joints** have a cylindrical segment of one bone that fits into a corresponding cavity of another. Pivot joints are also uniaxial in that they only allow rotational

▶ TABLE 2-2. STRUCTURE AND FUNCTION OF JOINTS

Joint Structure	Joint Function	Joint Mobility	Examples
Fibrous	Synarthrotic	Immovable	Sutures of skull
			Tibiofibular syndesmosis of lower leg
			Gomphosis of teeth
Cartilaginous	Amphiarthrotic	Slightly movable	Intervertebral joints
			Costochondral junctions of ribcage
			Pubic symphysis of pelvis
Synovial	Diarthrotic	Freely movable	Glenohumeral joint of shoulder
			Humeroulnar joint of elbow
			Tibiofemoral joint of knee

▌ TABLE 2-3. TYPES OF SYNOVIAL JOINTS

Type of Joint	Number of Planes/Axes	Movements Possible	Examples
Ball and socket	Triaxial	Flexion Extension Abduction Adduction Internal rotation External rotation Circumduction (combination movement)	Glenohumeral joint Sternoclavicular joint Coxal joint
Hinge	Uniaxial	Flexion Extension	Temporomandibular joint (modified) Humeroulnar joint Interphalangeal joints Tibiofemoral joint (modified) Talocrural joint
Pivot	Uniaxial	Rotation	Atlantoaxial joint Radioulnar joints
Ellipsoid/condyloid	Biaxial	Flexion Extension Abduction Adduction (or lateral flexion in spine)	Atlantooccipital joint Radiocarpal joints Metacarpophalangeal joints

Ball and socket illustration labels: Hip bone, Femur

Hinge illustration labels: Humerus, Ulna

Pivot illustration labels: Atlas, Axis

Ellipsoid/condyloid illustration labels: Metacarpal, Phalanges

▶ TABLE 2-3. TYPES OF SYNOVIAL JOINTS (continued)

Type of Joint	Number of Planes/Axes	Movements Possible	Examples
Saddle	Biaxial	Flexion Extension Abduction Adduction	1st Carpometacarpal joint (thumb)
Gliding	Nonaxial	N/A	Acromioclavicular joint Intercarpal joints

(longitudinal) movements at that joint. There are pivot joints at the atlantoaxial joint of the cervical spine and the radioulnar joints of the forearm.

- **Ellipsoid** (or *condyloid*) **joints** are similar to ball and socket joints, but have oval-shaped joint surfaces that resemble a flattened circle or ellipse (*ellip-* means shortened). Some resemble a condyle, which we defined earlier as a prominence that forms joints, giving them their alternate name. Ellipsoid joints are **biaxial** because they can move on two planes. The radiocarpal joints of the wrist and the metacarpophalangeal joints of the hand are examples.
- **Saddle joints** are made up of two bony surfaces that are concave in one direction and convex in the other. They fit together like a rider sitting in a saddle, hence their name. These joints are also biaxial and found only in the carpometacarpal joint of the thumbs. This allows unique movements in the thumbs that are found in none of the other digits.
- **Gliding joints** have flat surfaces that allow small, planar movements. These joints are considered **nonaxial** because they are the least mobile of all synovial joints. Limited movement is allowed between the articular processes of the vertebrae, the bones of the shoulder girdle, and the carpal bones of the hand.

ACCESSORY MOTIONS

In Chapter 1, we described joint movement through the cardinal planes (flexion, extension, abduction, etc.). These gross movements are called **physiological movements**. In contrast, the term **accessory motion** describes movement of a joint's articulating surfaces relative to each other. Full-range physiological movement depends on normal, healthy accessory motion. This in turn depends on a certain amount of "give" in the joint capsule and ligaments that surround that joint. This "give" is called **joint play**.

The terms *roll*, *glide*, and *spin* describe what happens between the joint surfaces as the joint is taken through physiological movements (Fig. 2-7). Each of these accessory motions helps maintain optimal joint position during physiological movements. This prevents compression and loss of contact between the articulating surfaces of the joint.

Roll

Rolling occurs when a series of points on one bony surface come in contact with a corresponding series of points on the other (Fig. 2-7A). This is similar to various points on a car tire contacting various points on the ground as a car rolls

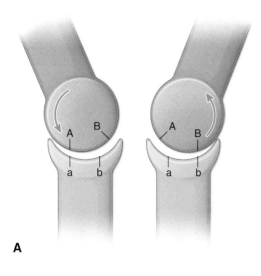

A

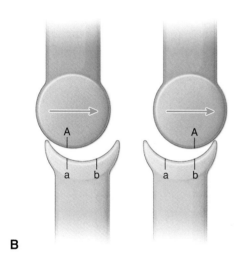

B

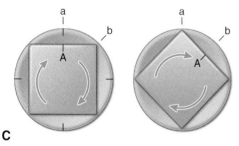

C

2-7. Accessory motions. Normal accessory motions are necessary for full-range physiological movement to occur. They prevent compression and loss of contact between the articulating surfaces of the joint. **A.** *Roll* occurs when a series of points on one bony surface (A and B) come in contact with a corresponding series of points on the other (a and b) (lateral view). **B.** *Glide* occurs when a point on one bony surface comes in contact with a series of points on another (lateral view). **C.** *Spin* occurs when one surface (A) rotates clockwise or counterclockwise around a stationary longitudinal axis (a and b) (superior view).

forward leaving a tread mark on the ground. For example, the rounded condyles of the femur roll on the depressed tibial plateau as the knee is flexed and extended.

Glide

Gliding occurs when a point on one bony surface comes in contact with a series of points on another (Fig. 2-7B). This is similar to a "skidding" motion: The tire isn't rolling, but the car still moves forward. Gliding is sometimes referred to as *translation*. Often, gliding and rolling occur together, maintaining optimal joint position. Let's use the tibiofemoral joint to illustrate (Fig. 2-8). Imagine you are moving to sit in a chair. As the knee moves through flexion, the femur rolls posteriorly and glides anteriorly (Fig. 2-8A). This maintains optimal contact between the articulating surfaces of both bones. Now imagine standing up from the chair. During extension, the femur rolls anteriorly and glides posteriorly (Fig. 2-8B).

The **convex–concave rule** determines the direction of glide and roll. This rule states that the shape of the joint surfaces will determine how they move. Most joint surfaces are either **convex** (rounded outward) or **concave** (rounded inward) (Fig. 2-9). If a concave joint surface (e.g., the proximal tibia) is moving on a fixed convex surface (e.g., the distal femur), gliding will occur in the same direction as rolling. Conversely, if a convex surface (e.g., the distal femur) is moving on a fixed concave surface (e.g., the proximal tibia), gliding and rolling will occur in opposite directions. According to this rule, the type of accessory motion at the tibiofemoral joint is dependent upon whether the subject is weight bearing (standing on a fixed tibia) or non–weight bearing (sitting or lying down with a fixed femur).

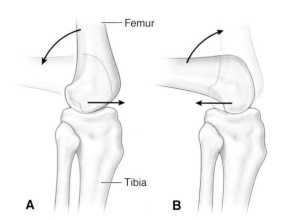

2-8. Roll and glide of the tibiofemoral joint. Often, gliding and rolling occur together, maintaining optimal joint position. **A.** In this lateral view, you can see that the femur rolls posteriorly and glides anteriorly on the tibia during knee flexion. **B.** The femur rolls anteriorly and glides posteriorly during knee extension. This accessory motion follows the *convex–concave rule* for a fixed tibia.

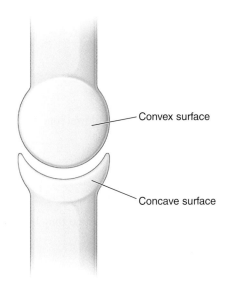

Convex surface

Concave surface

2-9. Convex–concave rule. This principle determines the direction of glide and roll and states that the shape of the joint surfaces will determine how they move. Most joint surfaces are either *convex* and rounded out (shown in blue) or *concave* and rounded in (shown in pink). Which end is fixed determines the direction of accessory motions.

Spin

Spinning occurs when one surface rotates clockwise or counterclockwise around a stationary longitudinal axis. This motion is similar to that of a tire rotating around its axle. Because the tibiofemoral joint is a "modified" hinge joint, it is able to rotate slightly. At the end of knee extension, the tibia spins laterally relative to the femur (Fig. 2-10). This

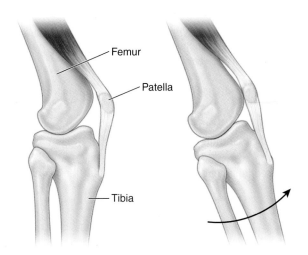

Femur

Patella

Tibia

2-10. Spin of the tibiofemoral joint. At the end of knee extension, the tibia spins laterally relative to the femur, allowing the joint to turn and "lock."

movement allows the tibiofemoral joint to turn and "lock," creating greater joint stability when fully extended. The spinning movement is reversed (the tibia rotates medially) to "unlock" the joint at the beginning of knee flexion.

SUMMARY

- Bones serve four primary functions in the human body, providing: support and protection of soft tissue; a system of levers for movement; a site for blood cell formation; and storage of minerals and fats.
- There are two type of bone tissue: spongy and compact. Spongy bone is porous, arranges its trabeculae according to lines of stress, and is the location of hematopoiesis. Compact bone is denser, tends to surround spongy bone, and has several unique features including a system of transport channels.
- Bones are surrounded by periosteum, which protects and nourishes the underlying structures.
- The typical human skeleton has 206 bones. The axial skeleton is the head and trunk, and the appendicular skeleton is the shoulder girdle, upper extremity, pelvic girdle, and lower extremity.
- Bones come in several shapes including long bones, short bones, flat bones, irregular bones, and Wormian bones. Each shape serves a unique purpose in the body.
- Bony landmarks indicate where nerves or vessels traverse a bone, where muscles, tendons or other structures reside, where joints are formed, and where tendons and ligaments attach. Each has a unique name that indicates its function and location.
- Bones come together to form joints. They are classified according to their structure and function.
- A specific system of naming joints has been established which combines the names of the two bones forming the joint, connecting them with an "o."
- Joint structures include fibrous, cartilaginous, and synovial, each having unique tissues binding them together.
- Joints can be classified as synarthrotic, amphiarthrotic, or diarthrotic. Each category has increasing space between joint surfaces and thus increased mobility.
- Synovial joints allow the most amount of movement in the human body.
- Synovial joint features include a thick joint capsule and a joint cavity containing synovial fluid.
- Synovial joints come in several shapes including ball-and-socket, hinge, pivot, ellipsoid (or condyloid), saddle, and gliding. Each shape has unique movement possibilities.
- Accessory motion describes movement between joint surfaces. It occurs in conjunction with physiological movements. Accessory motion decreases compression and maintains optimal joint alignment as the body moves.
- Roll, glide, and spin are the three types of accessory motion.

FOR REVIEW

Multiple Choice

1. The term that describes blood cell formation is:
   A. homeostasis
   B. hematopoiesis
   C. hemodynamics
   D. hemorrhage

2. A mineral that is stored in bones and assists with maintaining acid-base balance of the blood, nerve impulse conduction, muscle contraction, maintenance of blood pressure, and blood clotting is:
   A. phosphorus
   B. manganese
   C. calcium
   D. carbon

3. Porous tissue that is a site for blood cell formation.
   A. spongy bone
   B. trabeculae
   C. compact bone
   D. periosteum

4. Tissue that surrounds bones, providing nourishment, protection, and regeneration following injury.
   A. spongy bone
   B. trabeculae
   C. compact bone
   D. periosteum

5. A rounded articular projection that forms a joint.
   A. foramen
   B. meatus
   C. condyle
   D. fossa

6. A sharp, slender prominence where a tendon or ligament attaches.
   A. ramus
   B. spine
   C. meatus
   D. facet

7. The process by which osteoblasts lay down bone to replace a fibrous or cartilaginous model.
   A. ossification
   B. hematopoiesis
   C. osteology
   D. arthrology

8. Fills the center of the diaphysis of a mature long bone.
   A. trabeculae
   B. calcium
   C. yellow marrow
   D. red marrow

9. Type of bone that fills the spaces between cranial bones.
   A. sesamoid bone
   B. Wormian bone
   C. irregular bone
   D. flat bone

10. Accessory motion described by a series of points on one bony surface coming in contact with a corresponding series of points on the other.
    A. spin
    B. glide
    C. roll
    D. convex

Matching

Different types of joints are listed below. Match them with their appropriate qualities.

11. _____ Pivot

12. _____ Fibrous

13. _____ Gliding

14. _____ Saddle

15. _____ Synovial

16. _____ Ellipsoid/Condyloid

17. _____ Cartilaginous

18. _____ Hinge

19. _____ Ball-and-socket

20. _____ Synostosis

A. Always contain a joint capsule, joint cavity, and synovial fluid, making them freely movable.
B. The only triaxial synovial joint.
C. Has bony surfaces tightly bound by connective tissue.
D. Can only be found in the 1st carpometacarpal joint (thumb).
E. Characterized by ossification between bones.
F. A uniaxial joint that rotates.
G. Bony surfaces are joined by pliable soft tissue allowing slight movement.
H. Found in the intercarpal joints of the hand.
I. Can be "modified" to include more motion than uniaxial flexion and extension.
J. Found at the metacarpophalangeal joints or "knuckles" of the hand.

Short Answer

21. Identify and describe all of the functions of bone.

22. Compare and contrast the axial and appendicular skeleton. List the bones that make up each.

23. Identify the different bone shapes in the body and give an example of each.

24. Compare and contrast accessory motion and physiological movement. Identify the three types of accessory motion.

25. Identify each structure pointed out in the diagrams below.

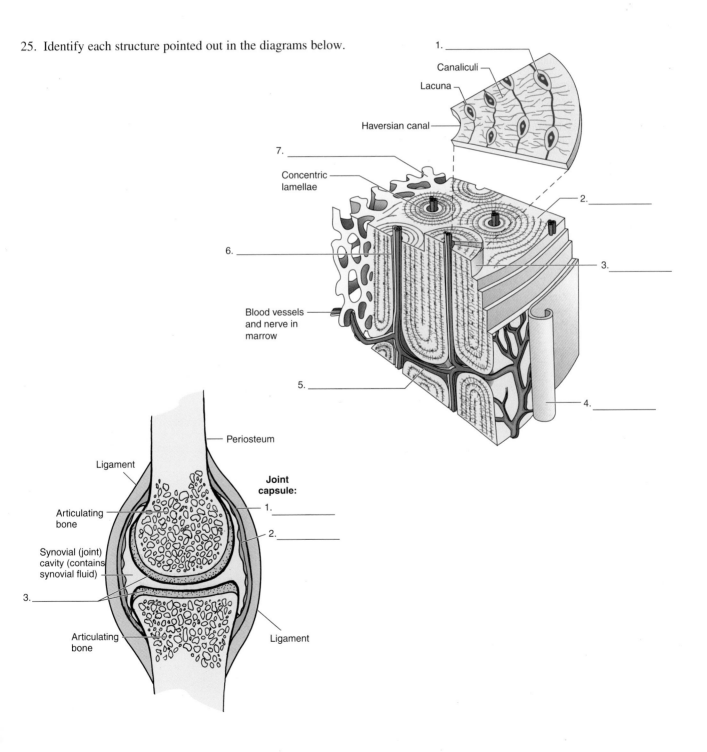

1. _____

Canaliculi

Lacuna

Haversian canal

7. _____

Concentric lamellae

2. _____

6. _____

3. _____

Blood vessels and nerve in marrow

5. _____

4. _____

Periosteum

Ligament

Joint capsule:

Articulating bone

1. _____

2. _____

Synovial (joint) cavity (contains synovial fluid)

3. _____

Articulating bone

Ligament

Try This!

Activity: Create a set of cards, each card indicating a type of joint (fibrous, cartilaginous, synovial). Also, have cards with the different types of synovial joints (ball-and-socket, hinge, pivot, ellipsoid/condyloid, saddle, and gliding). Shuffle your cards and draw one. Point out on your own body (or that of a partner) a joint that fits the category you chose. Practice using the joint's proper name (glenohumeral joint rather than shoulder) as you point it out. If you can't remember the joint name, use the bone + o + bone formula. Say the name out loud even if you are working by yourself.

Further challenge yourself by identifying the joint as uniaxial, biaxial, triaxial, or nonaxial (if you chose a synovial joint). Once you have done that, perform the movements possible at the joint. Say the movements as you do them.

SUGGESTED READINGS

Clarkson H. *Joint Motion and Function: A Research-Based Practical Guide*. Baltimore, MD: Lippincott, Williams & Wilkins; 2005.

Frost HM. From Wolff's law to the Utah paradigm: insights about bone physiology and its clinical applications. *Anat Rec.* 2001;262(4):398–419.

Moore KL, Dalley AF II. *Clinical Oriented Anatomy*. 4th Ed. Baltimore, MD: Lippincott Williams, & Wilkins; 1999.

Oatis CA. *Kinesiology—The Mechanics and Pathomechanics of Human Movement*. Baltimore, MD: Lippincott, Williams & Wilkins; 2004.

Prekumar K. *The Massage Connection Anatomy & Physiology*. 2nd Ed. Baltimore, MD: Lippincott, Williams, & Wilkins; 2004.

Prentice WE. *Techniques in Musculoskeletal Rehabilitation*. New York, NY: McGraw-Hill; 2001.

Ruff C, Holt B, Trinkaus E. Who's afraid of the big bad Wolff? "Wolff's law" and bone functional adaptation. *Am J Phys Anthropol.* 2006;129(4):484–498.

Myology

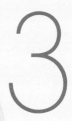

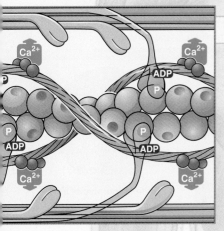

Learning Objectives

After working through the material in this chapter, you should be able to:

- Compare and contrast the three types of muscle tissue in the human body.
- Discuss the five functions of skeletal muscle.
- Compare and contrast parallel and pennate fiber arrangements and give an example of each.
- Identify the six factors that make up muscle names. Give examples using each factor.
- Explain the contribution of each of the five properties of skeletal muscle tissue to human movement.
- Identify the major macroscopic and microscopic structures of muscle tissue and describe the function of each.
- List the events that lead to a skeletal muscle contraction and identify all chemicals necessary in the process.
- Discuss the factors that influence the amount of force produced by a muscle.

- Compare and contrast slow twitch, fast twitch, and intermediate muscle fibers.
- Compare and contrast isometric and isotonic muscle contractions.
- Compare and contrast concentric and eccentric muscle contractions.
- Discuss the functional interrelationships between agonist, synergist, and antagonist muscles.
- Identify the major skeletal muscles of the human body.
- Identify the components of a lever and give an example of each type of lever in the human body.
- Identify and describe the anatomical structures of proprioception in the human body.
- Define and demonstrate active, passive, and resisted range of motion.
- Explain the purpose of performing active, passive, and resisted range of motion.

Chapter Outline

Now that we have discussed *osteology* (the study of bones) and *arthrology* (the study of joints), we are ready to examine **myology** (the study of muscles). All movements, from blinking an eye to jumping a hurdle, require the participation of muscles. Although there are three types of muscle tissue in the human body, in this chapter we focus on one: skeletal muscle, the type that generates movement. We will look at its functions and unique properties, and then explore the relationship between its structure and its ability to contract to produce the force behind human movement.

Once myology has been explored, concepts from Chapters 1 through 3 will be fused to examine more complex components of human movement. We will examine levers, where they are found in the human body, and their purpose. Next, we will explore the structures of proprioception and how they work. The chapter will finish with an examination of range of motion: the types, purpose, and guidelines for performing range of motion assessment.

TYPES OF MUSCLE TISSUE

The three types of muscle tissue in the human body are smooth, cardiac, and skeletal. Each type is found in specific locations and serves individual functions (Fig. 3-1).

Smooth Muscle

Smooth muscle is present in the walls of hollow organs, vessels, and respiratory passageways, where it functions in digestion, reproduction, circulation, and breathing. This type of muscle is called *involuntary* because it is not under our conscious control. For example, we don't have to think about pushing food through our digestive tract. Instead, in response to the presence of food, smooth muscle automatically generates the wavelike contractions (called *peristalsis*) that move digestion forward. Smooth muscle within blood vessels and bronchioles (found in the respiratory system) dilates and contracts these structures to increase or decrease the flow of blood or air. The pupil of the eye is also able to dilate and contract in response to changing light thanks to smooth muscle. Finally, smooth muscle surrounding hair follicles allows our hair to "stand on end," trapping warm air close to the body when we are cold.

Smooth muscle is so named because it has no **striations**, visible alternating dark and light fibers within other types of muscle tissue. Striations are indicative of tightly arranged proteins responsible for strong muscle contractions. In smooth muscle, these contractile proteins are scattered rather than aligned, and thus it appears unstriated. True striations are not necessary because smooth muscle contractions are slow, steady, and somewhat weaker than the contractions produced by striated cardiac and skeletal muscles.

Cardiac Muscle

Cardiac muscle makes up the wall of the heart, creating the pulsing action necessary to circulate blood. As with smooth muscle, it is involuntary: we do not consciously in-

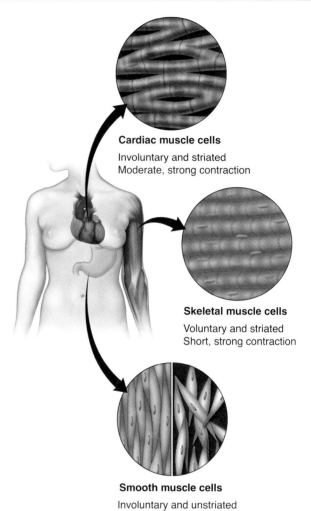

Cardiac muscle cells
Involuntary and striated
Moderate, strong contraction

Skeletal muscle cells
Voluntary and striated
Short, strong contraction

Smooth muscle cells
Involuntary and unstriated
Slow, steady contraction

3-1. Muscle types. Cardiac, smooth, and skeletal muscles are the three types in the human body. Each has a unique structure and location reflecting its function.

struct the muscle fibers in the heart to beat and push blood through the body. Unlike smooth muscle, cardiac muscle is striated, its bands of contractile proteins generating its steady, powerful contractions.

Cardiac muscle is unique in that the electrical impulse necessary for its fibers to contract travels from cell to cell. This trait allows the muscle fibers of the heart to synchronize and function as a single unit. Thus, the unified action of the cardiac muscle creates the powerful pumping action that drives the circulatory system.

Skeletal Muscle

Skeletal muscles are connected to bones and produce movement at joints. This is the only muscle type that is *voluntary* (under conscious control): we decide how and when our skeletal muscles contract to produce movement. Involuntary movement is possible, too: sometimes **reflexes**, protective mechanisms that occur without thought, activate skeletal muscles. Like cardiac muscle, skeletal muscle is striated, producing very strong, rapid contractions when activated. However, its fibers fatigue more rapidly than those of smooth or cardiac muscle.

Skeletal muscle fibers are fragile, and thus vulnerable to damage, and they have a very limited ability to regenerate themselves following injury. Fortunately, they are bundled together and reinforced with connective tissue (discussed shortly), which protects them during strong muscle contractions. These connective tissue envelopes converge to form tendons, attaching skeletal muscles to the bones they move.

SKELETAL MUSCLE FUNCTIONS

Since our focus in this text is human movement, we will direct our attention primarily to skeletal muscle. Skeletal muscle has several functions in the body, including initiation of motion, maintenance of posture, protection, heat production, and fluid pumping.

Motion

The primary function of skeletal muscles is to exert a pull on the bones, creating motion. Contracting muscles lift the feet off the ground, swing the arms back and forth, and even purse the lips for whistling while you walk. Skeletal muscles also expand the ribcage when you take a deep breath and contract it when you exhale. All of these movements of the body are initiated, modified, and controlled by skeletal muscle contractions.

Posture

Skeletal muscles maintain upright posture against gravity. They keep your head up and centered, your trunk straight and erect, and your hips and knees aligned over your feet. Skeletal muscles also adjust and respond to changes in posture, as when you lean over or stand up from a chair. These postural muscles cannot rest as long as you are awake and upright.

Protection

Skeletal muscles protect underlying structures in areas where bones do not. For example, the abdomen is unprotected by the skeleton, making the underlying organs vulnerable. Strong abdominal muscles protect the deep structures while allowing free movement of the trunk.

Thermogenesis

As the skeletal muscles contract to create movement, they also produce body heat. This heat production is called **thermogenesis**. Approximately three-quarters of the energy created by muscle tissue is heat. We can see this function when it's cold and the body begins to shiver. These involuntary muscle contractions produce heat and warm the body.

Vascular Pump

We know that cardiac muscle is responsible for driving the circulatory system, but the skeletal muscles also play a role. Specifically, contractions of skeletal muscles help propel the circulation of lymph and venous blood. The pumping of the heart keeps the pressure within arteries high, but both lymphatic vessels and veins have relatively low pressure. They require help from the contraction of surrounding muscles to keep their fluids moving forward. This is particularly important where these fluids must flow upward against gravity, as with venous blood returning to the heart from the lower limbs.

FIBER DIRECTION AND NAMING MUSCLES

Recall from our discussion about palpation of muscles (Chapter 1) that skeletal muscle cells, called muscle *fibers*, line up in parallel formations. On a larger scale, bundles of muscle fibers are arranged to achieve specific actions (Table 3-1). The two major divisions of fiber arrangements are parallel and pennate.

Parallel Arrangements

Parallel muscles have fibers equal in length that do not intersect. This arrangement enables the entire muscle to shorten equally and in the same direction. Parallel arrangement maximizes range of motion. Configurations include fusiform, circular, and triangular.

Fusiform Muscles

Fusiform fiber arrangements have a thick central belly with tapered ends. These tapered ends focus force production into specific bony landmarks. The *brachialis* and *biceps brachii* in the arm are examples of fusiform muscles. The biceps brachii in particular has very specific attachment points and a large range of motion.

Circular Muscles

Circular fiber arrangements surround an opening to form a sphincter. These muscles are designed to contract and close passages or relax and open them. The *orbicularis oris* around the mouth and the *sphincter ani* of the anus are both circular muscles. Each of these muscles regulates what passes in and out of the digestive system.

Triangular Muscles

Triangular fiber arrangements start at a broad base then converge to a single point. This fan-shaped arrangement allows them to diversify their actions, creating multiple movement possibilities. Both the *pectoralis major* and *trapezius* are triangular muscles with multiple, sometimes opposing, actions. These muscles can pull in different directions depending upon which fibers are recruited.

▶ TABLE 3-1. FIBER ARRANGEMENTS

	Appearance	Purpose	Examples
Parallel Arrangements		Shorten equally and in the same direction to maximize range of motion.	
Fusiform		Focus force production into specific bony landmarks.	Brachialis Biceps brachii
Circular		Contract and close passages or relax and open them.	Orbicularis oris Sphincter ani
Triangular		Diversification of actions, creating multiple movement possibilities.	Pectoralis major Trapezius
Pennate Arrangements		Maximize the number of fibers in an area for greater force production.	
Unipennate		Strong force production from one direction.	Tibialis posterior Biceps femoris
Bipennate		Strong force production from two directions.	Rectus femoris
Multipennate		Weaker force production from many directions.	Deltoid

Pennate Arrangements

Pennate muscles are feather-shaped (*penna* means feather) with shorter muscle fibers intersecting a central tendon. This arrangement maximizes the number of fibers in an area. More muscle fibers mean greater cross-sectional area and greater force production by these types of muscles. Pennate muscles, like parallel ones, come in several different types including unipennate, bipennate, and multipennate.

Unipennate Muscles

Unipennate muscle fibers run obliquely from one side of a central tendon. These muscles look like half of a feather. This arrangement allows strong force production from one direction. The *tibialis posterior* and *biceps femoris* are examples of unipennate muscles.

Bipennate Muscles

Bipennate muscle fibers run obliquely along both sides of a central tendon. These muscles look like a full feather. Very strong muscle contractions are possible from bipennate muscles as the central tendon is pulled from two directions. The *rectus femoris* is an example of a bipennate muscle.

Multipennate Muscles

Multiple tendons with oblique muscle fibers on both sides characterize **multipennate** muscles. The muscle fibers connect the tendons and pull from many directions. Of the three types of pennate muscles, this type produces the least amount of force. The multipennate design of the *deltoid* allows it to wrap around the outside of the shoulder and perform many different actions.

Naming Muscles

A muscle's name can reflect any of several characteristics, including its fiber direction, location, action, size, shape, and number of heads.

Box 3-1   CHARACTERISTICS USED TO NAME MUSCLES

- Fiber direction (*oblique, rectus, transverse*)
- Location (*brachii, femoris, pectoralis, abdominus*)
- Action (*flexor, extensor, adductor, abductor, pronator, supinator*)
- Size (*major, minor, maximus, medius, minimus, magnus, longus, brevis*)
- Shape (*trapezius, rhomboid, deltoid, serratus, quadratus*)
- Number of heads (*biceps, triceps, quadriceps*)

Fiber Direction

We have already discussed muscle fiber direction as the configuration of muscle fibers relative to their tendon (see above). Terms such as *oblique* (slanting) and *rectus* (straight) identify a muscle's fiber direction. The *external oblique* and *rectus abdominus* are both abdominal muscles, but are distinguished by their fiber direction.

Location

Often a muscle name will include its location or relative position in the body to differentiate it from a similar-looking muscle in a different area. Terms such as *brachii* (arm), *femoris* (thigh), *pectoralis* (chest), and *abdominus* (abdomen) identify regional location. We utilize this strategy when identifying the *biceps brachii* and *triceps brachii*, the *rectus femoris* and *rectus abdominus*, and the *pectoralis major*.

The location of muscle attachments is also reflected in muscle names. We see this with the *coracobrachialis*, which attaches to the coracoid process of the scapula, and the *iliacus*, which attaches to the iliac fossa of the pelvis. Similarly, the spinalis group of muscles attaches to the spinous processes of the vertebrae. In contrast, *supraspinatus* has no attachment to the vertebrae. Instead, it attaches to the supraspinous fossa of the scapula: *supra* means above, and here *spina* refers to the spine of the scapula.

Action

Sometimes it's useful to identify a muscle's action or movement in its name. Terms such as *flexor, extensor, adductor,* and *abductor* give insight into a muscle's purpose. Muscles named by their action include the *flexor carpi radialis, extensor digitorum,* and *pronator teres*.

Size

When muscles of similar shape and function reside in the same location, it is useful to distinguish them by size or bulk. The following muscles are all differentiated by size:

- *pectoralis major* and *minor*
- *gluteus maximus, medius,* and *minimus*
- *peroneus longus, brevis,* and *tertius*
- *adductor magnus, longus,* and *brevis*.

Shape

Sometimes a muscle has a unique shape or appearance, which reminded early anatomists of certain objects. For example, the kite-shaped *trapezius* is reminiscent of a geometric trapezoid. The triangular-shaped *deltoid* looks like the Greek letter *delta*. And jagged-edged *serratus anterior* has a shape that corresponds to a saw (*serratus* is Latin for saw-shaped).

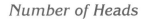

Number of Heads

Finally, a muscle may have more than one division or *head*. Using the suffix *–ceps*, which means "head," anatomists identify such muscles as *biceps* (two heads), *triceps* (three heads), and *quadriceps* (four heads). Examples include the *biceps brachii* and *triceps brachii* of the upper extremity. Four anterior thigh muscles that extend the knee are typically grouped together as the *quadriceps*. Three posterior lower leg muscles that share the Achilles tendon are sometimes referred to as the *triceps surae* (literally translated, "three-headed calf muscle").

By putting together certain qualities, we can glean information from a muscle's name. We know, for example, that the *pectoralis major* is a large chest muscle. We can guess that there is a smaller muscle in the same region (*pectoralis minor*). From its name we can tell that the *latissimus dorsi* is a broad muscle on the back of the body (*lati* means broad and *dors* means back). A *flexor carpi ulnaris* is a muscle that attaches to the ulna and flexes the wrist. We can discover all of this just from a muscle's name!

SKELETAL MUSCLE PROPERTIES

Now that we have a clearer idea of why we need skeletal muscles, how they are arranged, and how to name them, let's look more closely at how they work. Muscle tissue is one of the four primary tissue types in the body (see Chapter 1). It is different from the others (nervous, epithelial, and connective) in that it possesses the properties of extensibility, elasticity, excitability, conductivity, and contractility. Together, these properties enable a skeletal muscle to generate movement.

Extensibility

Extensibility is the ability to stretch without sustaining damage. This property allows muscles to lengthen when relaxed. This is important because muscles usually work in opposite directions as they produce movement while maintaining stability and balance at joints. If one muscle is shortening, its opposite must relax and lengthen to allow the joint to move in the intended direction. For example, when the anterior muscles of your upper arm (flexors) shorten, the posterior muscles of your upper arm (extensors) must relax and lengthen. Without extensibility, the lengthening muscles would be damaged.

Elasticity

Elasticity is the ability to return to original shape after lengthening or shortening. As muscle tissue performs its various functions, its shape changes or *deforms*. Once its work is completed, the muscle tissue can rest and resume its original form. This property maintains a specific shape and geometry in muscles despite their malleable nature. Using our previous example, once the flexors of the arm have finished contracting and the corresponding lengthening has occurred in the extensors, both will return to a resting length. This return to original length is possible because of elasticity.

Excitability

Excitability (also called *irritability*) means muscle tissue can respond to a stimulus by producing electrical signals. In response to an event such as a touch or a decision to move, nerves at their junction with muscles release specialized chemicals called *neurotransmitters*. The neurotransmitters prompt propagation (spread) of an electrical signal called an **action potential** that in turn triggers a series of events that lead to muscle contraction (see Sliding Filament Mechanism). Without this ability to respond to the nervous system, muscles would not be able to contract and function.

Conductivity

Conductivity describes muscle tissue's ability to propagate electrical signals, including action potentials. Once muscle tissue is "excited" by the nervous system, it must carry the electrical signal to the inner cell structures. Conductivity allows the action potential to be transmitted along the muscle cell, activating the tissue, and initiating a muscle contraction.

Contractility

Contractility is the ability to shorten and thicken—thus producing force—in response to a specific stimulus. Here, that stimulus is an action potential initiated by the nervous system. This ability to shorten is a unique feature of muscle tissue and responsible for its force-production ability. Specialized proteins within muscle tissue interact to shorten and thicken muscles, generating force. The human body depends on this force to move.

Box 3-2	SKELETAL MUSCLE PROPERTIES

- Extensibility: ability to stretch without damaging tissue
- Elasticity: ability to return to original shape after stretching or shortening
- Excitability: ability to respond to stimulus by producing electrical signals
- Conductivity: ability to propagate an electrical signal
- Contractility: ability to shorten and thicken in response to a stimulus

ANATOMY OF SKELETAL MUSCLE TISSUE

In order to understand how muscles generate force and produce movement, we must look at their macroscopic and microscopic anatomy.

Macroscopic Anatomy

Connective tissue wrappings support, protect, and separate portions of muscle and whole muscles (FIG. 3-2). Individual muscle cells, called *fibers*, are each wrapped in a sheath of connective tissue called the **endomysium** (*endo-* means within). Many muscle fibers group into bundles called **fascicles**, which are held together and encircled by a layer of connective tissue called the **perimysium** (*peri-* means around). Finally, these "bundles of bundles" are enveloped by the **epimysium** (*epi-* signifies a covering), part of the network of deep fascia (discussed in Chapter 1). All of these connective tissue layers work together to help transmit force while protecting the muscle fibers from damage during muscle contraction.

As shown in Figure 3-2, the epimysium surrounding a whole muscle converges to form a tendon that connects the muscle to bone. The **musculotendinous junction** describes the point at which this connective tissue convergence begins. The portion of the muscle between tendons is called the **muscle belly**. Larger blood vessels and nerves are enclosed within the epimysium, and capillaries and nerve fiber endings are wrapped within the endomysium where they interact with individual muscle fibers.

Microscopic Anatomy

If we were to look at muscle fibers under the microscope, we would see several specialized structures (see Fig. 3-2). The entire fiber is surrounded by the **sarcolemma**, which serves as the cell membrane and regulates chemical transport into and out of the fiber. Surrounding the structures within the fiber is a gelatinous substance called the **sarcoplasm**, the cytoplasm of muscle cells.

Important structures within the muscle fiber are the nuclei and the myofibrils. Most cells in the human body have a single nucleus, but muscle fibers have multiple **nuclei** that contain the functional information for the cell and control its operations. The **myofibrils** are the specialized contractile proteins that make skeletal muscle tissue appear striated. The stripes of the myofibrils reflect their two types of filaments: **Thin filaments** (seen in light blue in Fig. 3-2) occur alone at the lighter I band. The darker A band is where thin and **thick filaments** (seen in red) overlap. The lighter I bands are interrupted by a zigzag line called the Z line. This line marks the borders of the functional units of the muscle fiber, called **sarcomeres**; that is, a sarcomere includes structures from one Z line to the next. As we'll explain in more detail shortly, sarcomeres are considered the functional units of muscle fibers because it is the shortening of sarcomeres that produces muscle contraction.

Other functional structures contained within the sarcolemma include **mitochondria**, which produce **adenosine triphosphate** (**ATP**), a compound that stores the energy needed for muscle contraction. A network of tubules is also present: these **transverse tubules** run at right angles to the sarcomeres and transmit nerve impulses from the sarcolemma to the cell interior. The **sarcoplasmic reticulum** is a network of fluid-filled chambers that covers each myofibril like a lacy sleeve. Its channels store calcium ions, an electrically charged form of the mineral calcium, which you learned in Chapter 2 helps trigger muscle contractions.

PHYSIOLOGY OF MUSCLE CONTRACTION

Remember that one of the properties of muscle tissue is excitability. Muscle cells must respond to stimuli from the nervous system in order to function. So before we can examine the events that cause a muscle to contract, we must first learn how nerves and muscles communicate.

Events at the Neuromuscular Junction

FIGURE 3-3 shows the connection between neurons and muscle fibers. It is called the **neuromuscular junction**.

Recall from Chapter 1 that neurons have a thin axon that reaches out from the cell body to transmit an action potential through its terminal branches toward other cells—in this case skeletal muscle fibers. Unlike other types of electrical signals, action potentials are strong, invariable, and capable of traveling long distances in the body—from a neuron in your brain that decides to turn a page of this book to the muscle fibers in your fingers that do the turning. The axon branches nearly touch the muscle fibers they innervate, but a gap called a **synapse** (or *synaptic cleft*) prevents the signal from crossing to the muscle on its own. The signal can jump this gap only with the help of **acetylcholine** (abbreviated ACh), which is a type of neurotransmitter. ACh is stored in little sacs called *synaptic vesicles* at the ends of axon branches, and is released when an action potential reaches the neuromuscular junction. Once across the synaptic cleft, ACh binds to receptors within the muscle fiber's sarcolemma. This stimulates chemical changes that initiate a new action potential, this time on the muscle fiber "side" of the neuromuscular junction. This new action potential in turn initiates the chemical processes of muscle contraction. As we noted earlier in the chapter, transmission of action potentials in skeletal muscles fibers is possible because of their property of conductivity.

To review the steps involved in initiating muscle contraction:

1. A neuron sends an electrical signal called an action potential down its axon.

2. The signal reaches the ends of the axon branches, where it stimulates synaptic vesicles to release the neurotransmitter acetylcholine (ACh).

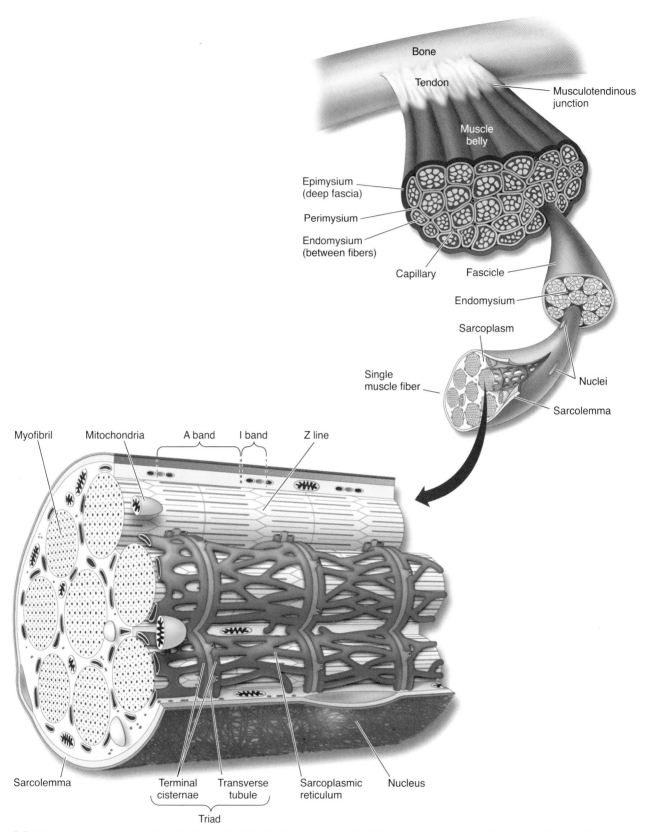

3-2. Macroscopic anatomy of skeletal muscle. Muscle fibers are organized into muscles by successive layers of connective tissue, including the epimysium, perimysium, and endomysium. This arrangement separates and protects fragile muscle fibers while directing forces toward the bone. The sarcolemma envelops the nucleus, mitochondria, and myofibrils. Myofibrils contain well-organized proteins that overlap and form Z lines, I bands, and A bands. The sarcoplasmic reticulum houses calcium and the transverse tubules transmit electrical signal from the sarcolemma inside the cell, both critical to muscle function.

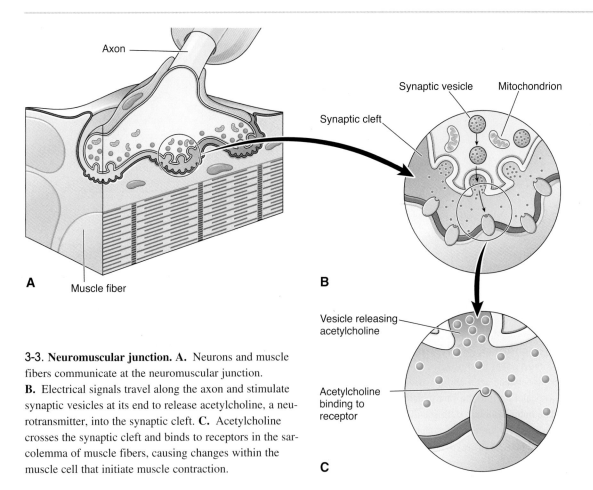

3-3. Neuromuscular junction. A. Neurons and muscle fibers communicate at the neuromuscular junction. **B.** Electrical signals travel along the axon and stimulate synaptic vesicles at its end to release acetylcholine, a neurotransmitter, into the synaptic cleft. **C.** Acetylcholine crosses the synaptic cleft and binds to receptors in the sarcolemma of muscle fibers, causing changes within the muscle cell that initiate muscle contraction.

3. Acetylcholine molecules cross the synaptic cleft and bind with receptors in the sarcolemma.
4. A muscle action potential travels along the sarcolemma and down the transverse tubules.

The remaining question is: How does the muscle action potential lead to muscle contraction?

Sliding Filament Theory

The events that follow production of the muscle action potential are described by the **sliding filament theory**. It explains how contractile proteins within the thin and thick filaments of the myofibrils bind and release to produce shortening in the sarcomere—that is, a muscle contraction. Four contractile proteins are involved (FIG. 3-4):

- Thin filaments are made up of strands of a globular protein called **actin**. Notice in Figure 3-4 that actin "beads" are assembled in long strands.
- The actin beads are covered with threads of **tropomyosin,** a protein that—as long as the muscle is relaxed—covers binding sites on the actin molecules, preventing them from participating in muscle contraction.
- The tropomyosin threads are in turn studded with and controlled by clusters of **troponin**. This protein keeps tropomyosin in place over actin's binding sites in relaxed muscle, and moves it out of the way to allow muscle contraction.

- Thick filaments are composed of a protein called **myosin** that forms shorter, thicker ropes with bulbous heads (see Fig. 3-4). These heads must bind with actin for muscle contraction to occur.

Now let's see how these four proteins contribute to muscle contraction.

After the action potential crosses the neuromuscular junction, it travels to the sarcoplasmic reticulum. From here, stored calcium ions are released into the sarcoplasm. The calcium ions bind with the studs of troponin on the thin filaments, thereby "moving aside" the tropomyosin protein strands covering the binding sites on the actin filament. With the binding sites of actin revealed, the thin filament is ready for contraction.

Meanwhile, the myosin heads on the thick filament are charged with energy from the breakdown of adenosine triphosphate (ATP). (Recall that the mitochondria in the muscle fibers synthesize ATP.) This energy is used to bind the myosin heads to the active receptor sites on the actin filament, making connections called **cross-bridges**.

Once cross-bridges are formed, a ratcheting action called the **power stroke** can occur as the myosin heads, bound to actin, pull the sarcomere together. Like a line of rowers in a long boat simultaneously pulling their oars against the water, myosin heads along the thick filaments pull and slide the thin filaments toward the center of the sarcomere, shortening the strand (FIG. 3-5).

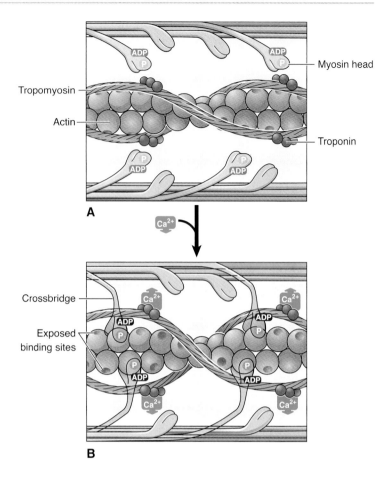

3-4. The events of muscle contraction. A. At rest, strands of tropomyosin proteins cover binding sites on actin and prevent interaction between actin and myosin. **B.** Action potentials release calcium into the sarcoplasm, which bind to troponin. The bound calcium deforms the tropomyosin protein, exposing actin binding sites and allowing cross-bridges to form between the myosin heads and actin.

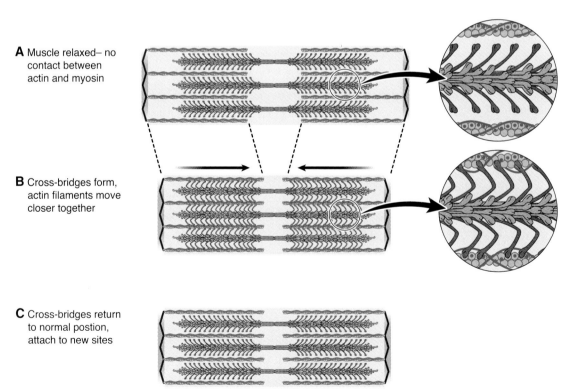

A Muscle relaxed– no contact between actin and myosin

B Cross-bridges form, actin filaments move closer together

C Cross-bridges return to normal postion, attach to new sites

3-5. Sliding filament mechanism. A. Prior to transmission of the action potential, no cross-bridges connect actin and myosin. **B.** Once the active sites are revealed and myosin heads bind to actin, the power stroke occurs. Synchronized movement of the myosin heads pulls the ends of the sarcomere together, shortening the muscle. **C.** Energy from ATP releases the myosin heads and positions them for another power stroke.

Box 3-3   EVENTS OF A MUSCLE CONTRACTION

1. Action potential crosses to sarcolemma.
2. Calcium ions released from sarcoplasmic reticulum.
3. Active sites on actin exposed as calcium ions bind to troponin.
4. Charged myosin heads bind to actin creating cross-bridges.
5. Power stroke pulls ends of sarcomere together creating muscle contraction.

As the myosin heads complete their power stroke, they bind more ATP. This provides the energy necessary for them to release their hold on the actin strand. The cross-bridges detach. This process is repeated by alternating myosin heads on both sides of the thin filament along the length of the muscle fiber, creating muscle contractions.

Once the sliding thick and thin filaments have accomplished muscle contraction, the nerve action potential stops. Any acetylcholine remaining in the synaptic cleft is broken down and deactivated. Calcium ions are released from troponin and actively pumped back into the sarcoplasmic reticulum (using additional energy from ATP). The tropomyosin threads realign with the actin binding sites, preventing further cross-bridge formation. The muscle then passively returns to its resting length.

Factors Affecting Force Production

All muscles generate force by the sliding filament mechanism, but how do the same muscles generate different amounts of force? How can we lift something light, like a piece of paper, and something heavy, like a paperweight, using the same muscle? Moreover, why are some muscles able to generate a much greater maximal force than others? The factors affecting force production include motor unit recruitment, cross-sectional area, fiber arrangement, and muscle length.

Motor Unit Recruitment

The relationship between neurons and muscle fibers is important in determining force production. Neurons responsible for initiating motion, called **motor neurons**, communicate with a specific number of muscle fibers. A motor neuron and all of the fibers it controls is called a **motor unit** (FIG. 3-6). Some motor units, like those in the hand and face, each have very few muscle fibers. They are therefore able to produce fine movements. Others, like those in the thigh, have thousands of muscle fibers, and therefore can produce powerful movements, but they lack fine control.

One muscle is typically composed of multiple motor units. The body can control the amount of force produced by a given muscle by varying the number and size of motor units recruited. Stimulation of a few motor units generates a small amount of force, whereas activating all motor units in a muscle generates maximal force. The process of recruiting more and more motor units is called **summation**. The larger the motor units and the more motor units recruited, the greater the potential force production.

Some motor units remain activated all the time, creating a minimal amount of tension in resting muscles that keeps them firm and in a state of readiness to contract. This tension from continual motor unit activation is called **muscle tone**, and indicates the strength of the connection between the nervous system and skeletal muscles. If muscles are utilized frequently, as with exercise, increased tone may result. Indeed, overworked muscles sometimes develop excessive tone, termed **hypertonicity**. Decreased use or injury can create less tone, or **flaccid** muscles. Muscle tone helps maintain posture and joint stability and decreases time needed for muscle force production.

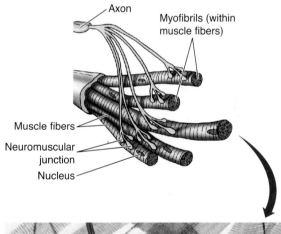

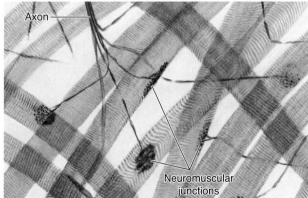

3-6. The motor unit. Motor units include a motor neuron and all of the muscle fibers it innervates. Some, like the one shown here, contain a few muscle fibers. Others contain thousands. The size of the motor unit will influence its force-production capability.

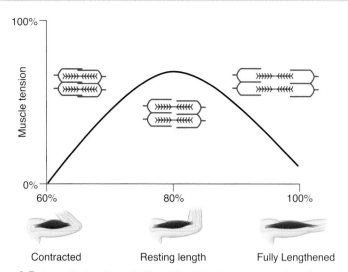

3-7. Length–tension relationship. Muscles at resting length are capable of generating the most force. Interaction between thick and thin filaments is limited in shortened and stretched muscles.

Cross-Sectional Area

Muscle cross-sectional area is a major factor influencing muscle force production. Indeed, force production correlates more closely with a muscle's thickness than its total volume. Thus, shorter, thicker muscles generate more force than longer, thinner muscles. Cross-sectional area is related to the size of myofibrils. As myofibrils become larger through use (hypertrophy), muscles increase in cross-sectional area and are able to generate more force.

Fiber Arrangement

Pennate fiber arrangements generate more total force than their parallel counterparts. This fiber arrangement allows more muscle fibers to reside in a given area. More muscle fibers effectively increase the muscle's cross-sectional area and ability to generate force. Pennate muscles sacrifice range of motion for increased strength and speed.

Muscle Length

The relationship between the thick and thin myofilaments is influenced by a muscle's length; that is, whether it is shortened, relaxed, or stretched beyond resting length (FIG. 3-7). In shortened muscles, there is less distance for the thick and thin filaments to overlap any farther. This decreases their ability to produce force. In contrast, a muscle at resting length has space to shorten as well as maximal interaction between thick and thin filaments. This allows the greatest force production. As a muscle stretches beyond resting length, the number of cross-bridges formed between actin and myosin is diminished. Fewer cross-bridges formed means less force production.

SKELETAL MUSCLE FIBER TYPES

Earlier we classified muscles by their fiber arrangement. We're now ready to classify them by their fiber type, which is determined not only by their anatomy, but also by the way they produce energy from ATP. These factors in turn influence the contraction speed of the three types, as reflected in their names: slow twitch fibers, fast twitch fibers, and intermediate fibers.

Slow Twitch Fibers

Slow twitch fibers, also called *slow oxidative fibers,* contract (or twitch) slowly but are resistant to fatigue (FIG. 3-8A). This is possible because slow twitch fibers rely on **aerobic** energy production. Aerobic energy production utilizes oxygen in generating ATP, hence the name *oxidative.* Slow twitch fibers are utilized for long-duration activities (greater than 2 minutes) such as walking and jogging. Postural muscles that must remain contracted for extended periods are primarily composed of slow twitch fibers.

Fast Twitch Fibers

Fast twitch fibers, also called *fast glycolytic fibers,* generate fast, powerful contractions but quickly fatigue (FIG. 3-8B). These fibers are larger in diameter than their slow twitch

3-8. Muscle fiber types.
A. Slow-twitch fibers contain more capillaries and myoglobin for aerobic energy production. These fibers are recruited for long-duration activities like walking, jogging, and leisurely swimming. **B.** Fast-twitch fibers are thicker, paler, and can make energy without oxygen. These fibers fatigue quickly and are recruited for lifting, jumping, and sprinting.

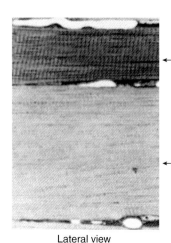

Lateral view

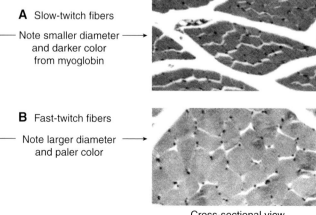

A Slow-twitch fibers

← Note smaller diameter → and darker color from myoglobin

B Fast-twitch fibers

← Note larger diameter → and paler color

Cross-sectional view

counterparts due to a greater number of myofilaments. More myofilaments produce greater amounts of force. Fast twitch fibers do not rely on oxygen for energy production. They utilize **anaerobic** energy production. Here, a form of fuel called glucose is converted to lactate in a process called *glycolysis.* These fibers are utilized for short-duration activities (less than 2 minutes) such as sprinting and lifting. Large, powerful muscles are composed primarily of fast twitch fibers.

Intermediate Fibers

Intermediate fibers, or *fast oxidative glycolitic fibers*, have characteristics of both the slow twitch and fast twitch fibers. Some evidence suggests that these fibers will adapt to the body's demands. For example, as a distance runner trains, the intermediate fibers begin to behave like slow twitch fibers and produce energy aerobically. In someone training as a powerlifter, these fibers adapt and produce energy anaerobically, assisting the fast twitch fibers. Thus, you can think of intermediate fibers as reservists waiting to be called up when and where the need arises.

Distribution of Fiber Types

The distribution of slow-twitch, fast-twitch, and intermediate fibers is intermingled and genetically determined. Some people's muscles have a high concentration of slow-twitch fibers. Their muscles tend to be long and lean. This predisposes them to excel at long-duration activities like marathons or distance biking. Others have high concentrations of fast-twitch fibers, making them great sprinters or body builders. Their muscles tend to be larger and thicker.

Fiber-type distribution is a continuum and varies greatly from one individual to the next.

TYPES OF MUSCLE CONTRACTIONS

Some muscle contractions initiate movement, others control movement, while still others stabilize joints and maintain position of the body. Isometric and isotonic contractions describe these different possibilities.

Isometric Contractions

Isometric contractions occur when tension is generated in a muscle, but the muscle length and joint angle don't change (FIG. 3-9A). This type of contraction is used to stabilize joints rather than create movement. Pushing or pulling against an immovable object or holding an object in a fixed position requires effort by the muscles, but no motion in the joints.

Isotonic Contractions

Isotonic contractions describe muscle contractions that change the length of the muscle and create movement (FIG. 3-9B,C). There are two different types: concentric and eccentric.

Concentric Contractions

In **concentric contractions,** the muscle shortens. This type of contraction initiates or accelerates movement and overcomes some external resistance like gravity (Fig. 3-9B).

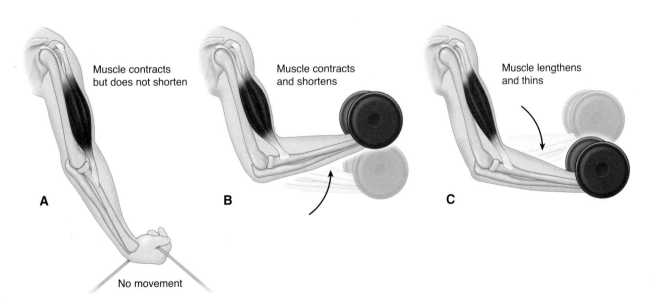

Muscle contracts but does not shorten

Muscle contracts and shortens

Muscle lengthens and thins

A

B

C

No movement

3-9. Contraction types. A. Isometric contractions involve no change in muscle length and are used to stabilize joints. In contrast, isotonic contractions involve changes in muscle length. **B.** Concentric contractions occur when the muscle shortens to initiate or accelerate movement or overcome external resistance. **C.** Eccentric contractions slow and control movements while the muscle lengthens.

Lifting a book off a table or standing up requires concentric contractions.

Eccentric Contractions

Eccentric contractions involve muscle lengthening. These contractions decelerate and control movements and produce greatest force at high speed (Fig. 3-9C). Eccentric contractions are the most powerful, followed by isometric, then concentric. Slowly lowering your book and placing it on the table or lowering yourself into a chair involves eccentric contractions. Injuries often occur with eccentric contractions when we try to prevent or control movements such as falling or dropping an object.

Integrating Contraction Types in Human Movement

Let's see if we can clarify how the body uses isometric, concentric, and eccentric contractions to accomplish everyday tasks. First, let's use the example of sitting in a chair. The quadriceps muscles on the front of your thighs play an important role in this activity. Imagine you are sitting and decide to stand up. The quadriceps muscles shorten to extend your knees, allowing you to rise from the chair. This is a concentric contraction of the quadriceps. The muscles of your trunk are keeping you steady as you rise. This is accomplished with isometric contractions of your trunk muscles. When you decide to sit back down, the quadriceps muscles must lengthen and slow your descent. This keeps you from flopping down in the chair.

Let's look at another example: filling a pot with water. Imagine (or try) standing at the sink holding a pot in one hand and filling it with water from the tap. You feel the muscles on the front of your upper arm (elbow flexors) working harder as the pot fills. This is an isometric contraction as you hold the pot steady. Once the pot is full, you lift it out of the sink using a concentric contraction of those same elbow flexors. You carry the pot to the stove and carefully lower it to the burner trying not to spill the water or drop the pot. Eccentric contraction of the elbow flexors controls this lowering movement.

MUSCLE RELATIONSHIPS

As we have seen in our examples of standing from a chair and filling a pot with water, muscles work together to achieve certain activities. Muscles group themselves into those responsible for a motion, those assisting with a motion, and those working against a motion. We can look at specific muscles and muscle groups (Fig. 3-10A,B) to understand how they interact and create movement.

Agonists

Agonist muscles are those most involved in creating a joint movement. Also called *prime movers*, they are primarily re-
sponsible for moving a joint through a given action such as flexion or abduction. The agonist also serves as a point of reference when describing relationships with other muscles or muscle groups. For example, the deltoid is primarily responsible for shoulder abduction; thus, it is the agonist for this movement.

Synergists

Synergist muscles assist in some way with the function of its agonist (*syn* means same). These muscles assist by stabilizing, steering, or contributing to a particular joint movement. Muscles that have the same action or actions are considered synergists. For example, the supraspinatus assists the deltoid in performing shoulder abduction, making this pair synergists. Some muscles have all of their actions in common and thus are **direct synergists**, whereas others have only one or a few actions in common, making them **relative synergists**. Here, relationships are motion-specific.

Antagonists

Muscles that perform opposite actions to the agonist are called **antagonists** (*anti* means against or opposite). The latissimus dorsi is an antagonist to the deltoid and supraspinatus because it performs shoulder adduction, the opposite of shoulder abduction. Opposite actions include flexion and extension, abduction and adduction, and internal and external rotation. The synergist or antagonist relationship is joint specific, meaning that muscles of the shoulder can be synergists or antagonists to each other, but not to muscles of the hip or knee.

The agonist–antagonist relationship is critical for balanced posture as well as for slowing and controlling movements initiated by the body. For example, the erector spinae group (trunk extensors) is counterbalanced by the antagonist rectus abdominus (trunk flexor). Proper development of each is critical for maintaining normal, upright trunk posture. The serratus anterior (scapular abductor, depressor, upward rotator) and the rhomboids (scapular adductor, elevator, downward rotator) of the shoulder girdle are also a good example, as together they maintain the position of the scapula on the ribcage by performing opposite actions.

During a movement such as walking the hip flexors and knee extensors swing the leg anteriorly, thereby helping to propel the body forward. The hip extensors and knee flexors are required to slow and stop this movement. Without proper balance between these muscle groups, the body would not be able to control and finish movements it initiated. As we examine individual muscles and muscle groups in future chapters, we will explore these relationships further.

MUSCLES OF THE HUMAN BODY

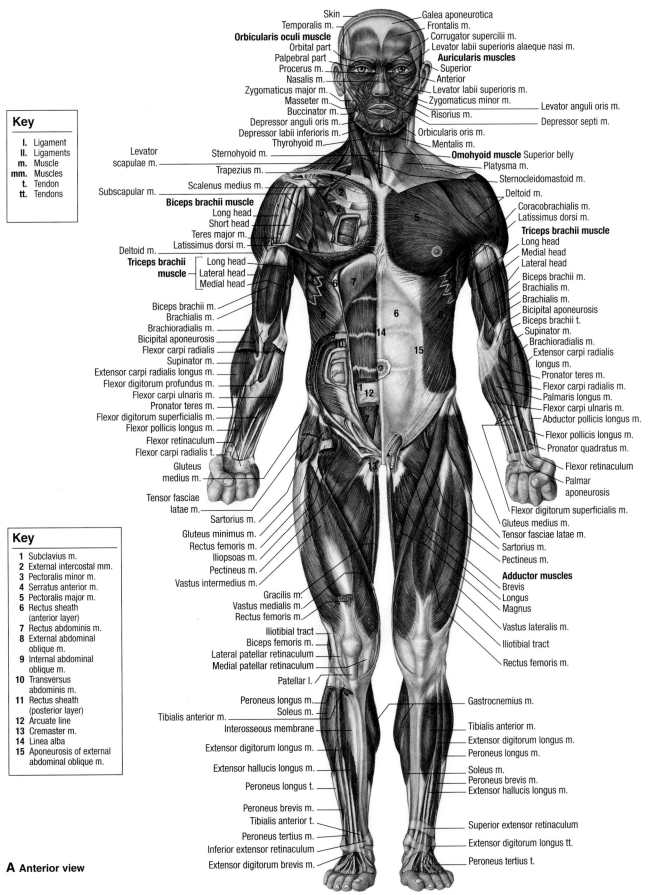

Skin
Temporalis m.
Orbicularis oculi muscle
Orbital part
Palpebral part
Procerus m.
Nasalis m.
Zygomaticus major m.
Masseter m.
Buccinator m.
Depressor anguli oris m.
Depressor labii inferioris m.
Thyrohyoid m.

Galea aponeurotica
Frontalis m.
Corrugator supercilii m.
Levator labii superioris alaeque nasi m.
Auricularis muscles
Superior
Anterior
Levator labii superioris m.
Zygomaticus minor m.
Risorius m.
Orbicularis oris m.
Mentalis m.

Levator anguli oris m.
Depressor septi m.

Levator scapulae m.
Sternohyoid m.
Trapezius m.
Scalenus medius m.
Subscapular m.
Biceps brachii muscle
Long head
Short head
Teres major m.
Latissimus dorsi m.
Deltoid m.
Triceps brachii muscle
Long head
Lateral head
Medial head

Omohyoid muscle Superior belly
Platysma m.
Sternocleidomastoid m.
Deltoid m.
Coracobrachialis m.
Latissimus dorsi m.
Triceps brachii muscle
Long head
Medial head
Lateral head
Biceps brachii m.
Brachialis m.
Brachialis m.
Bicipital aponeurosis
Biceps brachii t.
Supinator m.
Brachioradialis m.
Extensor carpi radialis longus m.
Pronator teres m.
Flexor carpi radialis m.
Palmaris longus m.
Flexor carpi ulnaris m.
Abductor pollicis longus m.
Flexor pollicis longus m.
Pronator quadratus m.
Flexor retinaculum
Palmar aponeurosis

Biceps brachii m.
Brachialis m.
Brachioradialis m.
Bicipital aponeurosis
Flexor carpi radialis
Supinator m.
Extensor carpi radialis longus m.
Flexor digitorum profundus m.
Flexor carpi ulnaris m.
Pronator teres m.
Flexor digitorum superficialis m.
Flexor pollicis longus m.
Flexor retinaculum
Flexor carpi radialis t.
Gluteus medius m.
Tensor fasciae latae m.
Sartorius m.
Gluteus minimus m.
Rectus femoris m.
Iliopsoas m.
Pectineus m.
Vastus intermedius m.

Flexor digitorum superficialis m.
Gluteus medius m.
Tensor fasciae latae m.
Sartorius m.
Pectineus m.
Adductor muscles
Brevis
Longus
Magnus
Vastus lateralis m.
Iliotibial tract
Rectus femoris m.

Gracilis m.
Vastus medialis m.
Rectus femoris m.
Iliotibial tract
Biceps femoris m.
Lateral patellar retinaculum
Medial patellar retinaculum
Patellar l.

Peroneus longus m.
Soleus m.
Tibialis anterior m.
Interosseous membrane
Extensor digitorum longus m.
Extensor hallucis longus m.
Peroneus longus t.
Peroneus brevis m.
Tibialis anterior t.
Peroneus tertius m.
Inferior extensor retinaculum
Extensor digitorum brevis m.

Gastrocnemius m.
Tibialis anterior m.
Extensor digitorum longus m.
Peroneus longus m.
Soleus m.
Peroneus brevis m.
Extensor hallucis longus m.
Superior extensor retinaculum
Extensor digitorum longus tt.
Peroneus tertius t.

Key

l.	Ligament
ll.	Ligaments
m.	Muscle
mm.	Muscles
t.	Tendon
tt.	Tendons

Key

1 Subclavius m.
2 External intercostal mm.
3 Pectoralis minor m.
4 Serratus anterior m.
5 Pectoralis major m.
6 Rectus sheath (anterior layer)
7 Rectus abdominis m.
8 External abdominal oblique m.
9 Internal abdominal oblique m.
10 Transversus abdominis m.
11 Rectus sheath (posterior layer)
12 Arcuate line
13 Cremaster m.
14 Linea alba
15 Aponeurosis of external abdominal oblique m.

A Anterior view

3-10. Muscles of the human body. A. Anterior view. *(continues)*

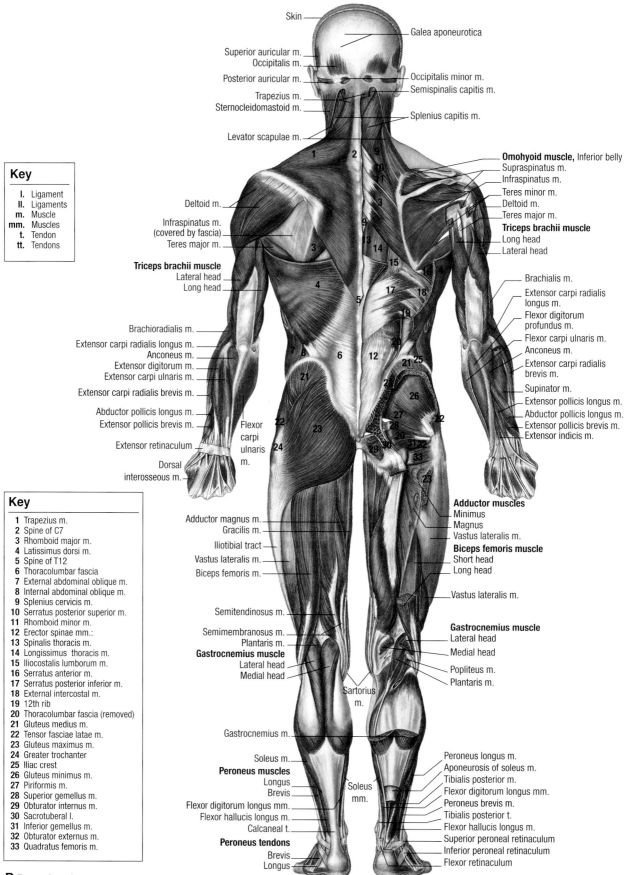

Skin
Galea aponeurotica
Superior auricular m.
Occipitalis m.
Posterior auricular m.
Occipitalis minor m.
Semispinalis capitis m.
Trapezius m.
Sternocleidomastoid m.
Splenius capitis m.
Levator scapulae m.

Omohyoid muscle, Inferior belly
Supraspinatus m.
Infraspinatus m.
Teres minor m.
Deltoid m.
Deltoid m.
Infraspinatus m.
(covered by fascia)
Teres major m.
Teres major m.
Triceps brachii muscle
Long head
Lateral head

Triceps brachii muscle
Lateral head
Long head

Brachialis m.
Extensor carpi radialis longus m.
Flexor digitorum profundus m.
Flexor carpi ulnaris m.
Anconeus m.
Extensor carpi radialis brevis m.

Brachioradialis m.
Extensor carpi radialis longus m.
Anconeus m.
Extensor digitorum m.
Extensor carpi ulnaris m.
Extensor carpi radialis brevis m.

Supinator m.
Extensor pollicis longus m.
Abductor pollicis longus m.
Extensor pollicis brevis m.
Extensor indicis m.

Abductor pollicis longus m.
Extensor pollicis brevis m.

Extensor retinaculum

Flexor carpi ulnaris m.

Dorsal interosseous m.

Adductor magnus m.
Gracilis m.
Iliotibial tract
Vastus lateralis m.
Biceps femoris m.

Adductor muscles
Minimus
Magnus
Vastus lateralis m.
Biceps femoris muscle
Short head
Long head

Vastus lateralis m.

Semitendinosus m.
Semimembranosus m.
Plantaris m.
Gastrocnemius muscle
Lateral head
Medial head

Gastrocnemius muscle
Lateral head
Medial head
Popliteus m.
Plantaris m.

Sartorius m.

Gastrocnemius m.

Soleus m.
Peroneus muscles
Longus
Brevis
Flexor digitorum longus m.
Flexor hallucis longus m.
Calcaneal t.
Peroneus tendons
Brevis
Longus

Soleus mm.

Peroneus longus m.
Aponeurosis of soleus m.
Tibialis posterior m.
Flexor digitorum longus mm.
Peroneus brevis m.
Tibialis posterior t.
Flexor hallucis longus m.
Superior peroneal retinaculum
Inferior peroneal retinaculum
Flexor retinaculum

Key

l.	Ligament
ll.	Ligaments
m.	Muscle
mm.	Muscles
t.	Tendon
tt.	Tendons

Key

1 Trapezius m.
2 Spine of C7
3 Rhomboid major m.
4 Latissimus dorsi m.
5 Spine of T12
6 Thoracolumbar fascia
7 External abdominal oblique m.
8 Internal abdominal oblique m.
9 Splenius cervicis m.
10 Serratus posterior superior m.
11 Rhomboid minor m.
12 Erector spinae mm.:
13 Spinalis thoracis m.
14 Longissimus thoracis m.
15 Iliocostalis lumborum m.
16 Serratus anterior m.
17 Serratus posterior inferior m.
18 External intercostal m.
19 12th rib
20 Thoracolumbar fascia (removed)
21 Gluteus medius m.
22 Tensor fasciae latae m.
23 Gluteus maximus m.
24 Greater trochanter
25 Iliac crest
26 Gluteus minimus m.
27 Piriformis m.
28 Superior gemellus m.
29 Obturator internus m.
30 Sacrotuberal l.
31 Inferior gemellus m.
32 Obturator externus m.
33 Quadratus femoris m.

B Posterior view

3-10. *(continued)* **Muscles of the human body. B.** Posterior view.

LEVERS IN THE HUMAN BODY

Now it's time to put things together to understand how human movement happens. As you may recall from Chapter 2, our examination of the skeleton revealed that the bones are a system of **levers**, rigid devices that transmit or modify forces to create movement.

Components of a Lever

To understand lever systems, we must examine all components. Every lever system must have an **axis** (or **fulcrum**). This is the part that the lever itself turns around. For example, in a pair of scissors, the axis is the pivot point between the handles and the blades. A wrench is a lever that uses the center of the bolt you are turning as an axis. In the body, joints serve as the axis. For example, the elbow joint serves as the pivot point between the upper arm and forearm.

Next, we need two sources of mechanical energy. One of these is internal, and is generated by pulling muscles. It is identified simply as the **force**. An external source of mechanical energy, such as gravity or friction, is the second. This we call **resistance**. Using our scissor example, the effort you generate at the handles is the force, and resistance is provided by the item you are cutting. In our wrench example the effort you use to turn the wrench is the force and the resistance is provided by the threads of the bolt.

Types of Levers

Lever systems can be arranged in different configurations to accomplish different tasks. Three different configurations found in the body include: first-class levers, second-class levers, and third-class levers. Let's examine each, using an everyday example (FIG. 3-11).

First-Class Levers

A **first-class lever** is characterized by a central axis with the force on one side and the resistance on the other. This type can be referred to as force–axis–resistance (FAR). If you have ever played on a teeter–totter (see–saw), you have experienced a first-class lever (see Fig. 3-11A). A plank is placed on a central stand and one person sits on each end. The two can balance on the central axis, or one can move skyward while the other moves down.

This type of lever is designed for balance. Moving the axis closer or farther away from the end can change the leverage or **mechanical advantage**. Range of motion and speed are increased as the axis moves toward the force (muscle). When the axis is close to the resistance, the lever can produce greater force.

First-class levers are utilized where the body needs balanced strength. Lifting your head up after looking down is a first-class lever at work. The weight of the head is forward relative to the vertebral column. This forms the resistance of the lever. The joint between the base of the skull and the first cervical vertebrae forms the axis. The *trapezius* muscle and its synergists that extend the head provide the force to move the lever. Resistance is on one side, the axis is in the middle, and the force is on the other side. This type of lever at this location allows your head to balance on your vertebral column.

Second-Class Levers

A **second-class lever** has the force on one end, the axis on the other end, and the resistance between the two (FRA). Wheelbarrows are a commonly used second-class lever (see Fig. 3-11B). Your body lifts the handles providing force on one end. The wheel serves as the axis. The bucket in the center is filled with dirt or other material providing resistance in the center. Second-class levers are very powerful, but at the cost of range of motion and speed.

A second-class lever is found in the ankle where power and propulsion is critical. The lever formed when you stand on your toes is an example. Here, the axis is the ball of the foot and strong calf muscles (plantar flexors) attaching to the heel provide the force. The resistance comes from the weight of the body compressing down through the tibia between the two. This powerful lever propels the body when walking, running, and jumping. It also helps explain why the calf muscles are so big compared to the smaller shin muscles. This lever is not meant to be balanced, just strong.

Third-Class Levers

Third-class levers are those with the resistance on one end, the axis on the other, and the force between the two (RFA). A shovel is a third-class lever (see Fig. 3-11C). The ground provides resistance when you dig the end in. Force is provided when you lift the middle of the handle. Your other hand provides the axis at the far end of the handle. These levers provide great speed and range of motion.

Third-class levers are the most common type of lever in the human body. Flexing the elbow to raise the hand toward the shoulder is a third-class lever at work. The elbow joint is the axis, the *biceps brachii* and *brachialis* muscles just distal provide the force. Resistance is the weight of the forearm and whatever is held in the hand.

PROPRIOCEPTION

We have seen how the motor neuron, part of the nervous system, initiates muscle contractions and contributes to force production. The nervous system also contributes to the health and function of muscles through proprioception. **Proprioception** is an overall awareness of body position. This awareness is independent of vision and critical in preventing injury and creating efficient movement. The nervous system communicates with muscles, tendons, and joints through different proprioceptors to sense and alter body position.

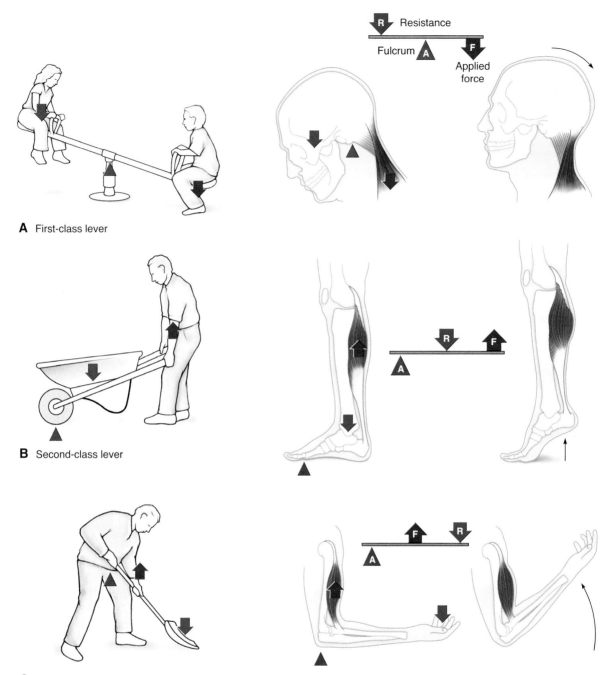

A First-class lever

B Second-class lever

C Third-class lever

3-11. **Types of levers.** Different configurations of the component of a lever serve different purposes in the body. **A.** First-class levers promote balanced strength and are found in the head and spine. **B.** Second-class levers are the most powerful and can be found in the ankle. **C.** Third-class levers are the most common and promote speed and range of motion.

Try raising your arm over your head with your eyes closed or without looking at your arm. Can you tell when it's raising and when it is fully overhead? How can you tell if you're not looking at it? What sensations tell you where it is? Try standing on one foot. Get yourself settled, then close your eyes. Do you feel your body adjusting? How does this happen? This is the function of the proprioceptors (Table 3-2).

Muscle Spindles

Muscle spindles are proprioceptors that are distributed throughout skeletal muscle tissue and monitor changes in tissue length. A muscle spindle includes specialized muscle fibers called *intrafusal fibers* surrounded by a coil of sensory nerve endings. The sensory nerves, or *afferent fibers,* monitor the rate and magnitude of stretch within the muscle.

▶ TABLE 3-2. PROPRIOCEPTORS

Structure	Location	Trigger	Response
Muscle spindle	Parallel to skeletal muscle fibers	Rapid or excessive muscle lengthening	Target muscle contraction
Golgi tendon organ	Within connective tissue of tendons	Excessive muscle contraction or passive stretch	Inhibition of target muscle contraction and contraction of opposite muscles
Vestibular apparatus	Inner ear	Change in head position	Reestablishes equilibrium
Pacinian corpuscle	Skin, connective tissue, muscles, and tendons	Vibration and deep pressure	Indicates direction and speed of movement
Ruffini corpuscle	Joint capsules	Distortion of joint capsule	Indicates joint position

If a stretch is strong or fast enough to potentially cause tissue damage, the *alpha motor neuron* prompts the surrounding *extrafusal fibers* to contract and shorten the muscle, thus protecting it from harm. This response is called the **myotatic reflex**. As the extrafusal fibers adjust their length to protect the muscle, *gamma motor neurons* adjust the tension of the muscle spindle to maintain its length-monitoring function.

If you have ever had a physician test your reflexes, you have witnessed the myotatic reflex. A reflex hammer is used to tap and quickly stretch the patellar tendon at the front of the knee. This action usually prompts the quadriceps muscles on the front of the thigh to contract. Your leg kicks out, telling the doctor that your muscle spindle is working correctly.

Golgi Tendon Organs

Golgi tendon organs are another important type of proprioceptor. These structures are woven into the connective tissue present in tendons and monitor changes in muscle tension. Muscle tension is created through either stretching or contraction.

If a muscle generates excessive tension, either through strong muscle contraction or excessive stretch, the Golgi tendon organ will inhibit muscle contraction and prompt the muscle to relax. It also prompts the opposite muscle group to contract. Both actions decrease tension on the affected muscle. This response is called the **inverse myotatic reflex**. We see this response in "cliffhanger" movies when the bad guy is hanging on for dear life and then his fingers just "let go." This "letting go" is a function of the Golgi tendon organs trying to protect his hand and arm muscles from damage.

Both muscle spindles and Golgi tendon organs are capable of reciprocal inhibition. **Reciprocal inhibition** describes the relaxation of one muscle while the opposite contracts. This allows the body to move and not fight against itself. Appropriate give and take must occur between opposing muscle groups in order for smooth, coordinated movement to take place.

Other Proprioceptors

The body relies on other proprioceptors besides the muscle spindles and Golgi tendon organs. Receptors deep within the inner ear, the skin, connective tissue, and joint capsule provide additional feedback regarding body position and movement.

Vestibular Apparatus

The **vestibular apparatus** of the inner ear provides feedback about head position. When you tilt your head, crystals of calcium carbonate housed in the apparatus move in response to gravity. This movement stimulates specialized cells that send signals to the brain indicating relative head position. Damage or infection in the inner ear can compromise balance and equilibrium and decrease proprioception.

Mechanoreceptors

Mechanoreceptors are specialized nerve endings that deform in response to pressure. This deformation is similar to squishing a rubber ball in your hand. By registering the speed and amount of deformation, they indicate position and movement of their associated structures. Two types of mechanoreceptors contribute to proprioception:

- **Pacinian corpuscles** reside in skin, connective tissue around muscles, and tendons. They detect the initial application of vibration or deep pressure in these tissues, and thereby help to monitor direction and speed of body movement.
- **Ruffini corpuscles** are scattered throughout joint capsules. Here they determine the exact position of the joint as the joint capsule distorts.

RANGE OF MOTION

Range of motion is a term used to describe the extent of movement possible at a joint. Each joint has a range of movement that is normally available at that joint. This normal range can be limited by several factors including the shape of the bones that form the joint, the ligaments that hold the bones together, the length of the muscles that cross that joint, the amount of tone or nervous system control in the same muscles, injury or a chronic response to injury such as swelling or scar tissue formation, and other factors like age and gender.

Range of motion can be divided into three categories: **active**, **passive**, and **resisted** range of motion.

Active Range of Motion

Active range of motion occurs when a person moves a given body part through its possible motions independently. It therefore demonstrates a client's willingness and ability to voluntarily perform available motions at that joint. All structures and systems must work together in order to accomplish active movement. Slightly less motion is possible actively compared to passively (discussed shortly) because the nervous system limits the range of movement to protect the muscles and tendons around the joints.

Guidelines for assessing active range of motion include:

1. Have the client assume a comfortable, upright position with well-aligned posture.

2. Position yourself where you can observe the motion as well as the client's facial expressions, which might reveal that the movement is causing the client pain.

3. Demonstrate the motion you want the client to perform. As you demonstrate, instruct the client to move within his or her own comfort range. Use common terminology. For example, ask the client to "Straighten your right arm and lift it above your head leading with your thumb."

4. Now ask the client to perform the movement. Observe for any limitation of motion or break in normal rhythm or symmetry.

5. When appropriate, have the client repeat the movement on the opposite side and compare the two.

6. Inquire about limiting factors, differentiating between sensations of stretch, approximation (body runs into itself), pain, and apprehension or guarding. These sensations are described shortly.

7. Document your findings for comparison.

Passive Range of Motion

Passive range of motion occurs when the client is resting and the therapist moves a joint through its possible motions. The joint is taken through its full possible motion, as the client remains relaxed. The practitioner is then able to determine the **endfeel** (or *limiting factor*) for that joint. Endfeel describes the perceived quality of movement at the end of a joint's available range of motion. The type of endfeel a joint displays provides insight into the health and function of passive or inert stabilizers such as ligaments and joint capsules, as well as the muscles and tendons being stretched during the movement. These would include the antagonist muscles from the performed movement (i.e., passive elbow flexion would assess the health and function of the elbow extensors).

There are four types of healthy endfeel.

- In **bony endfeel**, the contact of two bones is limiting. This is sometimes described as a *hard endfeel* and can be found at the end of elbow extension (FIG. 3-12A).
- In **capsular endfeel**, the joint capsule provides a firm limitation. For example, if you internally rotate the client's thigh you will encounter a "leathery" feel at the end of the movement (FIG. 3-12B).
- In **springy** (or *muscular*) **endfeel**, the stretching of muscles and tendons limits joint motion. For example, the latissimus dorsi and teres major muscles are stretched with shoulder abduction creating a more elastic feel compared to the leathery capsular endfeel (FIG.3-12C).
- **Approximation** is a fourth type of healthy endfeel, in which the body runs into itself, as when the forearm meets the upper arm, limiting elbow flexion (FIG. 3-12D).

Abnormal endfeel is possible when a joint is injured or diseased. **Muscle spasm** (also called **guarding**), is characterized by jerky or shaky movements prior to expected end range. This can result from muscle or joint injury prompting the nervous system to limit movement. **Springy block** is a

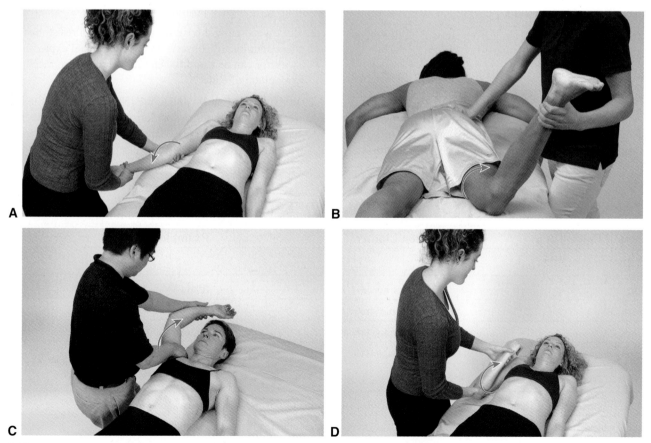

3-12. Different types of normal endfeel. The blue arrow indicates direction of movement. **A.** Bony or hard endfeel of elbow extension. **B.** Capsular endfeel of hip internal rotation. **C.** Springy endfeel of shoulder abduction. **D.** Approximation endfeel of elbow flexion.

rubbery or bouncy stoppage that occurs prior to end range. It usually results from torn cartilage such as the meniscus of the knee occluding joint movement. **Loose** or **empty** endfeel occurs where abnormal motion is allowed where a ligament or joint capsule should prevent it. Finally, **spongy** endfeel is squishy or boggy and indicates swelling in a joint. Each abnormal endfeel indicates injury or pathology in the joint and should be evaluated by a physician. Examples of normal and abnormal endfeel are summarized in Table 3-3.

Guidelines for performing passive range of motion include:

1. Place your client in a comfortable and supported position where you can observe joint movement as well as the client's facial expression.

2. Support surrounding joints in order to protect them and maximize relaxation.

3. Instruct the client to relax fully as you take the joint through the appropriate range of motion.

4. Inquire about discomfort or pain as you perform the movement.

5. Take the joint to endfeel and identify the type as normal (bony, capsular, springy, or approximation) or abnormal (muscle spasm/guarding, springy block, loose/empty, or spongy).

6. When appropriate, repeat movement on other side and compare the two.

7. Document your findings including amount of motion as well as corresponding endfeel.

Resisted Range of Motion

Resisted range of motion occurs when the client meets the resistance of the practitioner in attempting to produce movement at a joint. It is used to assess the health and

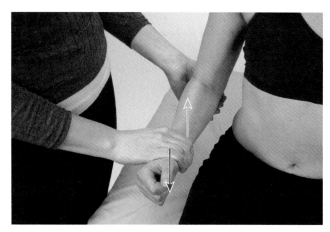

3-13. Resisted range of motion. Performance and observation of resisted range of motion for elbow flexion. Red arrow indicates direction of practitioner's pressure and green arrow indicates direction of client's resistance.

function of contracting muscles and their corresponding tendons. The nervous system, muscle fibers, and tendons all work together to generate force against gravity and the practitioner's resistance.

Guidelines for performing resisted range of motion include:

1. Have the client assume a comfortable, upright position with well-aligned posture.

2. Place yourself in a position where you can resist movement and, ideally, observe the client's facial expression. A mirror can be useful when you are unable to face your client directly.

3. When appropriate, stabilize the joint proximal to the one being tested either positionally or with your other hand. This helps decrease compensation and maximize your ability to target specific muscles.

▶ TABLE 3-3. NORMAL AND ABNORMAL ENDFEEL

Type of Endfeel	Motion Limiter	Example
Normal endfeel		
Bony	Contact of bones	Elbow extension
Capsular	Joint capsule stretch	Hip rotation
Springy	Muscle/tendon stretch	Shoulder abduction
Approximation	Body contact	Elbow flexion
Abnormal endfeel		
Muscle spasm/guarding	Injured muscle, tendon, or joint	Pain, muscle strain
Springy block	Torn cartilage, foreign body in joint	Torn meniscus in knee
Loose/empty	Lack of limitation	Torn ligament or joint capsule (sprain)
Spongy	Swelling	Acute ligament sprain or inflamed bursa

▶ TABLE 3-4. GRADING RESISTED RANGE OF MOTION

Numerical Grade	Description
5	Able to maintain test position against gravity and maximal resistance.
4+	Able to resist maximal resistance, but unable to maintain this resistance.
4	Able to maintain test position against gravity and moderate resistance.
4−	Able to maintain test position against gravity and less-than-moderate resistance.
3+	Able to maintain test position against gravity and minimal resistance.
3	Able to maintain test position against gravity.

Resisted range of motion scores below "3" are indicative of pathology and should be evaluated by a physician.

4. Demonstrate the movement you will be resisting. Instruct the client to meet the resistance you apply.

5. Apply resistance, and ask the client to attempt the joint movement (Fig. 3-13). The muscle contraction your client generates will typically be static (isometric); that is, no movement will usually occur. The client need only meet your resistance, not try to overcome it.

6. Inquire about discomfort or pain as the client performs the movement.

7. When appropriate, repeat the movement on the other side and compare the two.

8. Grade the client's resistance according to Table 3-4. Note your findings in the client's record.

The ranges of motion possible at all joints and procedures for evaluating each will be discussed in each regional chapter of this book.

SUMMARY

- Muscle tissue is one of the four primary tissue types in the human body. Three types of muscle tissue are cardiac, smooth, and skeletal. Each has a specialized function reflecting its anatomical configuration and location.
- Skeletal muscles serve several purposes in the body including initiation of motion, maintenance of posture, protection of underlying structures, generation of heat, and fluid pumping.
- Skeletal muscle fibers have parallel or pennate fiber arrangements depending on the location and function of the muscle. Parallel arrangements maximize range of motion while pennate arrangements maximize force production.
- Factors that may influence skeletal muscle names include fiber direction, location, action, size, shape, and number of heads.
- Skeletal muscle tissue has several properties essential to its function. These include extensibility, elasticity, excitability, conductivity, and contractility. Contractility is unique to muscle tissue.

- Muscles and muscle fibers are organized into multiple levels by layers of connective tissue including the epimysium, perimysium, and endomysium. This arrangement protects fragile muscle fibers and directs forces toward the bones.
- Muscle cells contain multiple nuclei, a sarcolemma or cell membrane, and a sarcoplasm that houses specialized organelles.
- Myofilaments are specialized proteins responsible for force production. Troponin, tropomyosin, and actin proteins form the thin filament while myosin proteins make up the thick filament.
- Thick and thin filaments interact according to the sliding filament mechanism to generate force within a muscle. This process is initiated and governed by the nervous system using electrical signals called action potentials.
- Factors that influence the amount of force produced by a muscle include the number of motor units recruited, muscle cross-sectional area, fiber arrangement, and muscle length.
- Slow twitch, fast twitch, and intermediate types of muscle fibers make energy differently and serve individual purposes in the body. The distribution and development of these fibers is scattered and dependent upon genetics, muscle function, and patterns of physical activity.
- Muscles generate isometric, concentric, and eccentric contractions. Together, these contraction types stabilize the body and generate and control movement.
- Muscles are organized as agonists responsible for movement, synergists working together, or antagonists balancing each other. Healthy relationships between muscle groups are critical to posture and functional movement.
- First-class, second-class, and third-class levers are present in the human body. Different arrangements of the axis, force, and resistance accomplish different goals including balance, power, speed, and range of motion.
- Proprioception describes awareness of body position in space, independently of vision. Muscle spindles and Golgi tendon organs monitor muscle length and tension. The vestibular apparatus monitors head position. Mechanoreceptors perceive joint position and movement.

Together, proprioceptors enhance movement and protect the structures involved.

- Active range of motion is voluntary movement without outside assistance. It requires coordinated effort between multiple systems of the body.
- Passive range of motion requires movement by an outside source. It is used to assess endfeel and inert structures such as ligaments and joint capsules.
- Resisted range of motion utilizes controlled opposition to movement to evaluate the health of dynamic structures like muscles and tendons.

FOR REVIEW

Multiple Choice

1. Characteristics of cardiac muscle cells include:
   A. voluntary control, striated
   B. voluntary control, unstriated
   C. involuntary control, striated
   D. involuntary control, unstriated

2. Characteristics of smooth muscle cells include:
   A. voluntary control, striated
   B. voluntary control, unstriated
   C. involuntary control, striated
   D. involuntary control, unstriated

3. Characteristics of skeletal muscle cells include:
   A. voluntary control, striated
   B. voluntary control, unstriated
   C. involuntary control, striated
   D. involuntary control, unstriated

4. The most powerful muscle fiber arrangement is:
   A. multipennate
   B. triangular
   C. unipennate
   D. fusiform

5. A tissue characteristic that is unique to muscle tissue is:
   A. conductivity
   B. contractility
   C. excitability
   D. elasticity

6. The *qudratus femoris* muscle is named for which properties?
   A. size and location
   B. number of heads and action
   C. location and fiber direction
   D. shape and location

7. The fiber type that can alter how it makes energy depending upon use is:
   A. slow-twitch fibers
   B. fast-twitch fibers
   C. intermediate fibers
   D. all of the above

8. Sprinting, jumping, and throwing primarily utilize which type of muscle fiber?
   A. slow-twitch fibers
   B. fast-twitch fibers
   C. intermediate fibers
   D. all of the above

9. Muscle contractions used to initiate movements in the body are:
   A. isometric contractions
   B. concentric contractions
   C. eccentric contractions
   D. all of the above

10. A muscle that assists another with its movement or function is called a(n):
    A. agonist
    B. antagonist
    C. prime mover
    D. synergist

Sequencing

Place the following events of muscle contraction into the correct order.

11. _____ Nerve cell sends action potential down its axon.

12. _____ Action potential reaches the transverse tubules.

13. _____ Synaptic vesicles release acetylcholine (ACh)

14. _____ Calcium ions bind to troponin.

15. _____ Acetylcholine (ACh) binds to receptors on the sarcolemma.

16. _____ Tropomyosin proteins distort and active sites on actin are exposed.

17. _____ Muscle relaxation occurs, returning sarcomere to resting length.

18. _____ Shortening of the sarcomere begins.

19. _____ Sarcoplasmic reticulum releases calcium ions.

20. _____ Cross-bridges form between actin binding sites and myosin heads.

Short Answer

21. List the functions of skeletal muscle.

22. Identify all of the properties of skeletal muscle tissue and explain the significance of each to movement.

23. Identify and describe all of the factors that influence force production by a muscle.

24. Briefly explain the purpose of intermediate fibers and how they will adapt to different types of sport training.

25. In your own words, define proprioception. Identify and describe specific anatomical structures that contribute to proprioception.

26. Identify the structures in the picture below.

A. _____
B. _____
C. _____
D. _____
E. _____
F. _____
G. _____

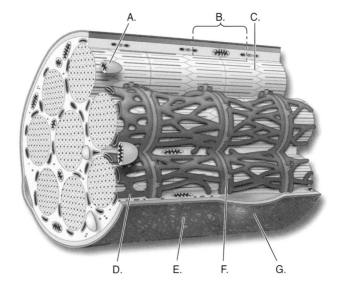

Try This!

Create a set of cards using muscle names from Figure 3-10. Each card should have the muscle name written on one side. Shuffle your cards and draw one. Say out loud everything you know about this muscle from its name. Remember, the name may tell you things like its fiber direction, location, action, size, shape, or number of heads.

To further challenge yourself, draw a picture of the muscle on the other side of the card. Include the muscle's unique fiber arrangement. Shuffle and draw a card without looking at the picture. Can you remember its fiber arrangement? Is it parallel or pennate? What shape is it: fusiform, circular, or triangular? If pennate, is it uni, bi, or multipennate?

As a final challenge, see if you can identify the muscle as primarily slow twitch or fast twitch dominant. Remember, small, deep, postural muscles tend to be slow twitch dominant while large powerful muscles tend to be fast twitch dominant. You can look up the muscle profile in Chapters 4–9 to see if you are correct.

SUGGESTED READINGS

Chandler J, Brown LE. *Conditioning for Strength and Human Performance.* Philadelphia: Lippincott, Williams & Wilkins, 2008.

Cohen BJ. *Memmler's the Structure and Function of the Human Body.* 8th Ed. Philadelphia: Lippincott, Williams & Wilkins, 2005.

McArdle WD, Katch FI, Katch VL. *Essentials of Exercise Physiology.* 2nd Ed. Baltimore: Lippincott, Williams and Wilkins, 2000.

Oatis CA. *Kinesiology—The Mechanics and Pathomechanics of Human Movement.* Baltimore: Lippincott, Williams & Wilkins, 2004.

Prekumar, K. *The Massage Connection Anatomy & Physiology.* 2nd Ed. Baltimore: Lippincott, Williams & Wilkins, 2004.

4

The Shoulder

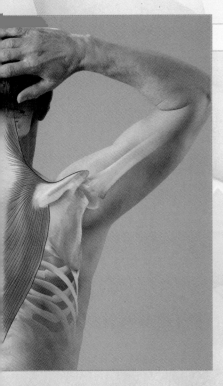

Learning Objectives

After working through the material in this chapter, you should be able to:

- Identify the main structures of the shoulder, including bones, joints, special structures, and deep and superficial muscles.
- Label and palpate the major surface landmarks of the shoulder.
- Draw, label, palpate, and fire the deep and superficial muscles of the shoulder.
- Locate the attachments and nerve supply of the muscles of the shoulder.
- Identify and demonstrate all actions of the muscles of the shoulder.
- Demonstrate passive and resisted range of motion of the shoulder.
- Describe the unique functional anatomy and relationships between each muscle of the shoulder.
- Identify both the synergists and antagonists involved in each movement of the shoulder (flexion, extension, etc.).
- Identify muscles used in performing four coordinated movements of the shoulder: reaching, lifting, throwing, and pushing.

▶ OVERVIEW OF THE REGION

The shoulders provide a sturdy base that supports movements of the head, neck, and arms. They are composed of paired bones and many powerful muscles that provide either increased stability or mobility, depending on body position and movement demands.

Some of the special structures of the shoulder, such as the ligaments, nerves, and bursae, are essential to healthy movement. Others, such as the lymphatic vessels and nodes and the blood vessels, help maintain the health and function of the shoulder and surrounding regions.

When all of its structures are healthy, balanced, and functionally sound, the shoulder is a dynamic, powerful tool that allows us to reach overhead, push and pull, cross our arms in front or behind us, support our body weight, and perform complex movements such as throwing. But, as you might guess, improper development, alignment, and use patterns can easily disrupt this functional equilibrium. Understanding the *function* of each muscle and its relationship with other structures helps us anticipate and prevent pathology and enhance performance of work tasks, exercise, sports, and activities of daily living, both for ourselves and for our clients.

▶ SURFACE ANATOMY OF THE SHOULDER

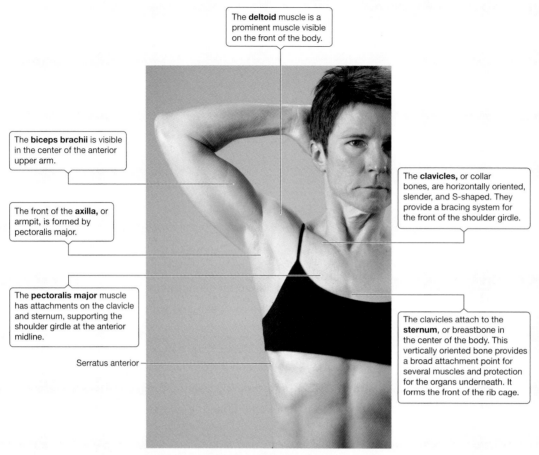

The **deltoid** muscle is a prominent muscle visible on the front of the body.

The **biceps brachii** is visible in the center of the anterior upper arm.

The front of the **axilla,** or armpit, is formed by pectoralis major.

The **pectoralis major** muscle has attachments on the clavicle and sternum, supporting the shoulder girdle at the anterior midline.

The **clavicles,** or collar bones, are horizontally oriented, slender, and S-shaped. They provide a bracing system for the front of the shoulder girdle.

The clavicles attach to the **sternum**, or breastbone in the center of the body. This vertically oriented bone provides a broad attachment point for several muscles and protection for the organs underneath. It forms the front of the rib cage.

Serratus anterior

4-1A. Anterior view.

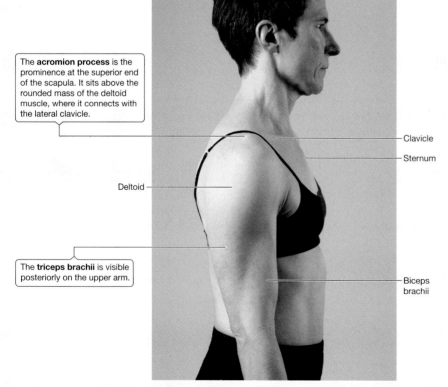

The **acromion process** is the prominence at the superior end of the scapula. It sits above the rounded mass of the deltoid muscle, where it connects with the lateral clavicle.

Deltoid

The **triceps brachii** is visible posteriorly on the upper arm.

Clavicle

Sternum

Biceps brachii

4-1B. Lateral view.

◗ SURFACE ANATOMY OF THE SHOULDER

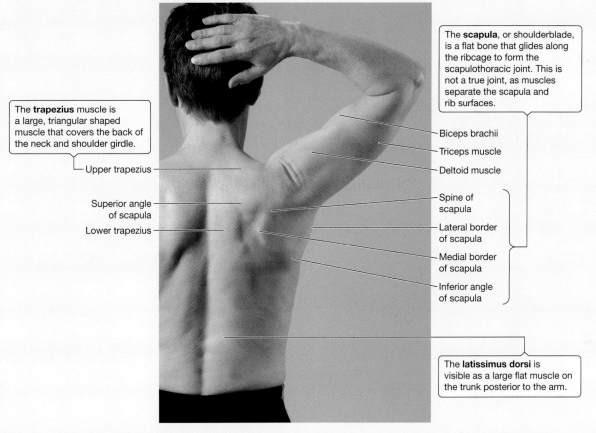

The **trapezius** muscle is a large, triangular shaped muscle that covers the back of the neck and shoulder girdle.

Upper trapezius

Superior angle of scapula

Lower trapezius

The **scapula**, or shoulderblade, is a flat bone that glides along the ribcage to form the scapulothoracic joint. This is not a true joint, as muscles separate the scapula and rib surfaces.

Biceps brachii

Triceps muscle

Deltoid muscle

Spine of scapula

Lateral border of scapula

Medial border of scapula

Inferior angle of scapula

The **latissimus dorsi** is visible as a large flat muscle on the trunk posterior to the arm.

4-1C. Posterior view.

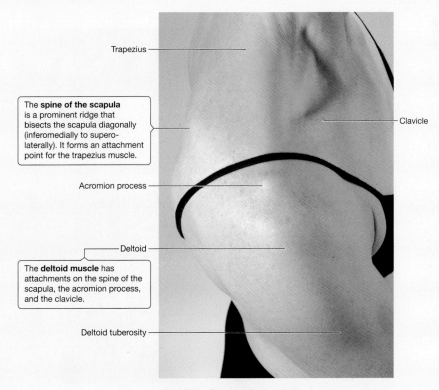

Trapezius

The **spine of the scapula** is a prominent ridge that bisects the scapula diagonally (inferomedially to superolaterally). It forms an attachment point for the trapezius muscle.

Acromion process

Clavicle

Deltoid

The **deltoid muscle** has attachments on the spine of the scapula, the acromion process, and the clavicle.

Deltoid tuberosity

4-1D. Superior view.

▶ SKELETAL STRUCTURES OF THE SHOULDER

The **acromioclavicular joint** is formed by the articulation of the acromion process of the superior scapula with the lateral clavicle.

Two bones comprise the **shoulder girdle**: the clavicle and the scapula. The shoulder girdle is also called the **pectoral girdle**.

The **coracoid process** of the scapula protrudes anteriorly and inferior to the clavicle, to form a strong bony attachment for several muscles of the shoulder.

The **sternoclavicular joint** is the articulation of the medial clavicle with the manubrium of the sternum.

The **manubrium** is the most superior portion of the sternum.

This shallow depression is the **glenoid fossa** of the scapula. It forms the socket of the **glenohumeral joint** which is the articulation of the glenoid fossa with the head of the humerus. The glenohumeral joint is commonly called the **shoulder joint**.

The **sternum** articulates with the ribs via costo-cartilage to form the anterior of the slightly moveable ribcage.

Humerus

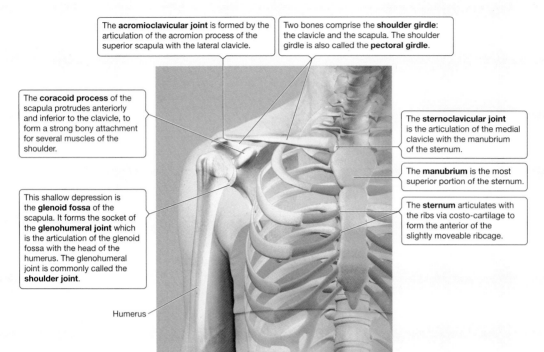

4-2A. Anterior view.

The fact that the scapula articulates with the axial skeleton only at the small **acromioclavicular joint** allows for a wide range of motion possible at the shoulder.

Spine of scapula

Clavicle

Acromion process

Head of the humerus

The combined motion of the **scapulothoracic joint** and the **glenohumeral joint** is called **scapulohumeral rhythm**.

The anterior surface (undersurface) of the scapula is somewhat concave, forming the subscapular fossa. This depression is the origin of the subscapularis muscle of the rotator cuff.

The **epicondyles of the humerus** form prominent attachment sites for muscles of the elbow and forearm.

Shaft of humerus

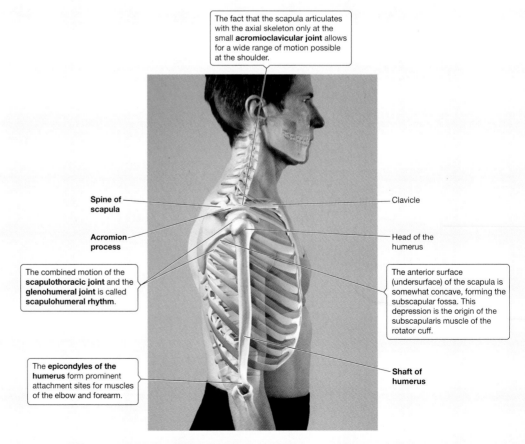

4-2B. Lateral view.

❯ SKELETAL STRUCTURES OF THE SHOULDER

Their are two depressions on the posterior scapula. The one superior to the spine of the scapula is called the **supraspinous fossa**, and the one inferior to the spine is the **infraspinous fossa**.

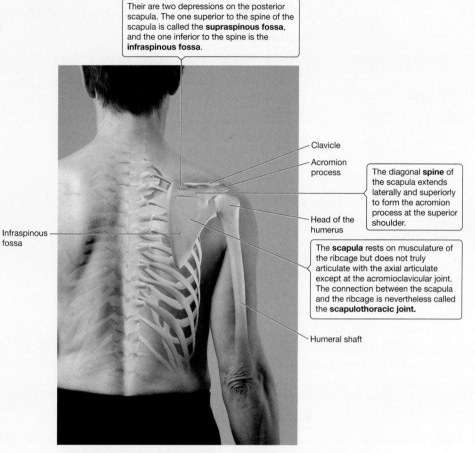

Clavicle

Acromion process

The diagonal **spine** of the scapula extends laterally and superiorly to form the acromion process at the superior shoulder.

Head of the humerus

Infraspinous fossa

The **scapula** rests on musculature of the ribcage but does not truly articulate with the axial articulate except at the acromioclavicular joint. The connection between the scapula and the ribcage is nevertheless called the **scapulothoracic joint.**

Humeral shaft

4-2C. Posterior view.

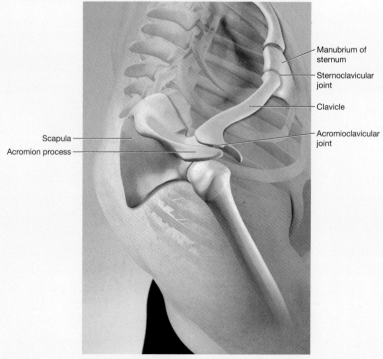

Manubrium of sternum

Sternoclavicular joint

Clavicle

Scapula

Acromion process

Acromioclavicular joint

4-2D. Superior view.

▶ BONY LANDMARKS OF THE SHOULDER

Palpating the Clavicle

Positioning: client supine.

1. Locate the horizontal prominence lateral to the midline at the base of the neck.
2. Palpate posteriorly and inferiorly locating the s-shaped bony ridge of the clavicle.

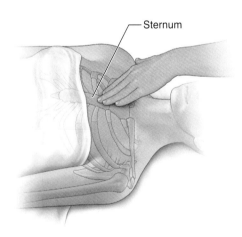

4-3A. **Clavicle.**

Palpating the Sternum

Positioning: client supine.

1. Locate the clavicle and palpate its most medial edge.
2. Palpate medially and inferiorly onto the flat, broad sternum at the center of the chest.

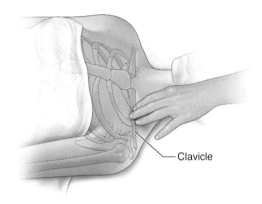

4-3B. **Sternum.**

Palpating the Acromion Process

Positioning: client supine.

1. Locate the clavicle and palpate its most lateral edge.
2. Palpate laterally and posteriorly onto the rounded point of the shoulder formed by the acromion.

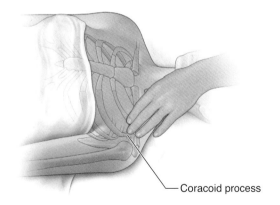

4-3C. **Acromion process.**

Palpating the Coracoid Process

Positioning: client supine.

1. Locate the lateral clavicle where its s-shape is most concave.
2. Palpate inferior and deep onto the pointed prominence of the coracoid just medial to the rounded humeral head.

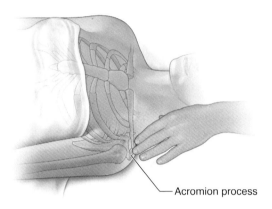

4-3D. **Coracoid process.**

▶ BONY LANDMARKS OF THE SHOULDER

Palpating the Greater Tubercle

Positioning: client supine with shoulder neutral.

1. Locate the lateral edge of the acromion process and palpate inferiorly onto the humeral head.
2. Palpate the rounded bump on the anterolateral humeral head.

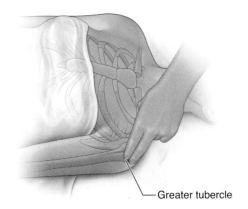

4-3E. **Greater tubercle.**

Palpating the Lesser Tubercle

Positioning: client supine with shoulder neutral.

1. Locate the greater tubercle of the humerus and maintain your contact as you passively rotate the client's shoulder externally.
2. Let your fingers slide past the bicipital groove and onto the small, rounded bump of the lesser tubercle.

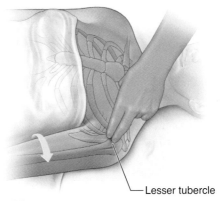

4-3G. **Lesser tubercle.**

Palpating the Bicipital Groove

Positioning: client supine with shoulder neutral.

1. Locate the greater tubercle of the humerus and maintain your contact as you passively rotate the client's shoulder externally.
2. Let your fingers slide into the bicipital groove just medial to the greater tubercle.

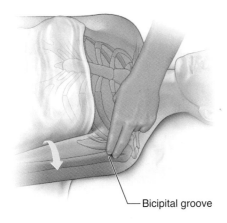

4-3F. **Bicipital groove.**

Palpating the Deltoid Tuberosity

Positioning: client supine.

1. Locate the lateral edge of the acromion process and palpate inferiorly about halfway down the lateral humerus.
2. Palpate medial and deep where the rounded mass of the deltoid muscle converges at the deltoid tuberosity.

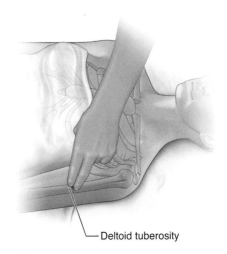

4-3H. **Deltoid tuberosity.**

▶ BONY LANDMARKS OF THE SHOULDER

Palpating the Spine of the Scapula

Positioning: client prone.

1. Locate the acromion process at the lateral tip of the shoulder and palpate medial and slightly inferior.
2. Follow the sharp posteriorly protruding scapular spine as it traverses the width of the scapula.

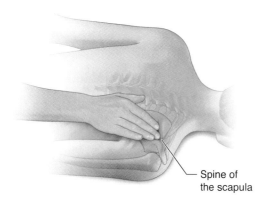

Spine of the scapula

4-3I. Spine of the scapula.

Palpating the Medial Border of the Scapula

Positioning: client prone.

1. Locate the spine of the scapula and palpate to its most medial edge.
2. Palpate the vertically oriented medial border as the spine expands superiorly and inferiorly.

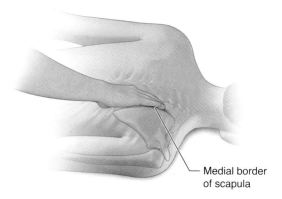

Medial border of scapula

4-3J. Medial border of the scapula.

Palpating the Superior Angle of the Scapula

Positioning: client prone.

1. Locate the medial border of the scapula and palpate superiorly past the spine.

2. Palpate the superior corner of the scapula as it curves laterally forming the superior angle.

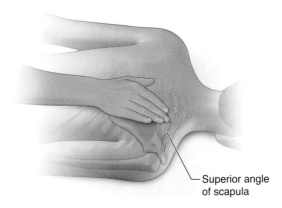

4-3K. Superior angle of the scapula.

Palpating the Lateral Border of the Scapula

Positioning: client prone.

1. Locate the medial border of the scapula and palpate inferiorly around the inferior angle.

2. Continue palpating superiorly onto the rounded lateral edge as it parallels the posterior axilla.

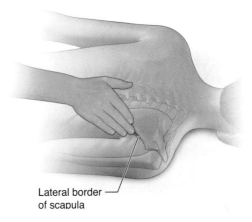

4-3L. Lateral border of the scapula.

▶ MUSCLE ATTACHMENT SITES

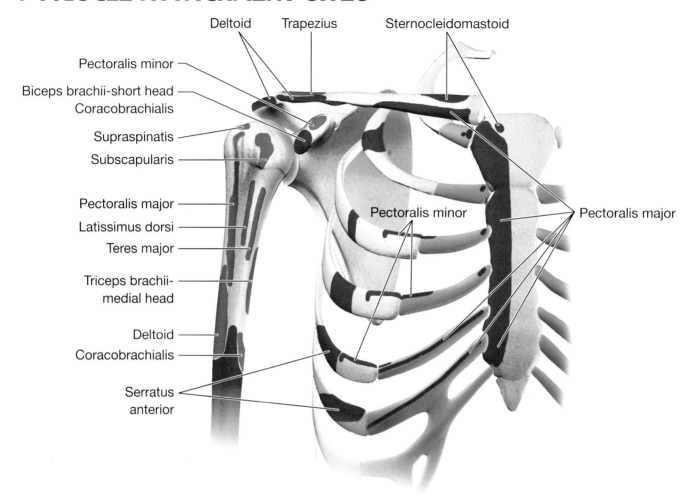

4-4. Axial muscle attachments: anterior view. The ribcage forms a stable attachment for several muscles of the shoulder. Large, prime mover muscles such as the pectoralis major have broad origins (areas in red) on the ribcage and smaller insertions (areas in blue) on the humerus.

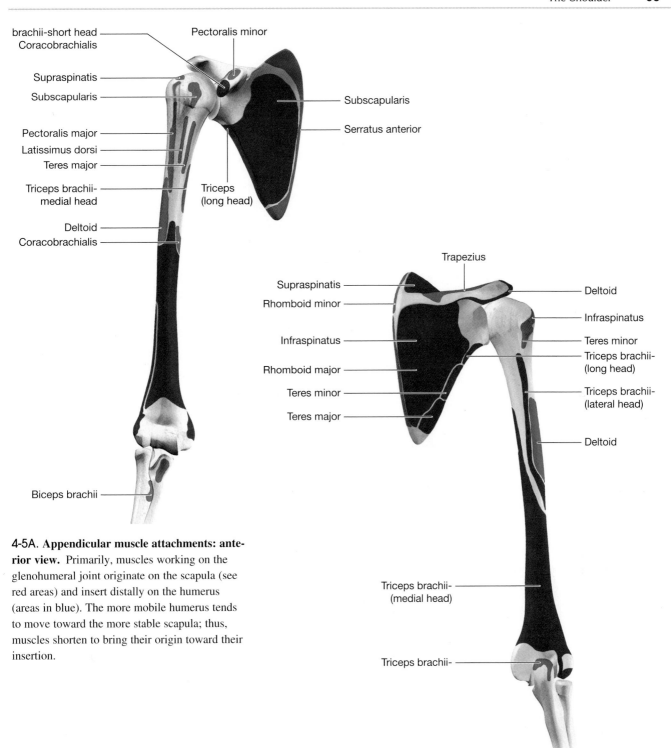

brachii-short head
Coracobrachialis

Pectoralis minor

Supraspinatis

Subscapularis

Pectoralis major
Latissimus dorsi
Teres major

Triceps brachii-
medial head

Deltoid
Coracobrachialis

Subscapularis

Serratus anterior

Triceps
(long head)

Biceps brachii

Trapezius

Supraspinatis
Rhomboid minor

Infraspinatus

Rhomboid major

Teres minor

Teres major

Deltoid

Infraspinatus

Teres minor
Triceps brachii-
(long head)

Triceps brachii-
(lateral head)

Deltoid

Triceps brachii-
(medial head)

Triceps brachii-

4-5A. Appendicular muscle attachments: anterior view. Primarily, muscles working on the glenohumeral joint originate on the scapula (see red areas) and insert distally on the humerus (areas in blue). The more mobile humerus tends to move toward the more stable scapula; thus, muscles shorten to bring their origin toward their insertion.

4-5B. Appendicular muscle attachments: posterior view. The posterior scapula provides several attachment sites for muscles of the shoulder. The prominent spine is leveraged by the large trapezius and deltoid. Rotator cuff muscles that stabilize the glenohumeral joint fill the fosses above and below the spine.

▶ LIGAMENTS OF THE SHOULDER

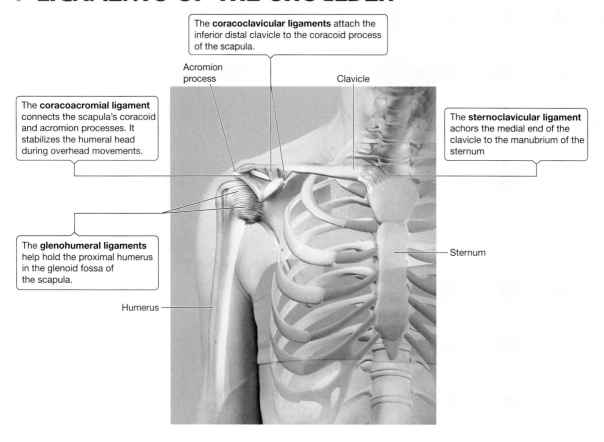

The **coracoclavicular ligaments** attach the inferior distal clavicle to the coracoid process of the scapula.

Acromion process

Clavicle

The **coracoacromial ligament** connects the scapula's coracoid and acromion processes. It stabilizes the humeral head during overhead movements.

The **sternoclavicular ligament** achors the medial end of the clavicle to the manubrium of the sternum

The **glenohumeral ligaments** help hold the proximal humerus in the glenoid fossa of the scapula.

Sternum

Humerus

4-6A. Anterior view.

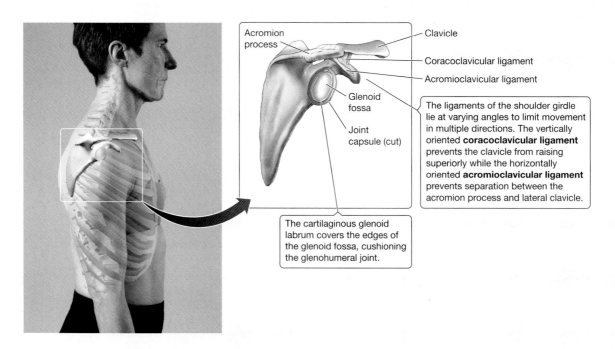

Acromion process

Clavicle

Coracoclavicular ligament

Acromioclavicular ligament

Glenoid fossa

Joint capsule (cut)

The ligaments of the shoulder girdle lie at varying angles to limit movement in multiple directions. The vertically oriented **coracoclavicular ligament** prevents the clavicle from raising superiorly while the horizontally oriented **acromioclavicular ligament** prevents separation between the acromion process and lateral clavicle.

The cartilaginous glenoid labrum covers the edges of the glenoid fossa, cushioning the glenohumeral joint.

4-6B. Lateral view.

▶ LIGAMENTS OF THE SHOULDER

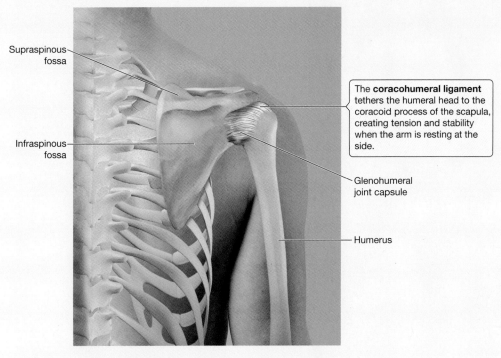

Supraspinous fossa

Infraspinous fossa

> The **coracohumeral ligament** tethers the humeral head to the coracoid process of the scapula, creating tension and stability when the arm is resting at the side.

Glenohumeral joint capsule

Humerus

4-6C. Posterior view.

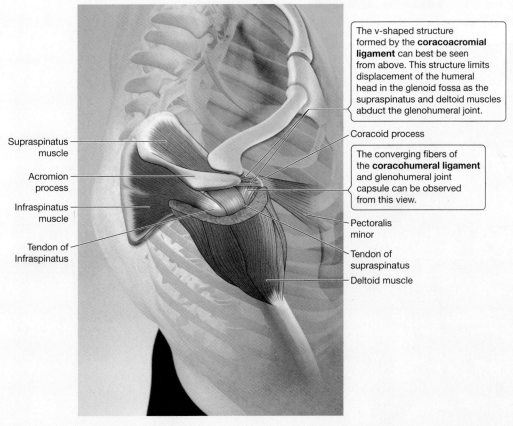

> The v-shaped structure formed by the **coracoacromial ligament** can best be seen from above. This structure limits displacement of the humeral head in the glenoid fossa as the supraspinatus and deltoid muscles abduct the glenohumeral joint.

Supraspinatus muscle

Acromion process

Infraspinatus muscle

Tendon of Infraspinatus

Coracoid process

> The converging fibers of the **coracohumeral ligament** and glenohumeral joint capsule can be observed from this view.

Pectoralis minor

Tendon of supraspinatus

Deltoid muscle

4-6D. Superior view.

▶ SUPERFICIAL MUSCLES OF THE SHOULDER

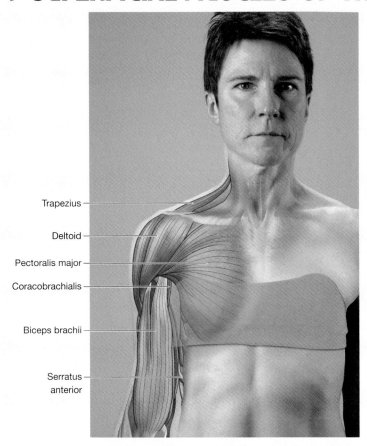

Trapezius

Deltoid

Pectoralis major

Coracobrachialis

Biceps brachii

Serratus
anterior

4-7A. Anterior view.

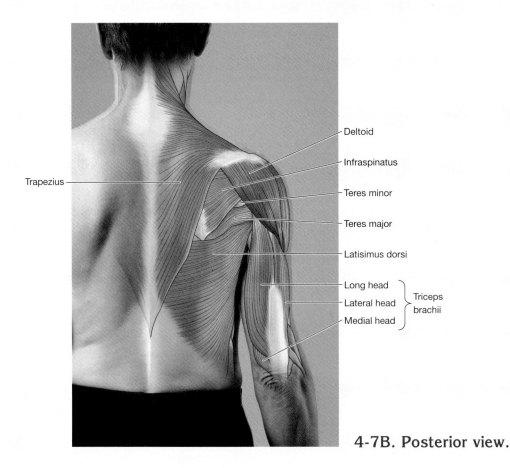

Trapezius

Deltoid

Infraspinatus

Teres minor

Teres major

Latisimus dorsi

Long head
Lateral head
Medial head

Triceps
brachii

4-7B. Posterior view.

▶ DEEP MUSCLES OF THE SHOULDER

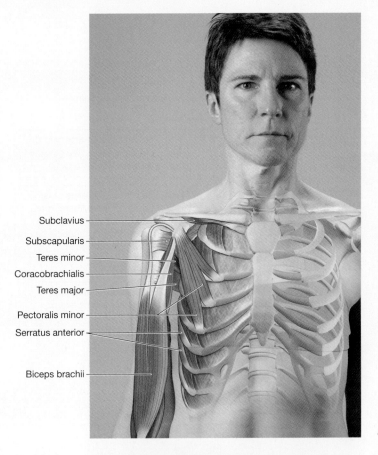

Subclavius
Subscapularis
Teres minor
Coracobrachialis
Teres major
Pectoralis minor
Serratus anterior

Biceps brachii

4-8A. Anterior view.

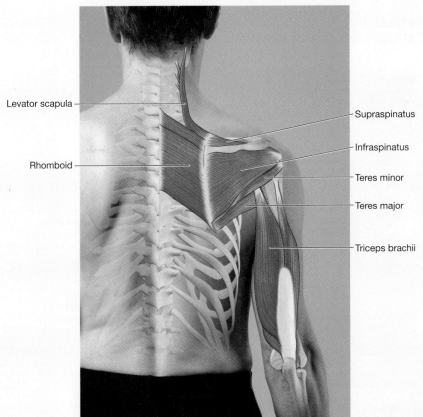

Levator scapula

Rhomboid

Supraspinatus

Infraspinatus

Teres minor

Teres major

Triceps brachii

48-B. Posterior view.

▶ SPECIAL STRUCTURES OF THE SHOULDER

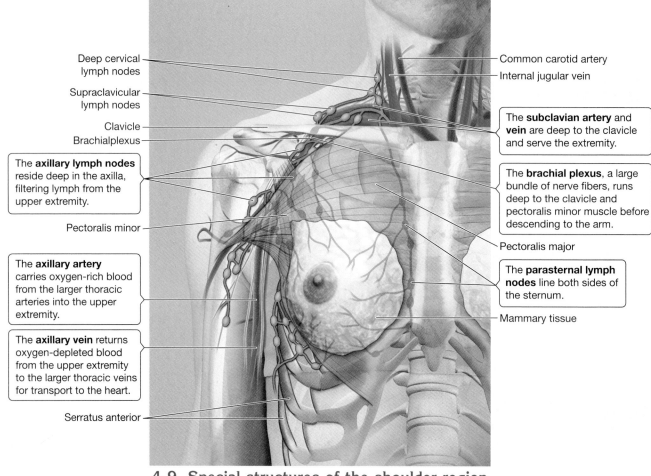

Deep cervical lymph nodes

Supraclavicular lymph nodes

Clavicle

Brachialplexus

The **axillary lymph nodes** reside deep in the axilla, filtering lymph from the upper extremity.

Pectoralis minor

The **axillary artery** carries oxygen-rich blood from the larger thoracic arteries into the upper extremity.

The **axillary vein** returns oxygen-depleted blood from the upper extremity to the larger thoracic veins for transport to the heart.

Serratus anterior

Common carotid artery

Internal jugular vein

The **subclavian artery** and **vein** are deep to the clavicle and serve the extremity.

The **brachial plexus**, a large bundle of nerve fibers, runs deep to the clavicle and pectoralis minor muscle before descending to the arm.

Pectoralis major

The **parasternal lymph nodes** line both sides of the sternum.

Mammary tissue

4-9. Special structures of the shoulder region.

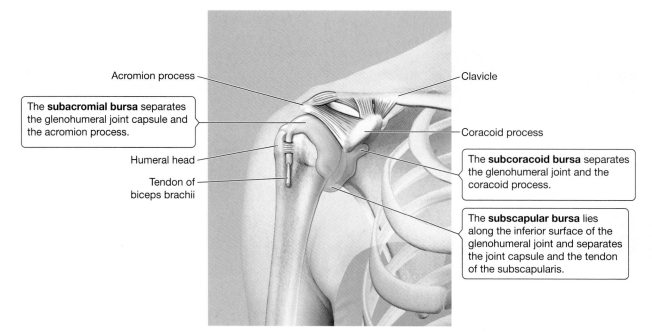

Acromion process

The **subacromial bursa** separates the glenohumeral joint capsule and the acromion process.

Humeral head

Tendon of biceps brachii

Clavicle

Coracoid process

The **subcoracoid bursa** separates the glenohumeral joint and the coracoid process.

The **subscapular bursa** lies along the inferior surface of the glenohumeral joint and separates the joint capsule and the tendon of the subscapularis.

4-10. Bursae of the shoulder region.

◗ MOVEMENTS AVAILABLE: SCAPULOTHORACIC JOINT

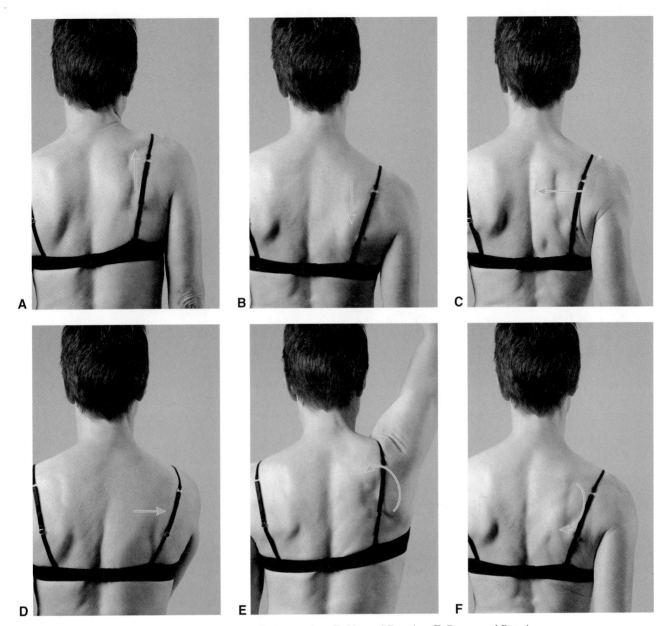

4-11 **A.** Elevation. **B.** Depression. **C.** Retraction. **D.** Protraction. **E.** Upward Rotation. **F.** Downward Rotation.

▶ MOVEMENTS AVAILABLE: GLENOHUMERAL JOINT

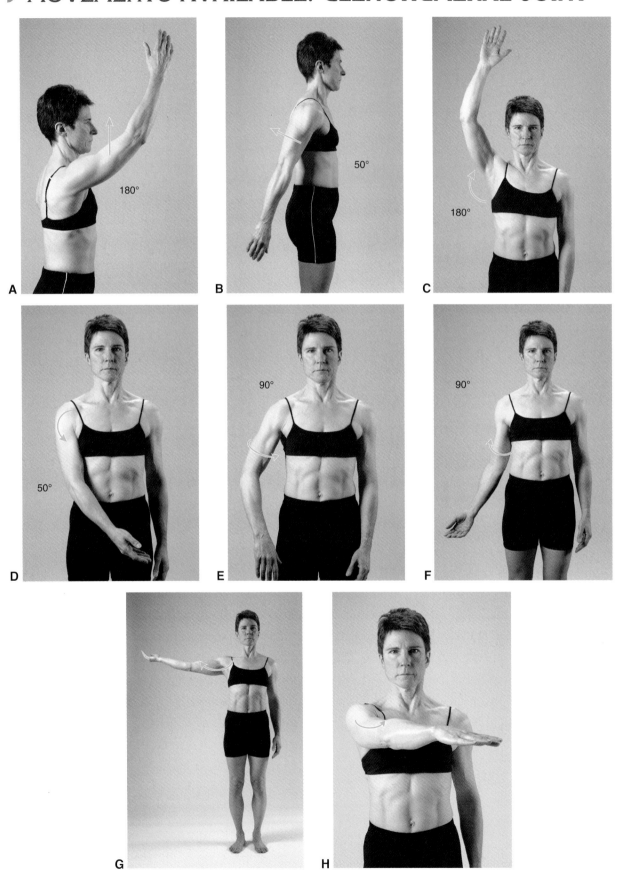

4-12 **A.** Flexion. **B.** Extension. **C.** Abduction. **D.** Adduction. **E.** Internal Rotation. **F.** External Rotation. **G.** Horizontal Abduction. **H.** Horizontal Adduction.

▶ PASSIVE RANGE OF MOTION

Performing passive range of motion (ROM) in the gleno-humeral joint helps establish the health and function of inert structures such as the glenohumeral joint capsule and the ligaments of the glenohumeral, acromioclavicular, and ster-noclavicular joints. It also allows you to evaluate the relative movements between the scapulothoracic and glenohumeral joints.

The client should be lying on a massage or examination table. Ask the client to relax and allow you to perform the ROM exercises without the client "helping." For each of the movements illustrated below, take the arm through to end-feel while watching for compensation (extraneous move-ment) in the scapulothoracic joint or trunk. Evaluate the scapula and shoulder together so that you can assess their in-tegrated functions. Procedures for performing passive ROM are described in Chapter 1.

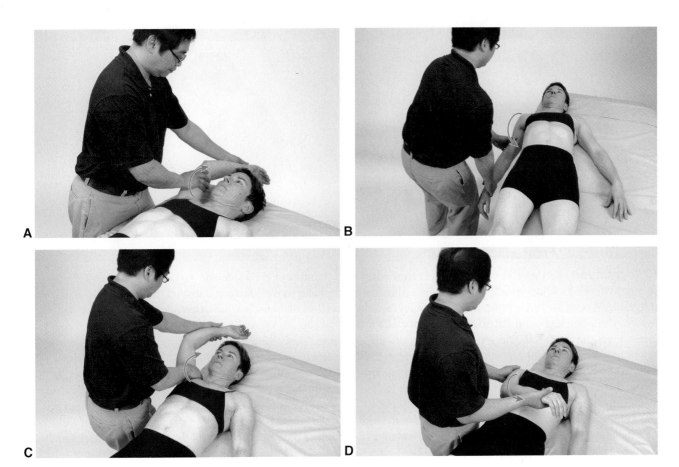

4-13 A. Passive shoulder flexion. The blue arrow indicates the direction of movement. Stand at head of the table. Hold the client's wrist with one hand and grasp the elbow with the other hand to stabilize the limb. Turn the client's palm inward, facing the client's body, and keep the elbow relatively straight. Then move the client's arm from the side of the body over the client's head. Assess the range of motion of the joint capsule as well as the muscles that extend the shoul-der. **B. Passive shoulder extension.** Stand at client's side and support the wrist and elbow in the same way as for passive shoulder flexion. With the client's palm turned inward and the elbow relatively straight, bring the arm back down to the client's side and toward the floor as far as is comfortable. Assess the range of motion of the joint capsule as well as the muscles that flex the shoulder. **C. Passive shoulder abduction.** Stand at client's side toward the head of the table. Support the wrist and elbow and turn the client's palm up toward the ceiling. Move the arm to the side, away from the body, as far as is comfortable. Assess the range of motion of the joint capsule as well as the muscles that adduct the shoulder. **D. Passive shoulder adduction.** Stand at client's side and support the wrist and elbow in the same way as for passive shoulder abduction. Move the arm down and across the front of the body as far as is comfortable. Assess the range of motion of the joint capsule as well as the muscles that abduct the shoulder. *(continues)*

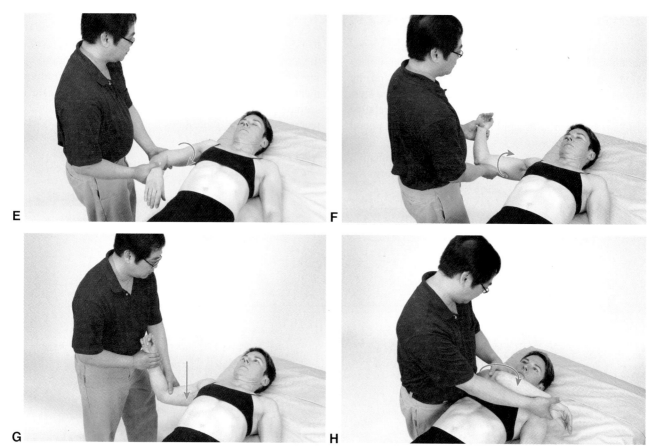

4-13 (continued) E. **Passive shoulder internal rotation.** Stand at client's side and support the wrist and elbow with elbow flexed to 90 degrees. Pivot the client's shoulder so the hand moves down and toward the floor as far as is comfortable. Assess the range of motion of the joint capsule as well as the muscles that externally rotate the shoulder. **F. Passive shoulder external rotation.** Stand at client's side and support the wrist and elbow with elbow flexed to 90 degrees. Pivot the client's shoulder so the hand moves up and toward the ceiling as far as is comfortable. Assess the range of motion of the joint capsule as well as the muscles that internally rotate the shoulder. **G. Passive shoulder horizontal abduction.** Stand at client's side and support the wrist and elbow. Move the arm until the elbow is even with the shoulder and then down toward the floor as far as is comfortable. Assess the range of motion of the joint capsule as well as the muscles that horizontally adduct the shoulder. **H. Passive shoulder horizontal adduction.** Stand at client's side and support the wrist and elbow. Move the arm until the elbow is even with the shoulder and then in and across the body as far as is comfortable. Assess the range of motion of the joint capsule and the muscles that horizontally abduct the shoulder.

▶ RESISTED ROM

Performing resisted ROM for both the scapulothoracic joint and glenohumeral joint helps establish the health and function of the dynamic stabilizers and prime movers in this region. Evaluating functional strength and endurance helps you to identify balance and potential imbalance between the muscles that steer the scapula, stabilize the humeral head, and move the humerus. Notice that you do not assess upward rotation and downward rotation of the scapula individually, as these motions are integral to and assessed during movements of the glenohumeral joint. Procedures for performing and grading resisted ROM are outlined in Chapter 1.

Resisted ROM: Scapula

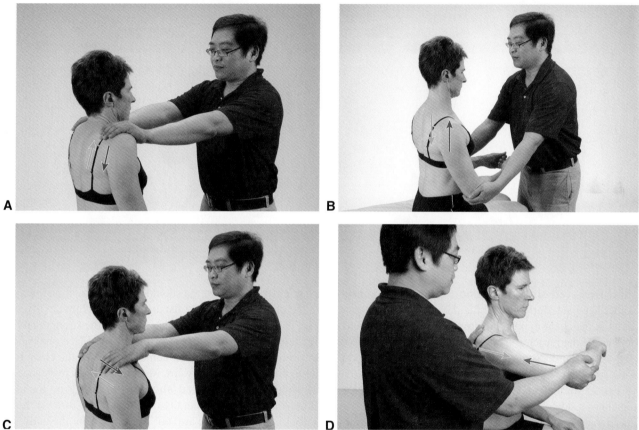

4-14 **A. Resisted scapular elevation.** The green arrow indicates the direction of movement of the client and the red arrow indicates the direction of resistance from the practitioner. Stand facing the client. Place the palms of your hands on top of the client's shoulders. Instruct the client to meet your resistance by shrugging the shoulders up as you gently but firmly press the shoulders down. Assess the strength and endurance of the muscles that elevate the scapulas.
B. Resisted scapular depression. Stand facing the client. Place the palms of your hands underneath the client's forearms. Ask the client to press his or her shoulders down as you gently but firmly press the client's arms up toward the ceiling. Assess the strength and endurance of the muscles that depress the scapulas. **C. Resisted scapular retraction.** Stand facing the client. Place the palms of your hands on the sides of the client's shoulders. Gently but firmly pull the client's shoulders forward toward you as the client meets your resistance by squeezing the shoulders back. Assess the strength and endurance of the muscles that retract the scapulas. **D. Resisted scapular protraction.** Stand behind the client. Have the client reach forward with one arm keeping the elbow bent to 90 degrees. Place your hand on the front of the client's bent elbow. Ask the client to push the whole arm forward as you gently but firmly pull the arm straight back toward you, meeting the client's resistance. Assess the strength and endurance of the muscles that protract the scapula.

Resisted ROM: Shoulder

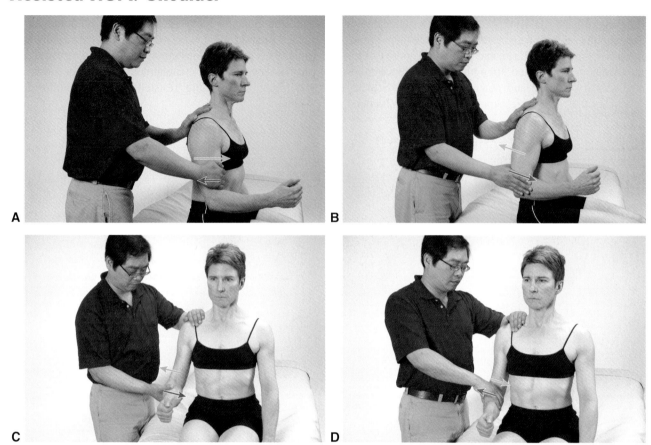

4-15 A. Resisted shoulder flexion. Stand behind client. Place one hand on top of the shoulder to stabilize it and wrap the other hand anteriorly around the middle of the humerus. Have the client make a loose fist and bend the elbow to 90 degrees. Ask the client to push the arm forward. As the client does so, meet the client's resistance to assess the strength and endurance of the muscles that flex the shoulder. **B. Resisted shoulder extension.** Stand behind client. Place one hand on top of the shoulder to stabilize it and the other hand posteriorly around the bottom of the humerus. Instruct the client to make a loose fist and bend the elbow to 90 degrees. Ask the client to push the arm backward. Meet the client's resistance to assess the strength and endurance of the muscles that extend the shoulder. **C. Resisted shoulder abduction.** Stand at the client's side. Place one hand on top of the shoulder to stabilize it and the other laterally on the forearm. Instruct the client to make a loose fist and bend the elbow to 90 degrees. Ask the client to push the arm out and away from the body. Meet the client's resistance to assess the strength and endurance of the muscles that abduct the shoulder. **D. Resisted shoulder adduction.** Stand at the client's side. Place one hand on top of the shoulder to stabilize it and the other medially on the forearm. Instruct the client to make a loose fist and bend the elbow to 90 degrees. Ask the client to pull the arm in toward the body. Meet the client's resistance to assess the strength and endurance of the muscles that adduct the shoulder. *(continued)*

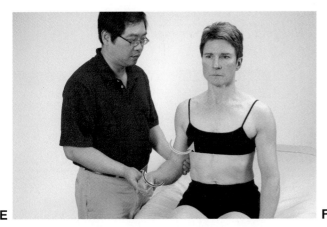
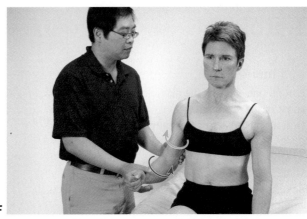

E   F

4-15 *(continued)* **E. Resisted shoulder internal rotation.** Stand at client's side. Place one hand around the elbow to stabilize it and the other on the medial forearm toward the wrist. Instruct the client to make a loose fist and bend the elbow to 90 degrees. Ask the client to pivot the arm and bring the forearm toward the body. Meet the client's resistance to assess the strength and endurance of the muscles that internally rotate the shoulder. **F. Resisted shoulder external rotation.** Stand at the client's side. Place one hand around the client's elbow to stabilize it and the other on the lateral forearm near the wrist. Instruct the client to make a loose fist and bend the elbow to 90 degrees. Ask the client to pivot the arm and rotate the forearm away from the body. Meet the client's resistance to assess the strength and endurance of the muscles that externally rotate the shoulder.

Deltoid ● del'toyd • "**delta**" Greek *the letter delta* "**oid**" Latin *resemblance*

Attachments
O: Lateral one-third of the clavicle, acromion process, and spine of the scapula
I: Deltoid tuberosity of the humerus

Actions
- Abducts the shoulder (all fibers)
- Flexes, internally rotates, and horizontally adducts the shoulder (anterior fibers)
- Extends, externally rotates, and horizontally abducts the shoulder (posterior fibers)

Innervation
- Axillary nerve
- C5–C6

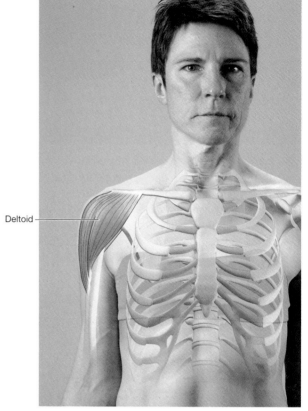

Deltoid

4-16

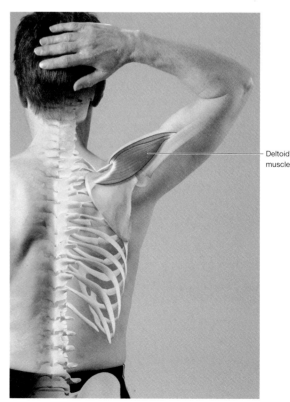

Deltoid muscle

4-17

Deltoid *(continued)*

Functional Anatomy

The deltoid is a prime mover for nearly all movements of the shoulder. Its pennate fiber arrangement, large cross-sectional area, and broad attachment points create excellent leverage on the glenohumeral joint. The deltoid also plays an important role in stabilizing the shoulder by wrapping itself around the glenohumeral joint and holding it together. When all fibers of the deltoid work together, it is a powerful abductor. The supraspinatus stabilizes the head of the humerus as the deltoid abducts the shoulder and prevents impingement of the humeral head on the acromion process. This function of the deltoid is essential for lifting and reaching below shoulder height and above the head.

The anterior fibers of the deltoid work with the pectoralis major to flex and internally rotate the humerus. This is a powerful combination and these muscles are utilized in pushing, reaching, and initiating throwing movements. As a result of this association with the pectoralis major, as well as the fact that most activities of daily living utilize movements in front of the body, the anterior fibers of the deltoid are often overdeveloped and the posterior fibers are typically underdeveloped.

Finally, the posterior fibers of the deltoid work with the latissimus dorsi and teres major to extend the shoulder and are the primary external rotators of the humerus. The posterior fibers are also strong agonists for pulling movements, such as rowing. In overhead movements, such as throwing and hitting, the posterior deltoid works synergistically with the pectoralis major, latissimus dorsi, and teres major to extend the humerus from its overhead, flexed position.

Palpating Deltoid

Anterior and Middle Fibers

Positioning: client supine with arm at side.

1. Locate acromion process.
2. Palpate inferiorly along muscle belly with palm of hand.
3. Continue palpating the muscle belly as it converges about half way down the lateral humerus.
4. Client resists shoulder flexion and/or abduction to ensure proper location.

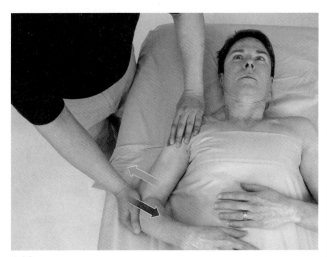

4-18

Posterior Fibers

Positioning: client prone with arm at side.

1. Locate spine of the scapula with tips of four fingers.
2. Follow spine of the scapula laterally to acromion process.
3. Palpate distally toward the deltoid tuberosity to find muscle belly.
4. Client resists shoulder extension to ensure proper location.

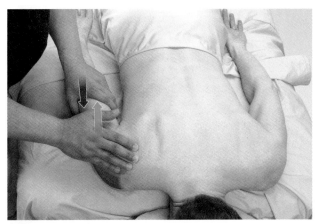

4-19

Pectoralis Major  pek *tor al* us *ma'jor* • **"pectoral"** Latin *chest* **"major"** Latin *larger*

Attachments

O: Medial clavicle, sternum, and costal cartilages of ribs
    1–7

I: Lateral lip of the bicipital groove of the humerus

Actions

- Flexes the shoulder (clavicular fibers)
- Extends the shoulder from overhead position (costal fibers)
- Adducts the shoulder from below shoulder height
- Abducts the shoulder from above shoulder height
- Internally rotates the shoulder
- Horizontally adducts the shoulder (all fibers)

Innervation

- Medial and lateral pectoral nerves
- C5–T1

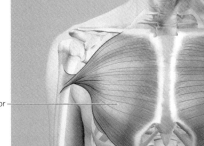

Pectoralis major

4-20

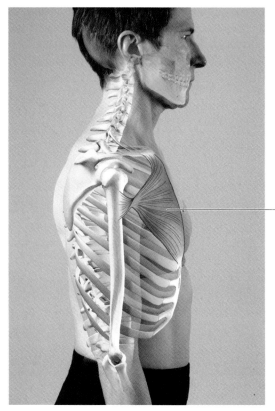

Pectoralis major

4-21

Functional Anatomy

The pectoralis major is a powerful chest muscle responsible for movements in front of the body, such as pushing, reaching, throwing, and punching. Pectoralis major has multiple segments with descending, horizontal, and ascending fiber directions. These different fiber arrangements allow various movement possibilities. The upper or clavicular fibers are primarily utilized during flexion of the humerus. The middle or sternal fibers are utilized in conjunction with all other fibers for horizontal adduction. The lower or costal fibers are activated during extension of the humerus from a flexed or overhead position.

The pectoralis major has a distinct twist in the muscle near its attachment on the humerus. This feature maintains the leverage of the different fibers in the various positions possible at the shoulder. Fully flexing the shoulder "unwinds" the twist near the distal attachment and prepares the muscle for its action of extending and internally rotating the humerus. This is particularly important for powerful overhead movements such as throwing, hitting, spiking, and swimming. There is a similar twist in the large latissimus dorsi muscle, which is a clue to the synergistic relationship between them. These two broad, strong muscles work together, along with the teres major and posterior deltoid, to generate tremendous power, forcibly lowering the arm from an overhead position.

Pectoralis major works with the muscles attached to the shoulder girdle to keep the chest erect when the arms are supporting the body's weight. This occurs when you push yourself up out of a chair or during athletic activities such as parallel bars. It also works with the latissimus dorsi and teres major to adduct the shoulder when pulling objects down from overhead or pulling the body up toward a fixed hand, such as when climbing a ladder or rope.

Palpating Pectoralis Major

Muscle Belly

Positioning: client supine with arm at side.

1. Locate inferior clavicle.
2. Palpate inferiorly along muscle belly with palm toward the sternum and costocartilage.
3. Follow the muscle belly to its attachments on the clavicle, costocartilage, and sternum.
4. Client resists shoulder internal rotation to ensure proper location.

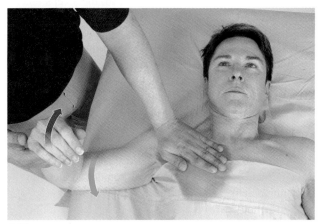

4-22

Anterior Border of Axilla

Positioning: client supine with arm abducted.

1. Locate inferior clavicle with fingertips.
2. Grasp lateral edge of pectoralis major inside the axilla with thumb and compress upwards toward fingers, below clavicle.
3. Client resists shoulder internal rotation to ensure proper location.

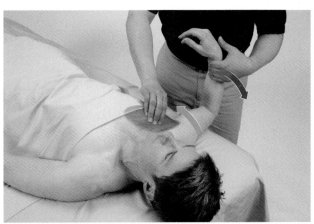

4-23

Coracobrachialis

kor'a ko bra ke al'is • **"coraco"** Greek *coracoid process*
"brachialis" Latin *arm*

Attachments

O: Coracoid process of the scapula
I: Medial shaft, middle one-third of the humerus

Actions

- Flexes and adducts the shoulder
- Innervation
- Musculocutaneous nerve
- C5–C7

Functional Anatomy

The coracobrachialis works strongly with the biceps brachii to flex and adduct the shoulder. It is like a third head of the biceps brachii. This muscle is also an antagonist to the deltoid and has a similar attachment site about halfway down the humerus, with the deltoid attaching laterally and the coracobrachialis attaching medially.

The coracobrachialis, latissimus dorsi, teres major, pectoralis major, and long head of the triceps brachii all work together to adduct the shoulder. Movements that involve pulling down and in toward the body, weight-bearing activities on the arms, and sports activities, such as gymnastics rings and parallel bars, involve shoulder adduction. The coracobrachialis is also utilized when bringing the arm across the body as with a golf swing or a pitching motion in fast-pitch softball.

Coracobrachialis is a strong stabilizer of the shoulder and assists with swinging the arms forward during walking gait.

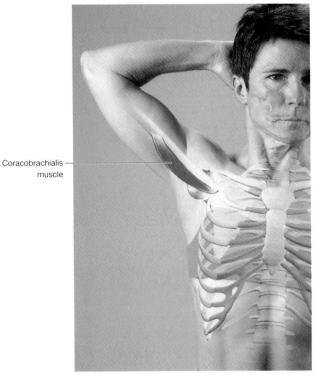

Coracobrachialis
muscle

4-24

Palpating Coracobrachialis

Positioning: client supine with arm at side.

1. Locate anterior border of axilla.

2. Palpate posteriorly and laterally along the medial surface of the humerus.

3. Locate the muscle belly deep to the biceps brachii and follow toward its insertion on the medial shaft of the humerus about the same distance distally as the deltoid.

4. Client resists shoulder adduction to ensure proper location.

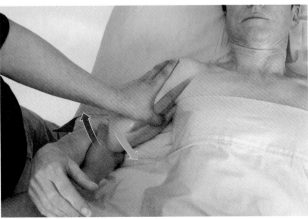

4-25

Biceps Brachii ● *bi'seps bra'ke i* • "**biceps**" Latin *two heads* "**brachii**" Latin *arm*

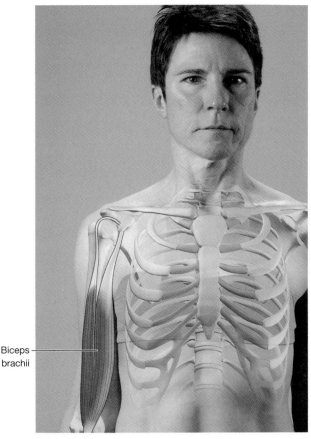

Biceps
brachii

4-26

Palpating Biceps Brachii

Positioning: client supine with arm at side and supinated.

1. Locate muscle belly in center of anterior upper arm.

2. Pincer grasp the muscle belly halfway between the shoulder and elbow.

3. Client resists elbow flexion and supination to ensure proper location.

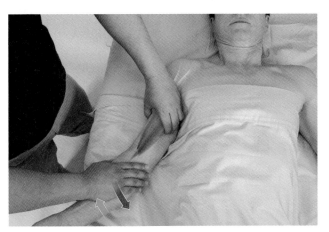

4-27

Attachments

O: Long head: supraglenoid tubercle of the scapula
O: Short head: coracoid process of the scapula
I: Radial tuberosity and bicipital aponeurosis overlying common flexor tendon

Actions

• Flexes, abducts (long head), and adducts (short head) the shoulder
• Flexes and supinates the forearm

Innervation

• Musculocutaneous nerve
• C5–C6

Functional Anatomy

The biceps brachii is one of the most superficial muscles in the upper arm and works on both the shoulder and forearm. Its fusiform shape and multijoint function limit its mechanical advantage compared with its powerhouse synergists deltoid and brachialis, which have pennate fiber arrangements and work on a single joint.

The opposing attachments of the long and short heads of the biceps brachii help stabilize the shoulder during flexion. In this way, it is working in collaboration with the deltoid, coracobrachialis, and triceps brachii. The short head of the biceps brachii also works in conjunction with the coracobrachialis to adduct the arm and swing it forward during walking.

Primarily, biceps brachii works to flex the forearm along with the brachialis, brachioradialis, and most of the wrist flexors. It has the additional movement of supinating the forearm, which makes it functional in twisting motions such as removing a cork from a bottle.

Pectoralis Minor • pek tor *al* us *mi'nor* • "**pectoris**" Latin *chest* "**minor**" Latin *smaller*

Attachments

O: Ribs 3–5
I: Coracoid process of the scapula

Actions

- Protracts and depresses the scapula
- Elevates ribs 3–5

Innervation

- Medial and lateral pectoral nerves
- C5–C8 and T1

Functional Anatomy

The pectoralis minor has a strong attachment to the coracoid process of the scapula and functions as a tether for the scapula to the front of the ribcage. This helps stabilize the scapula anteriorly when bodyweight or external force is placed through the arms. Pectoralis minor works in tandem with the serratus anterior to hold the scapula against the body when you push yourself up with your arms. This anchoring of the scapula is necessary when you push yourself up out of a chair or off the ground when doing pushups. These muscles, in conjunction with the subclavius, dynamically stabilize the shoulder girdle and maintain its posture.

Pectoralis minor also serves as a secondary respiratory muscle: by fixing the scapula and elevating ribs 3–5, it helps expand the ribcage and increase space in the thoracic cavity. In this function, pectoralis minor is working synergistically with the diaphragm, external intercostals, scalenes, serratus anterior, serratus posterior superior and inferior, and quadratus lumborum. All of these muscles have attachments on the ribcage and can be recruited for thoracic expansion during labored breathing.

Overuse and tightness of the pectoralis minor contribute to the rounded-shoulder postural deviation. This is commonly seen in people who do repetitive activities in front of the body such as computer work, driving, pushing, and lifting.

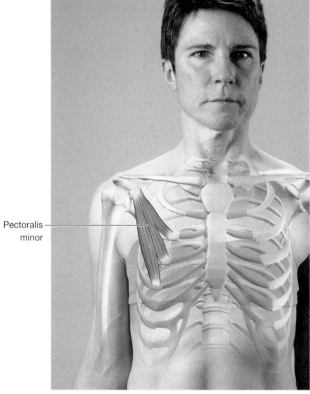

Pectoralis minor

4-28

Palpating Pectoralis Minor

Positioning: client supine.

1. Passively abduct humerus to slack tissue.

2. Slide fingers into axilla from lateral to medial.

3. Find the coracoid process of the scapula and slide medially and inferiorly along the anterior ribs and onto the fibers of pectoralis minor.

4. Client resists scapular depression to assure proper location.

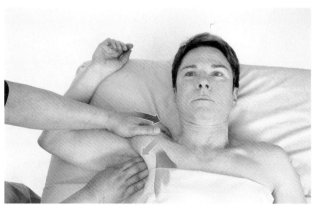

4-29

Subclavius • sub *cla* vee us • "**sub**" Latin *under* "**clavius**" Latin *key*

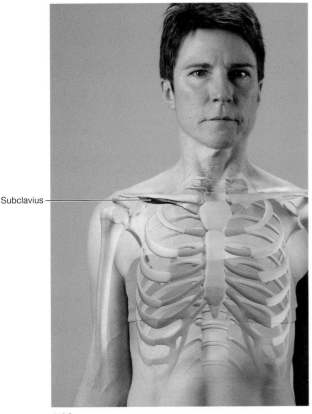

Subclavius

4-30

Palpating Subclavius

Positioning: client supine.

1. Find the inferior edge of the clavicle halfway between the medial and lateral ends.

2. Slide thumb inferiorly and deep to the clavicle.

3. Client resists scapular depression to assure proper location.

Attachments
O: 1st rib at the junction with the costocartilage
I: Clavicle, the middle one-third of the inferior surface

Actions
- Fixes the clavicle inferiorly or elevates the first rib
- Helps protract the scapula, drawing the shoulder inferiorly and anteriorly

Innervation
- A nerve from the brachial plexus
- C5–C6

Functional Anatomy

The function of the subclavius muscle is controversial and somewhat unclear. Most agree that it functions mainly to stabilize or fix the clavicle during movements of the arm and/or shoulder girdle. Thus, the subclavius muscle works on the sternoclavicular joint and acromioclavicular joint, both of which have strong ligaments that greatly limit their mobility. Most of the movement occurs at the sternoclavicular joint, which is a ball and socket joint allowing slight rotation of the clavicle during overhead movements.

The subclavius muscle assists other stabilizing muscles such as the pectoralis minor and serratus anterior. These muscles work together to dynamically stabilize the shoulder girdle. Both the scapula and the clavicle must be strongly fixed whenever the arms are bearing bodyweight or pushing an external load. These activities strengthen the subclavius and its stabilizing synergists.

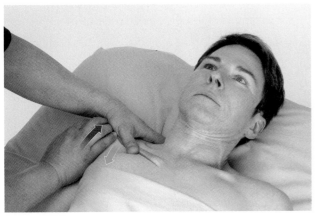

4-31

Trapezius   tra pe´ze us • "**trapezius**" Greek *little table*

Attachments

O: Entire muscle: occiput, nuchal ligament and spinous processes of C7–T12

O: Upper fibers: the external occipital protuberance, the medial one-third of the superior nuchal line of the occiput, the nuchal ligament and spinous process of C7

O: Middle fibers: spinous processes of T1–T5

O: Lower fibers: spinous processes of T6–T12

I: Lateral one-third of the clavicle, acromion process, and spine of the scapula

Actions

• Extends, laterally flexes, and rotates the head and neck to the same side (contralaterally)
• Elevates and upwardly rotates the scapula (upper fibers)
• Retracts the scapula (entire muscle)
• Depresses and upwardly rotates the scapula (lower fibers)

Innervations

• Medial and lateral pectoral nerves
• C5–T1

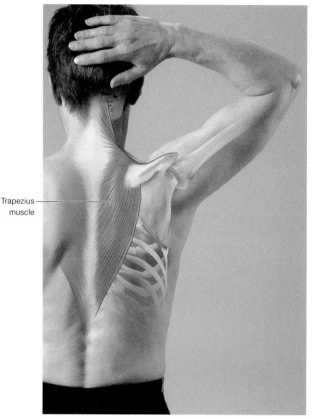

Trapezius muscle

4-32

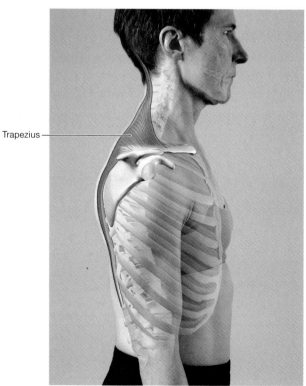

Trapezius

4-33

Functional Anatomy

The trapezius is the most superficial muscle on the back and covers a large, kite-shaped area starting at the base of the skull, extending laterally across the scapulas, and overlapping the superior portion of the latissimus dorsi on the spine. It can be divided into three distinct fiber directions, including the upper fibers, middle fibers, and lower fibers.

The upper fibers have an ascending fiber direction and are responsible for shrugging motions or elevation of the scapula along with the levator scapulae and rhomboids. They also perform extension, lateral flexion, and contralateral rotation of the head and neck.

The middle fibers have a horizontal fiber direction. They work with the rhomboids to retract the scapula.

The lower fibers have a descending fiber direction and depress the scapula. The upper and lower fibers work together to upwardly rotate the scapula.

When all fibers of the trapezius work together, the scapula is fixed on the ribcage, allowing strong support during weight-bearing and pushing activities. When the upper extremity is not fixed, the different fibers of the trapezius work with other synergist muscles to accomplish specific movements of the scapula such as elevation, retraction, or depression. The trapezius' function in upward rotation of the scapula helps optimally position the glenoid fossa during overhead motions, thereby enhancing ROM in the glenohumeral joint.

Despite the ability of the trapezius fibers to work together as a unit, the lower fibers are often weak and underutilized and the upper fibers are often tight and overutilized for lifting, carrying, and pulling. This contributes to the commonly encountered elevated shoulder postural deviation. Balanced flexibility and strength between the upper and lower fibers of trapezius helps optimally position the head and shoulder girdle against gravity.

Palpating Trapezius

Muscle Belly

Positioning: client supine with arm at side.

1. Locate medial border of the scapula.

2. Palpate medially along muscle belly with edge of hand toward the spine.

3. Follow the broad muscle belly along each of its three separate fiber directions: upwardly toward the occiput, horizontally toward the upper thoracic spine, and at a downward diagonal toward the lower thoracic spine.

4. Client resists scapular retraction to ensure proper location.

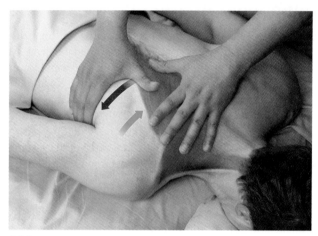

4-34

Upper Fibers

Positioning: client prone with arm at side.

1. Locate spine of the scapula with your thumb.

2. Move thumb superior to spine and wrap fingers anteriorly around muscle to just above the clavicle.

3. Pincer grasp with the thumb and fingers together to locate the fibers of the upper trapezius.

4. Client resists scapular elevation to ensure proper location.

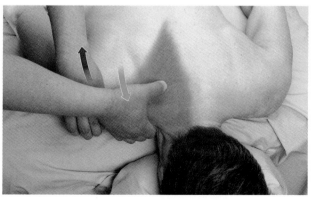

4-35

Levator Scapula

le va'tor skap'yu le • "**levator**" Latin *raiser* "**scapula**" Latin *shoulder blade*

Attachments

O: Transverse processes of C1–C4
I: Superior angle of the scapula

Actions

• Elevates and downwardly rotates the scapula
• Extends, laterally flexes, and rotates the neck to the same side (ipsilaterally)

Innervation

• Dorsal scapular nerve
• C3–C5

Functional Anatomy

The levator scapula and the upper fibers of the trapezius work together to elevate the scapula and extend the head. At other times, the levator scapula opposes the upper and lower fibers of trapezius to rotate the scapula inferiorly while the trapezius rotates it superiorly. The rhomboid major and minor assist the levator scapula with this downward rotation, helping to position the glenoid fossa during movements of the upper extremity. This "steering" of the glenoid enhances the motion of the glenohumeral joint, particularly in adduction.

Cocontraction of these and the other scapular stabilizers (pectoralis minor and serratus anterior) help anchor the scapula to the ribcage during weight-bearing activities such as pushing. The distinctive twist near its attachment on the transverse processes of the cervical vertebrae helps the levator scapula maintain tension and force-production throughout its ROM.

The levator scapula is commonly overused and hypertonic as a result of asymmetrical carrying, lifting, and reaching with the upper extremity. It typically works in conjunction with other muscles such as the trapezius or rhomboids; thus, any dysfunction often will be paralleled in these synergistic groups.

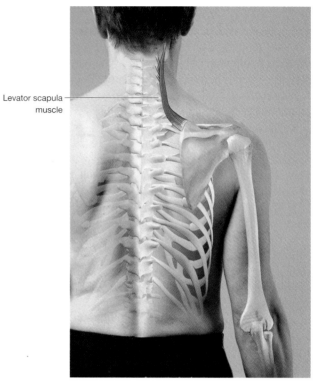

Levator scapula muscle

4-36

Palpating Levator Scapula

Positioning: client prone.

1. Stand beside client's head and find the superior angle of the scapula on the same side.

2. Find the transverse processes of the upper cervical vertebrae with the fingertips of your other palpating hand.

3. Follow the muscle belly of levator scapula toward the scapula.

4. Client resists scapular elevation to assure proper location.

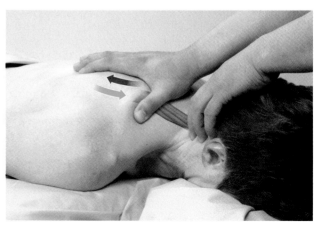

4-37

Rhomboid Major and Minor

rom boyd *ma'jor,* rom boyd *mi'nor* "**rhombos**"
Greek *rhombus (a geometric shape)* "**oid**"
Latin *resemblance*

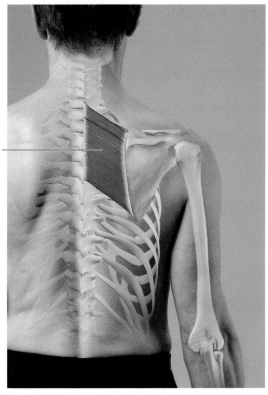

Rhomboid muscle

4-38

Attachments

O: Spinous processes C7–T1 (Minor)
O: Spinous processes T2–T5 (Major)
I: Medial border of scapula from the root of the spine to the inferior angle (Major and Minor)

Actions

• Retracts, elevates, and downwardly rotates the scapula

Innervation

• Dorsal scapular nerve
• C4–C5

Functional Anatomy

The rhomboids work with the trapezius, levator scapulae, and serratus anterior to stabilize the scapula on the ribcage during weight-bearing movements. There is a clear antagonistic relationship between the rhomboids and the serratus anterior in particular, as both muscles attach to the medial border of the scapula, but their fibers extend in opposite directions. Cocontraction of these two powerful muscles helps stabilize the scapula against the ribcage. The rhomboids, levator scapula, and serratus anterior also steer the glenoid in downward rotation to enhance the ROM of motion of the glenohumeral joint. Pulling motions, such as rowing, are the result of the rhomboids and trapezius working together to retract the scapula.

Along with the middle trapezius, the rhomboids are commonly underdeveloped. This can contribute to a rounded-shoulder posture. When the rhomboids are out of balance with the powerful serratus anterior, the scapula is held in a protracted and depressed position, which creates tension and decreased mobility in the cervical spine. Maintaining comparable strength in the muscles attached to the scapula and shoulder girdle contributes to healthy alignment and mobility in the upper body.

Palpating Rhomboids

Positioning: client prone with arm at side.

1. Locate spinous processes of C7–T5.
2. Palpate to the medial border of the scapula with tips of the four fingers.
3. Notice that the muscle belly is flat and the fiber direction is oblique and inferior.
4. Client resists scapular retraction and elevation to ensure proper location.

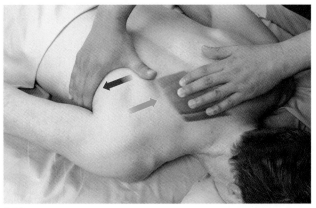

4-39

Latissimus Dorsi  *la* tis'i *mus* dor'si • "**latissimus**" Latin *wide* "**dorsi**" Latin *back*

Attachments

O: Spinous processes of T7–L5, posterior iliac crest and posterior sacrum (via thoracolumbar aponeurosis)

I: Medial lip of the bicipital groove of the humerus

Actions

• Adducts, extends, and internally rotates the shoulder

Innervation

• Thoracodorsal nerve
• C6–C8

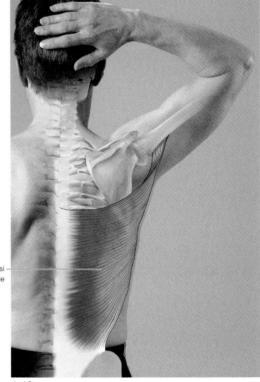

Latissimus dorsi
muscle

4-40

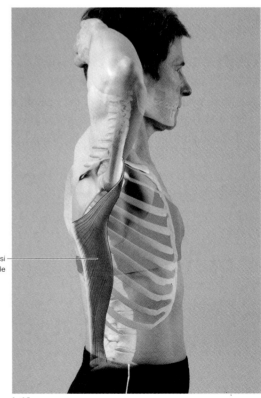

Latissimus dorsi
muscle

4-41

Functional Anatomy

The latissimus dorsi is a large back muscle that primarily moves the humerus. Its broad attachment into the thoracolumbar aponeurosis and specific attachment on the humerus create the potential for producing a tremendous amount of force on the glenohumeral joint. In a small percentage of people, the latissimus dorsi also has an attachment on the lateral, inferior portion of the scapula, near the teres major.

The latissimus dorsi has a distinct twist in the muscle near its attachment on the humerus. There is a similar twist in the large pectoralis major muscle. This common feature is a clue to the synergistic relationship of these two broad, strong muscles. They work together, along with the teres major and posterior deltoid, to pull the raised arm downward during throwing and hitting motions (a position that "unwinds" the twist near the distal attachment). The latissimus dorsi also works with pectoralis major to adduct the arm or raise the body when the arm is fixed, such as during climbing. Finally, these muscles work together to prevent downward displacement of the trunk when bearing weight on the arms, like when pushing up from a chair, walking with crutches, or performing on the rings or parallel bars in gymnastics.

Adequate ROM in the latissimus dorsi is critical for proper performance of overhead movements. When this muscle is tight, the back arches to compensate, creating compression of the posterior structures of the spinal column. This is a common source of low back pain in athletes and others performing repetitive overhead movements, such as lifting or pushing.

Palpating Latissimus Dorsi

Muscle Belly

Positioning: client prone with arm at side.

1. Locate spinous processes of lumbar vertebrae with palm of hand.
2. Palpate laterally toward the inferior angle of the scapula.
3. Locate the broad muscle belly, beginning on the posterior iliac crest and sacrum and ending on the proximal humerus.
4. Client resists shoulder extension and adduction to ensure proper location.

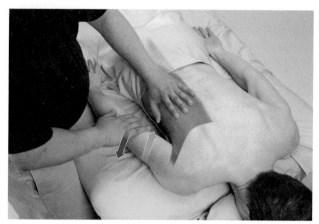

4-42

Posterior Axilla

Positioning: client prone with arm abducted.

1. Locate lateral border of the scapula with pads of four fingers.
2. Pincer grasp from inside the axilla onto the posterior, lateral musculature between thumb and fingers.
3. Client resists shoulder extension to ensure proper location.

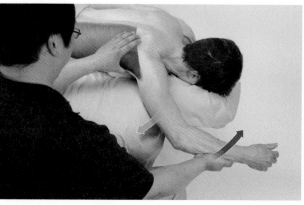

4-43

Teres Major • *ter'ez ma'jor* • "**teres**" Latin *round* "**major**" Latin *large*

Attachments

O: Inferior lateral border of the scapula
I: Medial lip of the bicipital groove on the humerus

Actions

• Adducts, extends, and internally rotates the shoulder

Innervation

• Lower subscapular nerve
• C5–C7

Functional Anatomy

The teres major is a direct synergist to the latissimus dorsi because they share all of the same actions: extension, adduction, and internal rotation of the shoulder. Both muscles wrap around the humerus anteriorly and insert on the lesser tubercle and bicipital groove. Teres major is often called "lat's little helper" because of the strong association between these two muscles.

Teres major works more strongly with the subscapularis than any other rotator cuff muscle as they perform internal rotation of the shoulder. Teres minor may have the same shape as teres major, but they do not share functions. In fact, teres minor is an antagonist to teres major as it wraps around the posterior humerus and functions as an external rotator.

When the arm is fixed, the teres major works with the latissimus dorsi to pull the trunk toward the arm, such as when climbing. When the arm is free, the teres major works with all of the shoulder internal rotators and extenders to pull the raised arm forward and downward, such as with swimming, throwing, and hitting overhead.

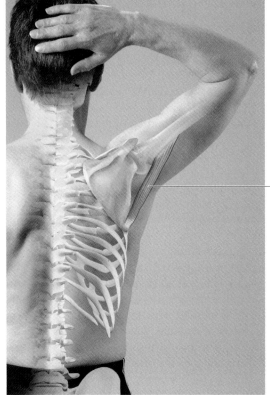

Teres major muscle

4-44

Palpating Teres Major

Positioning: client prone with arm at side.

1. Locate lateral border of the scapula with thumb.
2. Palpate muscle belly just inferior and lateral to the lateral border of the scapula.
3. Follow the thick, round muscle belly as it helps form the posterior border of the axilla.
4. Client resists shoulder extension to ensure proper location.

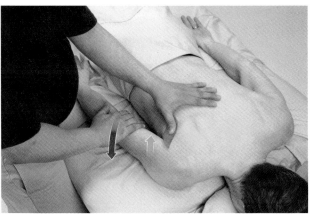

4-45

Serratus Anterior

ser a'tus an te're or • **"serra"** Latin *saw* **"anterior"** Latin *toward the front*

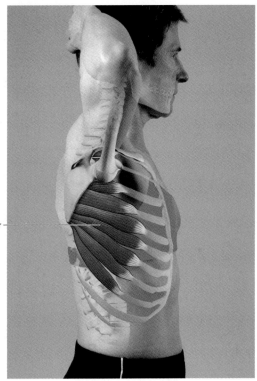

Serratus anterior muscle

4-46

Palpating Serratus Anterior

Positioning: client side-lying with arm forward.

1. Stand behind client and find the most lateral portion of the scapula.

2. Use your four fingers to palpate from the lateral edge of the scapula anteriorly and inferiorly toward the ribs.

3. Follow each section of the muscle belly toward its insertion on individual ribs.

4. Client resists scapular protraction to assure proper location.

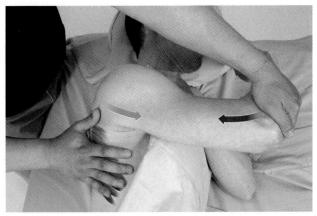

4-47

Attachments

O: Outer surfaces of upper 8 or 9 ribs
I: Costal surface of medial border of the scapula

Actions

• Protracts, depresses, and upwardly rotates the scapula
• Assists with forced inspiration when the insertion is fixed

Innervation

• Long thoracic nerve
• C5–C8

Functional Anatomy

The serratus anterior has multiple functions in the body. Primarily, it works with the pectoralis minor to fix the scapula against the thoracic cavity, particularly during weight-bearing activities on the arms. This function is utilized in activities that involve pushing. Serratus anterior resides deep to the subscapularis, between the scapula and thoracic cavity, and has a common anchor on the medial border of the scapula with the rhomboids.

Serratus anterior also works with the trapezius to steer the glenoid fossa into position for maximal ROM in overhead activities. This function is critical to healthy scapulohumeral rhythm during movements such as reaching, throwing, and pushing. Scapulohumeral rhythm is the coordinated movement between the scapulothoraic and glenohumeral joints.

Finally, the serratus anterior can be utilized for forced inspiration along with the diaphragm, external intercostals, pectoralis minor, scalenes, and other muscles that have attachments on the thoracic cavity. It is recruited, for example, during the labored breathing commonly associated with exercise, but only if the medial border of the scapula is fixed to the ribcage.

Supraspinatus • *su pra spi na'tus* • "**supra**" Latin *above* "**spina**" Latin *spine (of the scapula)*

Attachments

O: Supraspinous fossa of the scapula
I: Greater tubercle of the humerus

Actions

• Initiates abduction of the shoulder

Innervation

• Suprascapular nerve
• C5–C6

Functional Anatomy

The supraspinatus is one of four muscles that make up the rotator cuff. The supraspinatus, infraspinatus, teres minor, and subscapularis all function as a unit to stabilize the humeral head in the glenoid fossa. Each muscle has a specific role in steering the head of the humerus as the arm moves into different positions. Without the rotator cuff working to dynamically stabilize this joint, the humeral head would collide with the surrounding bony structures such as the acromion or coracoid processes. This would result in impingement of bursae, tendons, nerves, and blood vessels.

Specifically, the supraspinatus maneuvers the humeral head inferiorly as prime movers such as the deltoid move the shoulder through shoulder abduction. This prevents the humerus from impinging on the acromion process and damaging the subacromial bursa and tendon of the supraspinatus.

The location of the tendon of the supraspinatus underneath the acromion makes this muscle particularly vulnerable to tendonitis, impingement, and tearing. Trauma to this muscle is common and debilitating to the function of the entire shoulder. Maintaining a strong, healthy supraspinatus in conjunction with the other rotator cuff muscles is essential to shoulder function.

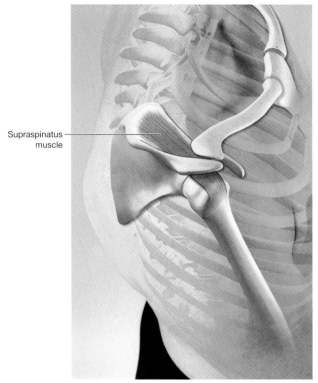

Supraspinatus muscle

4-48

Palpating Supraspinatus

Positioning: client prone with arm at side.

1. Palpate the spine of the scapula with thumb.

2. Move thumb superiorly above the spine to locate the supraspinous fossa.

3. Locate the muscle belly in the supraspinous fossa.

4. Follow the tendon of supraspinatus under the acromion process to the greater tubercle of the humerus.

5. Client resists shoulder abduction to ensure proper location.

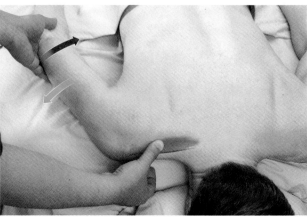

4-49

Infraspinatus ● in'fra spi na'tus • "**infra**" Latin *below* "**spina**" Latin *spine (of the scapula)*

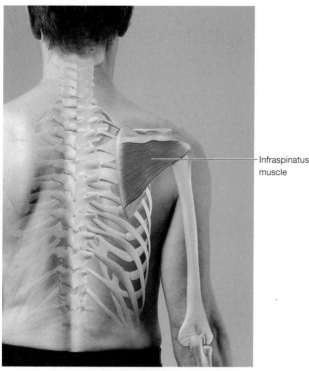

Infraspinatus muscle

4-50

Palpating Infraspinatus

Positioning: client prone with arm off edge of table.

1. Palpate the lateral border of the scapula with your thumb.

2. Place fingers of that same hand medially and superiorly to find infraspinatus.

3. Locate the muscle belly in the infraspinous fossa of the scapula.

4. Follow the tendon of infraspinatus superiorly and laterally around the head of the humerus to the greater tubercle of the humerus.

5. Client resists shoulder external rotation to ensure proper location.

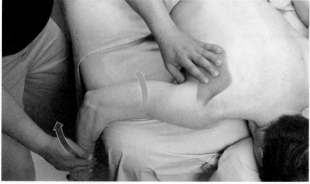

4-51

Attachments

O: Infraspinous fossa of the scapula
I: Greater tubercle of the humerus

Actions

• Externally rotates, adducts, extends, and horizontally abducts the shoulder

Innervation

• Suprascapular nerve
• C5–C6

Functional Anatomy

The infraspinatus is one of four muscles that make up the rotator cuff. The supraspinatus, infraspinatus, teres minor, and subscapularis all function as a unit to stabilize the humeral head in the glenoid fossa. Each muscle has a specific role in steering the head of the humerus as the arm moves into different positions. Specifically, the infraspinatus works with the teres minor to seat the humeral head posteriorly in the glenoid fossa and prevent impingement on the coracoid process of the scapula.

The infraspinatus is one of the most powerful external rotators of the glenohumeral joint and is essential in "preloading" the upper extremity in backward extension and external rotation for shoulder movements, such as pitching and hitting overhead. Infraspinatus is also recruited eccentrically to slow the upper extremity during the follow-through or deceleration phase of these powerful movements.

Imbalances often develop between the powerful internal rotators of the shoulder (pectoralis major, latissimus dorsi, teres major, anterior deltoid, and subscapularis) and the smaller external rotators (posterior deltoid, infraspinatus, and teres minor), creating faulty mechanics in the glenohumeral joint.

Teres Minor • *ter'ez mi'nor* • "**teres**" Latin *round* "**minor**" Latin *small*

Attachments
O: Superior lateral border of the scapula
I: Greater tubercle of the humerus

Actions
• Externally rotates, adducts, extends, and horizontally abducts the shoulder

Innervation
• Axillary nerve
• C5–C6

Functional Anatomy

The teres minor is one of four muscles that make up the rotator cuff. The supraspinatus, infraspinatus, teres minor, and subscapularis all function as a unit to stabilize the humeral head in the glenoid fossa. Each muscle has a specific role in steering the head of the humerus as the arm moves into different positions. Specifically, the teres minor works with the infraspinatus to seat the humeral head posteriorly in the glenoid fossa and prevent impingement on the coracoid process of the scapula.

Teres minor also assists in lowering the raised arm along with the teres major, latissimus dorsi, and costal fibers of the pectoralis major. This function contributes to proper mechanics for complex movements such as pulling, throwing, and hitting from overhead.

Teres minor is recruited synergistically with the infraspinatus to externally rotate the shoulder during the "wind-up" or preload phase for overhead activities and eccentrically to decelerate the upper extremity during the follow-through phase of the same activities.

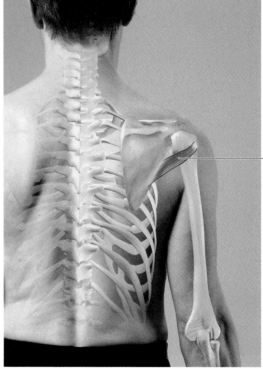

Teres minor muscle

4-52

Palpating Teres Minor

Positioning: client prone with arm off side of table.

1. Palpate the lateral border of the scapula with thumb.
2. Move thumb medially and superiorly to locate teres minor.
3. Locate the small, round muscle belly below the infraspinous fossa.
4. Follow tendon of teres minor along lateral border of scapula, superiorly and laterally around the head of the humerus to the greater tubercle of the humerus.
5. Client resists shoulder external rotation to ensure proper location.

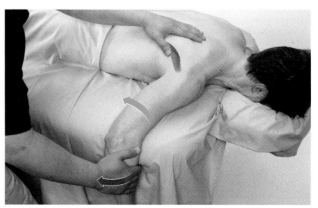

4-53

Subscapularis

*sub'*skap yu *la'*ris • **"sub"** Latin *under* **"scapula"** Latin *shoulder blade*

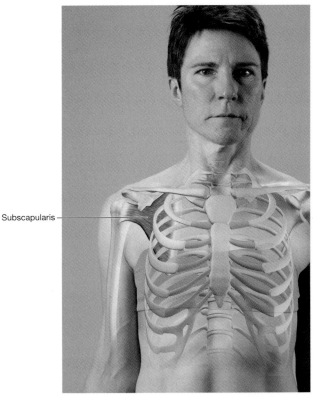

Subscapularis

4-54

Palpating Subscapularis

Positioning: client prone with arm at side.

1. Palpate the lateral border of the scapula with the palmar side of the four fingers.

2. Press posteriorly and medially to the latissimus dorsi, which forms the posterior border of the axilla.

3. Use your other hand to scoop the scapula laterally, improving access to the anterior surface of the scapula.

4. Client resists shoulder internal rotation to ensure proper location.

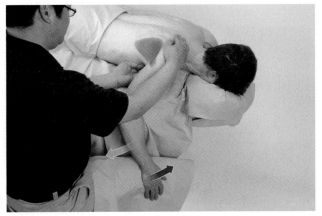

Attachments

O: Subscapular fossa of the scapula
I: Lesser tubercle of the humerus

Actions

• Internally rotates the shoulder

Innervation

• Upper and lower subscapular nerves
• C5–C6

Functional Anatomy

The subscapularis is one of four muscles that make up the rotator cuff. The supraspinatus, infraspinatus, teres minor, and subscapularis all function as a unit to stabilize the humeral head in the glenoid fossa. Each muscle has a specific role in steering the head of the humerus as the arm moves into different positions. The subscapularis is the largest rotator cuff muscle and the only internal rotator of the four.

Specifically, the subscapularis stabilizes the humeral head during the powerful movements of the pectoralis major, latissimus dorsi, teres major, and anterior deltoid as they lower the raised arm downward during pulling movements, such as throwing and hitting overhead. For proper execution, this overhead position requires a precise balance between all four rotator cuff muscles; the subscapularis is particularly vulnerable to impingement during these types of movements when the rotator cuff is dysfunctional.

The subscapularis is also primarily responsible for the backward arm swing motion during normal walking gait.

Triceps Brachii ● *tri'seps bra'kei* • "**triceps**" Latin *three heads* "**brachii**" Latin *arm*

Attachments

O: Long head: infraglenoid tubercle of the scapula
O: Lateral head: proximal one-half of posterior shaft of the
 humerus
O: Medial head: distal one-half of posterior shaft of the
 humerus
I: Olecranon process of the ulna

Actions

• Extends and adducts the shoulder (long head)
• Extends the elbow

Innervation

• Radial nerve
• C6–C8

Functional Anatomy

The triceps brachii is a multijoint muscle like its counter-part, the biceps brachii. Both muscles work on both the shoulder and forearm and primarily are antagonistic to each other. The triceps brachii works with the latissimus dorsi, teres major, and posterior deltoid to extend the shoulder during pulling motions such as rowing.

The long head of triceps brachii draws the raised or anteriorly extended arm posteriorly toward the body or into extension. It also pulls the shoulder toward and behind the body during motions like tucking in a shirt.

The strongest function of triceps brachii is extension of the forearm, which is accomplished by all fibers of the muscle. The anconeus muscle assists with this motion by pulling the synovial membrane of the elbow joint out of the way of the advancing olecranon process. This function of triceps brachii is utilized in pushing movements of the arm and shoulder.

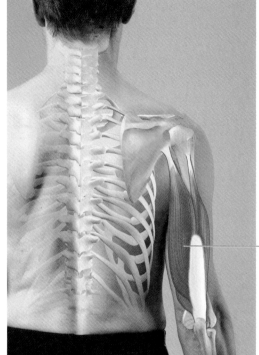

Triceps brachii muscle

4-56

Palpating Triceps Brachii

Positioning: client prone with arm at side and pronated.

1. Locate olecranon process.

2. Palpate superiorly along muscle belly with thumb and fingers toward the shoulder.

3. Locate the muscle belly in a pincer grasp where it becomes horseshoe-shaped as the three heads merge.

4. Follow the medial and lateral heads to their attachments on the humerus, and the long head until it continues under the deltoid and onto the scapula.

5. Client resists shoulder extension and elbow extension to ensure proper location.

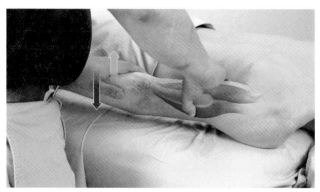

4-57

▶ SYNERGISTS/ANTAGONISTS: SCAPULA

Scapular Motion		Muscles Involved	Scapular Motion		Muscles Involved
Elevation		Trapezius (upper fibers) Levator scapula Rhomboids	Depression		Trapezius (lower fibers) Pectoralis minor Serratus anterior
Retraction		Trapezius (all fibers) Rhomboids Levator scapula	Protraction		Pectoralis minor Serratus anterior
Upward Rotation		Trapezius (all fibers) Serratus anterior	Downward Rotation		Levator scapula Pectoralis minor Rhomboids

▶ SYNERGISTS/ANTAGONISTS: SHOULDER

Shoulder Motion		Muscles Involved	Shoulder Motion		Muscles Involved
Flexion		Deltoid (anterior fibers) Pectoralis major (clavicular fibers) Coracobrachialis Biceps brachii	Extension		Deltoid (posterior fibers) Latissimus dorsi Teres major Pectoralis major sternal fibers) Triceps brachii (long head)
Abduction		Deltoid (all fibers) Supraspinatus Pectoralis major (overhead)	Adduction		Pectoralis major Latissimus dorsi Teres major Teres minor Coracobrachialis Biceps brachii (short head)
Internal Rotation		Deltoid (anterior fibers) Pectoralis major Latissimus dorsi Teres major Subscapularis	External Rotation		Deltoid (posterior fibers) Infraspinatus Teres minor
Horizontal Abduction	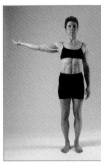	Deltoid (posterior fibers) Infraspinatus Latissimus dorsi Teres minor	Horizontal Adduction	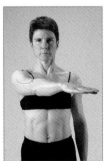	Pectoralis major Deltoid (anterior fibers)

▶ PUTTING IT IN MOTION

Muscles of the scapulothoracic and glenohumeral joints work together to perform common movements such as reaching, lifting, throwing, and pushing. As mentioned earlier, this co-ordinated action is called *scapulohumeral rhythm*. Smooth movement relies on proper timing of muscle contractions of multiple muscle groups. Some of these movements require moving body parts or objects through space while others involve moving the whole body against gravity. Concentric muscle contractions generate movement, whereas eccentric contractions serve to slow and control movements of the arm.

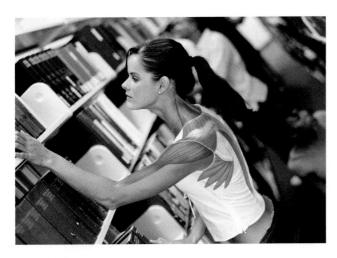

Reaching. Several muscles must work to pull the arm up over-head and lower objects against gravity. These include the muscles that stabilize the humeral head such as the supraspinatus, infra-spinatus, teres minor, subscapularis, and biceps brachii as well as prime movers such as the anterior deltoid, pectoralis major, and trapezius.

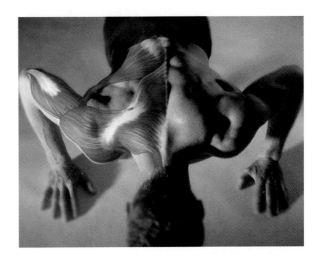

Lifting. The shoulder girdle and glenohumeral joint must work in concert with the core of the body and arm to lift objects from the ground. The rhomboids and trapezius retract the scapula while the deltoid, latissimus dorsi, teres major, and biceps brachii stabilize, abduct, and extend the humerus.

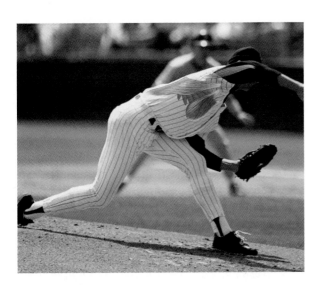

Throwing. One of the most complex motions of the upper body, throwing requires coordinated powerful muscle contractions along with deep stabilization of the glenohumeral joint. The rotator cuff muscles stabilize the humeral head while the powerful pectoralis major, latissimus dorsi, anterior deltoid, and triceps brachii pull the arm forward and across the body. Once the ball is released, the posterior deltoid, teres minor, infraspinatus, rhomboids, and trapezius must eccentrically contract to slow the motion of the arm. These agonist and antagonist muscles work together to make this motion fluid and effective.

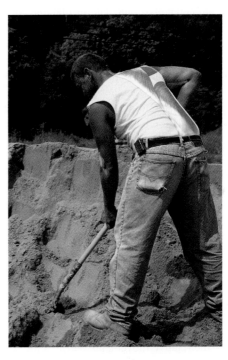

Push-Ups. Because the hands are planted on the ground, activities such as push-ups require fixation of the scapulae on the thorax while the glenohumeral joint moves through its range of motion. The trapezius, rhomboids, pectoralis minor, and serratus anterior anchor the scapula while the anterior deltoid and pectoralis major move the body up and down.

SUMMARY

- Six bones contribute to the shoulders. These include the paired clavicles, the scapulae, and the right and left humerus.
- The two main divisions of the shoulder are the shoulder girdle and the glenohumeral joint. The shoulder girdle is made up of the clavicle and scapula, which articulate at the acromioclavicular joint. The medial ends of the clavicles meet the manubrium of the sternum, a bone of the thorax. The glenohumeral joint is the articulation of the glenoid fossa of the scapula with the head of the humerus, the bone of the upper arm. This joint is also commonly called the shoulder joint.
- The scapulothoracic joint is not a true joint, as there is no bony articulation between the scapula and the thoracic cage. Instead, the scapula glides on thoracic musculature.
- Muscles that attach to the scapula enable several motions including elevation, depression, retraction, protraction, upward rotation, and downward rotation.
- The potential movements of the glenohumeral joint include flexion, extension, abduction, adduction, internal rotation, external rotation, horizontal abduction, and horizontal adduction.
- Passive ROM helps establish the health and function of inert structures, such as the glenohumeral joint capsule and the ligaments of the glenohumeral, acromioclavicular, and sternoclavicular joints. It also allows you to evaluate the relative movements between the scapulothoracic and glenohumeral joints.
- Resisted ROM helps establish the health and function of the dynamic stabilizers and prime movers of the scapulothoracic and glenohumeral joints. Evaluating functional strength and endurance helps you to identify balance and potential imbalance between the muscles that steer the scapula, stabilize the humeral head, and move the humerus.
- The deeper, smaller muscles in the shoulder region, such as the rotator cuff muscles, tend to stabilize the joints. The larger, more superficial muscles, such as the pectoralis major, create powerful movements.
- Coordinated movement of the muscles of the shoulder girdle and glenohumeral joint is called scapulohumeral rhythm.
- Muscles of the shoulder girdle and glenohumeral joint must work in harmony to create movements such as throwing, reaching, lifting, and pushing.

FOR REVIEW

Multiple Choice

1. The bones that make up the acromioclavicular joint are:
   A. the scapula and the sternum
   B. the scapula and the clavicle
   C. the clavicle and the sternum
   D. none of the above

2. The glenohumeral joint is a:
   A. hinge joint
   B. gliding joint
   C. immovable joint
   D. ball and socket joint

3. The scapulothoracic joint is a:
   A. ball and socket joint
   B. saddle joint
   C. hinge joint
   D. none of the above

4. The structure underneath the acromion that reduces friction between the acromion process and the humeral head is the:
   A. subacromial bursa
   B. joint capsule
   C. acromioclavicular ligament
   D. rotator cuff

5. The four muscles that make up the rotator cuff are:
   A. supraspinatus, infraspinatus, teres major, and subscapularis
   B. supraspinatus, infraspinatus, teres minor, and subscapularis
   C. subclavius, infraspinatus, teres minor and subscapularis
   D. subclavius, infraspinatus, teres major and subscapularis

6. All of these muscles move the scapula:
   A. pectoralis minor, levator scapula, and serratus anterior
   B. pectoralis major, latissimus dorsi, and teres major
   C. pectoralis minor, rhomboids, and teres minor
   D. subscapularis, serratus anterior, and rhomboids

7. Three muscles that extend the humerus are:
   A. coracobrachialis, biceps brachii, and latissimus dorsi
   B. biceps brachii, triceps brachii, and deltoid
   C. triceps brachii, deltoid, and latissimus dorsi
   D. latissimus dorsi, teres major, and supraspinatus

8. Three muscles that externally rotate the humerus are:
   A. latissimus dorsi, pectoralis major, and deltoid
   B. pectoralis major, teres major, and deltoid
   C. subscapularis, infraspinatus, and teres minor
   D. deltoid, infraspinatus, and teres minor

9. Three muscles that depress the scapula are:
   A. levator scapula, supraspinatus, and trapezius
   B. serratus anterior, pectoralis minor, and trapezius
   C. trapezius, latissimus dorsi, and teres major
   D. serratus anterior, pectoralis minor, and latissimus dorsi

10. Two muscles of the shoulder that cross two joints are:
    A. coracobrachialis and teres minor
    B. coracobrachialis and biceps brachii
    C. biceps brachii and triceps brachii
    D. triceps brachii and subscapularis

Matching

Different muscle attachments are listed below. Match the correct muscle with its attachment.

11. _____ Occiput, ligamentum nuchae, and spinous processes C7–T12

12. _____ Coracoid process of the scapula

13. _____ Lateral clavicle, acromion process, and spine of the scapula

14. _____ Greater tubercle of the humerus

15. _____ Costal surface of medial border of the scapula

16. _____ Lateral lip of the bicipital groove of the humerus

17. _____ Infraglenoid tubercle of the scapula

18. _____ Medial lip of the bicipital groove of the humerus

19. _____ Superior angle of the scapula

20. _____ Spinous processes of C7–T5

A. Serratus anterior

B. Infraspinatus

C. Trapezius

D. Rhomboids

E. Deltoid

F. Latissimus dorsi

G. Levator scapula

H. Pectoralis minor

I. Triceps brachii

J. Pectoralis major

Different muscle actions are listed below. Match the correct muscle with its action. Answers may be used more than once.

21. _____ Elevates the scapula

22. _____ Depresses the scapula

23. _____ Downwardly rotates the scapula

24. _____ Retracts the scapula

25. _____ Protracts the scapula

26. _____ Flexes the shoulder

27. _____ Extends the shoulder

28. _____ Abducts the shoulder

29. _____ Adducts the shoulder

30. _____ Horizontally abducts the shoulder

A. Coracobrachialis

B. Deltoid (posterior fibers)

C. Serratus anterior

D. Supraspinatus

E. Levator scapula

F. Rhomboids

G. Triceps brachii

H. Biceps brachii

I. Pectoralis minor

J. Trapezius (upper fibers)

Short Answer

31. Define scapulohumeral rhythm.

32. Describe the general structure of the sternoclavicular joint and compare it to that of the glenohumeral joint.

Try This!

Activity: Find a partner and have him or her perform one of the skills identified in the *Putting It in Motion* segment. Identify the specific actions of the shoulder that make up this skill. Write them down. Use the synergist list to identify which muscles work together to create this movement. Make sure you put the actions in the correct sequence. See if you can discover which muscles are stabilizing or steering the joint into position and which are responsible for powering the movement.

Suggestions: Switch partners and perform a different skill from *Putting It in Motion*. Repeat the steps above. Confirm your findings with the *Putting It in Motion* segment on the student CD included with your textbook. To further your understanding, practice this activity with skills not identified in *Putting It in Motion*.

SUGGESTED READINGS

Bernasconi SM, Tordi NR, Parratte BM, et al. Effects of two devices on the surface electromyography responses of eleven shoulder muscles during azarian in gymnastics. *J Strength Cond Res.* 2006;20(1):53–57.

Bongers PM. The cost of shoulder pain at work: variation in work tasks and good job opportunities are essential for prevention. *BMJ.* 2001;322(7278):64–65.

Brumitt J, Meira E. Scapula stabilization rehab exercise prescription. *J Strength Cond Res.* 2006;28(3):62–65.

Cogley RM, Archambault TA, Fiberger JF, et al. Comparison of muscle activation using various hand positions during the push-up exercise. *J Strength Cond Res.* 2005;19(3):628–633.

Davies GJ, Zillmer DA. Functional progression of a patient through a rehabilitation program. *Orthopaedic Physical Therapy Clinics of North America.* 2000;9:103–118.

Grezios AK, Gissis IT, Sotiropoulos AA, et al. Muscle-contraction properties in overarm throwing movements. *J Strength Cond Res.* 2006;20(1):117–123.

Jeran JJ, Chetlin RD. Training the shoulder complex in baseball pitchers: a sport-specific approach. *J Strength Cond Res.* 2005;27(4):14–31.

McMullen J, Uhl TL. A kinetic chain approach for shoulder rehabilitation. *J Athl Train.* 2000;35(3):329–337.

Myers JB, Pasquale MR, Laudner KG, et al. On-the-field resistance-tubing exercises for throwers: an electomyographic analysis. *J Athl Train.* 2005;40(1):15–22.

Ronai P. Exercise modifications and strategies to enhance shoulder function. *J Strength Cond Res.* 2005;27(4):36–45.

Terry GC, Chopp TM. Functional anatomy of the shoulder. *J Athl Train.* 2000;35(3):248–255.

Tyson A. Identifying and treating rotator cuff imbalances. *J Strength Cond Res.* 2006;28(2):92–95.

Tyson A. The importance of the posterior capsule of the shoulder in overhead athletes. *J Strength Cond Res.* 2005;27(4):60–62.

Tyson A. Rehab exercise prescription sequencing for shoulder external rotators. *J Strength Cond Res.* 2005;27(6):39–41.

Voight ML, Thomson BC. The role of the scapula in the rehabilitation of shoulder injuries. *J Athl Train.* 2000;35(3):364–372.

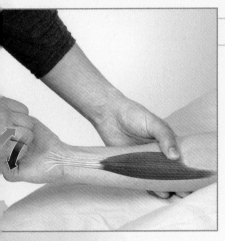

5

The Elbow, Forearm, Wrist, and Hand

Learning Objectives

After working through the material in this chapter, you should be able to:

- Identify the main structures of the elbow, forearm, wrist, and hand, including bones, joints, special structures, and deep and superficial muscles.
- Label and palpate the major surface landmarks of the elbow, forearm, wrist, and hand.
- Locate the attachments and nerve supply of the muscles of the elbow, forearm, wrist, and hand.
- Identify and demonstrate all actions of the muscles of the elbow, forearm, wrist, and hand.
- Demonstrate passive and resisted range of motion of the elbow, forearm, wrist, and hand.
- Draw, label, palpate, and fire the superficial and deep muscles of the elbow, forearm, wrist, and hand.
- Describe the unique functional anatomy and relationships between each muscle of the elbow, forearm, wrist, and hand.
- Identify both the synergists and the antagonists involved in each movement of the elbow, forearm, wrist, and hand (flexion, extension, etc.).
- Identify muscles used in performing four coordinated movements of the elbow, forearm, wrist, and hand: lifting, twisting, shooting, and grasping.

▶ OVERVIEW OF THE REGION

The elbow, forearm, wrist, and hand move in a variety of ways and serve many important functions. Some of these, such as grasping and lifting, are very powerful. Others, such as twisting and plucking, are more precise and even delicate. Many are complex, revealing the multifunctionality of the main joints of this region. For example, the elbow is capable of hinging as well as rotating. Two distinct joints at the elbow and one at the wrist work together to make this versatility possible. The wrist and hand are also multifunctional as a result of their multiple joints and many small muscles. Finally, joints from the elbow to the fingers work together to accomplish some of the tasks most characteristic of the human species—those of the human hand.

Long tendons connect muscle bellies in the elbow and forearm to bones in the wrist and hand. This pulley system requires a complex network of ligaments, connective tissue, and nerves to maintain optimal function, and blood and lymphatic vessels to keep the region nourished. Bursae and tendon sheaths reduce friction between the structures within the joints.

Given its structural complexity, you can readily appreciate why improper alignment and use patterns could easily disrupt this region's function. An understanding of the information in this chapter will help you promote healthy functioning for yourself and your clients.

▶ SURFACE ANATOMY OF THE ELBOW, FOREARM, WRIST, AND HAND

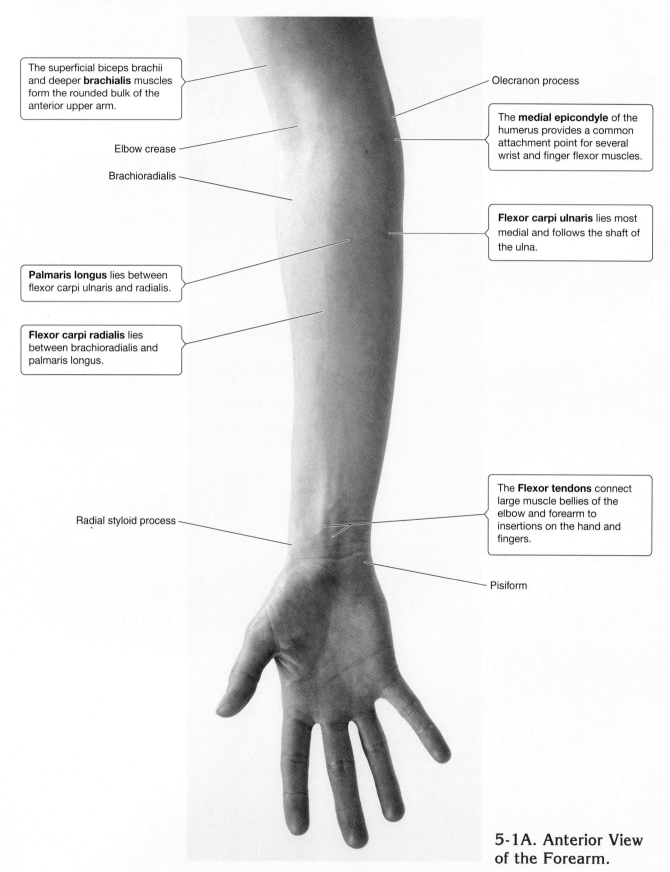

The superficial biceps brachii and deeper **brachialis** muscles form the rounded bulk of the anterior upper arm.

Elbow crease

Brachioradialis

Palmaris longus lies between flexor carpi ulnaris and radialis.

Flexor carpi radialis lies between brachioradialis and palmaris longus.

Radial styloid process

Olecranon process

The **medial epicondyle** of the humerus provides a common attachment point for several wrist and finger flexor muscles.

Flexor carpi ulnaris lies most medial and follows the shaft of the ulna.

The **Flexor tendons** connect large muscle bellies of the elbow and forearm to insertions on the hand and fingers.

Pisiform

5-1A. Anterior View of the Forearm.

▶ SURFACE ANATOMY OF THE ELBOW, FOREARM, WRIST, AND HAND

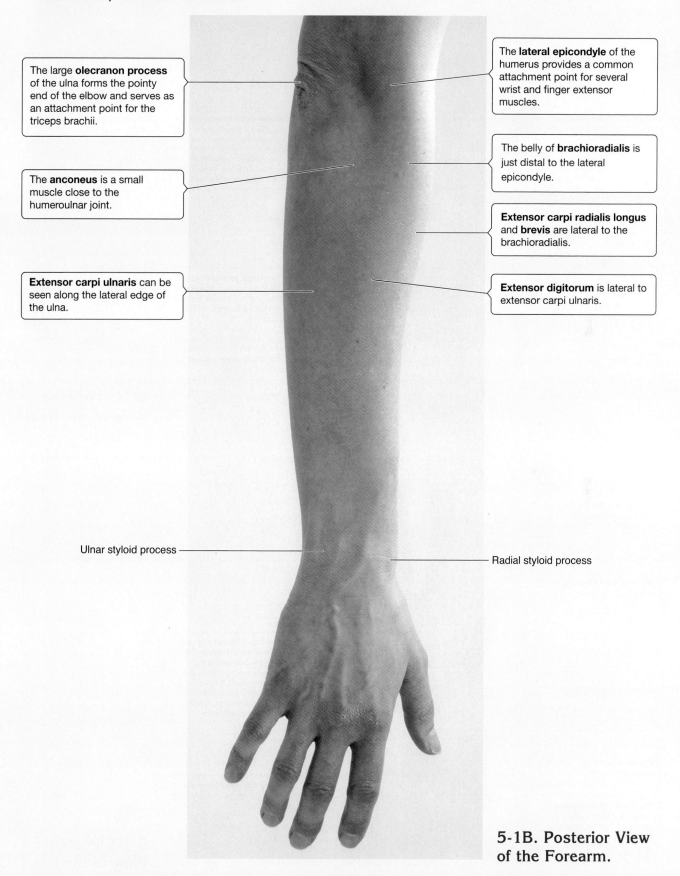

The large **olecranon process** of the ulna forms the pointy end of the elbow and serves as an attachment point for the triceps brachii.

The **anconeus** is a small muscle close to the humeroulnar joint.

Extensor carpi ulnaris can be seen along the lateral edge of the ulna.

The **lateral epicondyle** of the humerus provides a common attachment point for several wrist and finger extensor muscles.

The belly of **brachioradialis** is just distal to the lateral epicondyle.

Extensor carpi radialis longus and **brevis** are lateral to the brachioradialis.

Extensor digitorum is lateral to extensor carpi ulnaris.

Ulnar styloid process

Radial styloid process

5-1B. Posterior View of the Forearm.

▶ SURFACE ANATOMY OF THE ELBOW, FOREARM, WRIST, AND HAND

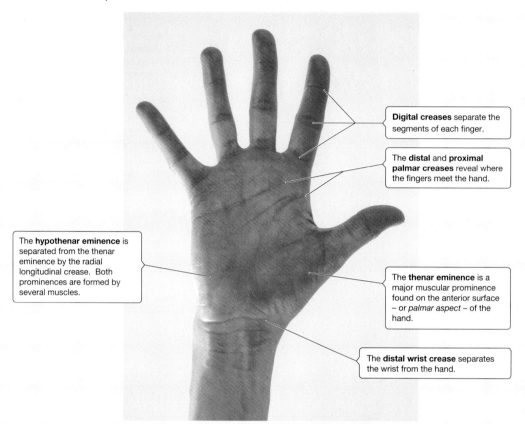

Digital creases separate the segments of each finger.

The **distal** and **proximal palmar creases** reveal where the fingers meet the hand.

The **hypothenar eminence** is separated from the thenar eminence by the radial longitudinal crease. Both prominences are formed by several muscles.

The **thenar eminence** is a major muscular prominence found on the anterior surface – or *palmar aspect* – of the hand.

The **distal wrist crease** separates the wrist from the hand.

5-1C. Anterior View of the Hand.

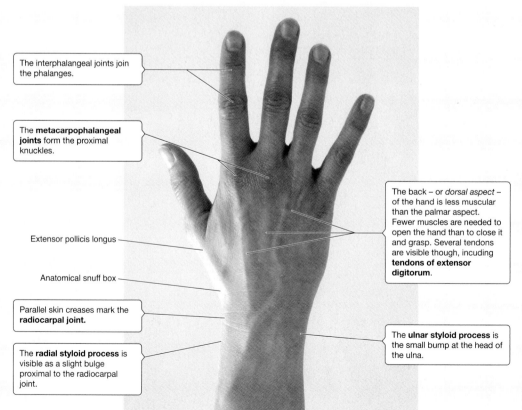

The interphalangeal joints join the phalanges.

The **metacarpophalangeal joints** form the proximal knuckles.

Extensor pollicis longus

Anatomical snuff box

Parallel skin creases mark the **radiocarpal joint.**

The **radial styloid process** is visible as a slight bulge proximal to the radiocarpal joint.

The back – or *dorsal aspect* – of the hand is less muscular than the palmar aspect. Fewer muscles are needed to open the hand than to close it and grasp. Several tendons are visible though, incuding **tendons of extensor digitorum**.

The **ulnar styloid process** is the small bump at the head of the ulna.

5-1D. Posterior View of the Hand.

SKELETAL STRUCTURES OF THE ELBOW, FOREARM, WRIST, AND HAND

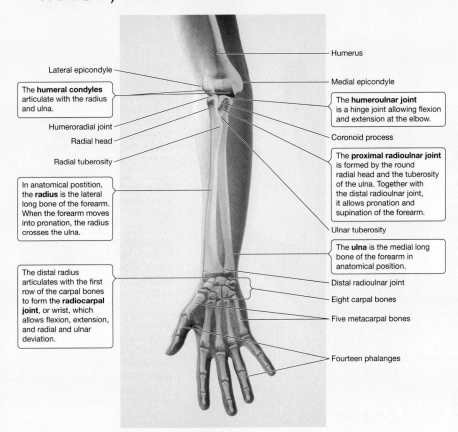

Lateral epicondyle

The **humeral condyles** articulate with the radius and ulna.

Humeroradial joint

Radial head

Radial tuberosity

In anatomical postition, the **radius** is the lateral long bone of the forearm. When the forearm moves into pronation, the radius crosses the ulna.

The distal radius articulates with the first row of the carpal bones to form the **radiocarpal joint**, or wrist, which allows flexion, extension, and radial and ulnar deviation.

Humerus

Medial epicondyle

The **humeroulnar joint** is a hinge joint allowing flexion and extension at the elbow.

Coronoid process

The **proximal radioulnar joint** is formed by the round radial head and the tuberosity of the ulna. Together with the distal radioulnar joint, it allows pronation and supination of the forearm.

Ulnar tuberosity

The **ulna** is the medial long bone of the forearm in anatomical position.

Distal radioulnar joint

Eight carpal bones

Five metacarpal bones

Fourteen phalanges

5-2A. Skeletal Structures of Forearm: Anterior View.

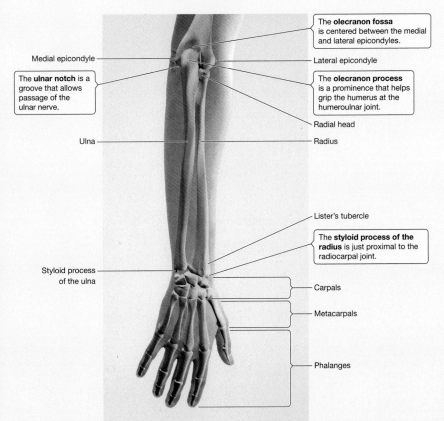

The **olecranon fossa** is centered between the medial and lateral epicondyles.

Medial epicondyle

The **ulnar notch** is a groove that allows passage of the ulnar nerve.

Ulna

Styloid process of the ulna

Lateral epicondyle

The **olecranon process** is a prominence that helps grip the humerus at the humeroulnar joint.

Radial head

Radius

Lister's tubercle

The **styloid process of the radius** is just proximal to the radiocarpal joint.

Carpals

Metacarpals

Phalanges

5-2B. Skeletal Structures of Forearm: Posterior View.

▶ SKELETAL STRUCTURES OF THE ELBOW, FOREARM, WRIST, AND HAND

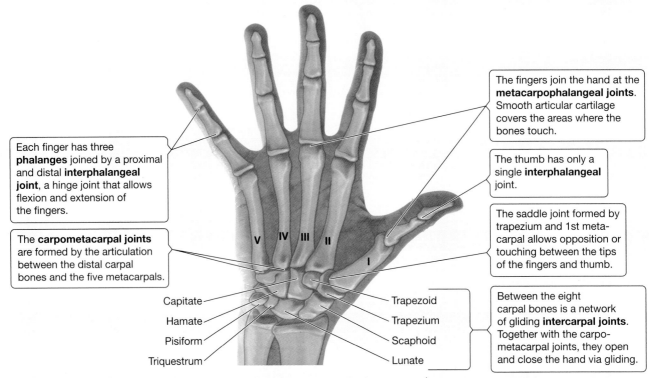

The fingers join the hand at the **metacarpophalangeal joints**. Smooth articular cartilage covers the areas where the bones touch.

Each finger has three **phalanges** joined by a proximal and distal **interphalangeal joint**, a hinge joint that allows flexion and extension of the fingers.

The thumb has only a single **interphalangeal** joint.

The saddle joint formed by trapezium and 1st metacarpal allows opposition or touching between the tips of the fingers and thumb.

The **carpometacarpal joints** are formed by the articulation between the distal carpal bones and the five metacarpals.

Capitate

Hamate

Pisiform

Triquestrum

Trapezoid

Trapezium

Scaphoid

Lunate

Between the eight carpal bones is a network of gliding **intercarpal joints**. Together with the carpometacarpal joints, they open and close the hand via gliding.

5-2C. Skeletal Structures of Hand: Anterior View.

▶ BONY LANDMARKS OF THE ELBOW, FOREARM, WRIST AND HAND

Palpating the Olecranon Process

Positioning: client supine with elbow flexed and forearm neutral.

1. Locate the posterior surface of the elbow.
2. Passively flex and extend the elbow while you palpate the rounded point of the olecranon process.

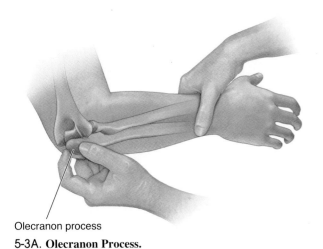

Olecranon process

5-3A. **Olecranon Process.**

Palpating the Lateral Epicondyle

Positioning: client supine with elbow flexed.

1. Locate the olecranon process of the ulna.
2. Slide fingers laterally and anteriorly onto the large, rounded bump of the lateral epicondyle.

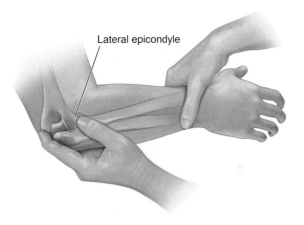

Lateral epicondyle

5-3C. **Lateral Epicondyle.**

Palpating the Olecranon Fossa

Positioning: client supine with elbow flexed.

1. Locate the olecranon process of the ulna.
2. Slide your fingers superiorly and deep into the depression that is the olecranon fossa.

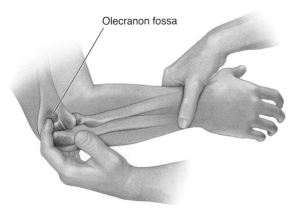

Olecranon fossa

5-3B. **Olecranon Fossa.**

Palpating the Medial Epicondyle

Positioning: client supine with elbow flexed and forearm supinated.

1. Locate the olecranon process of the ulna.
2. Slide fingers medially and anteriorly onto the large, rounded bump of the medial epicondyle.

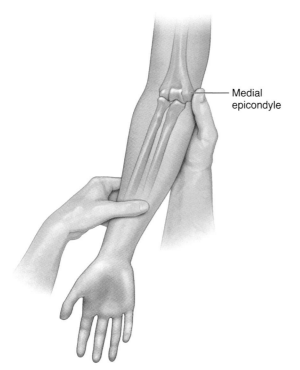

5-3D. **Medial Epicondyle**.

Palpating the Radial Head

Positioning: client supine with elbow bent and forearm neutral.

1. Locate the lateral epicondyle of the humerus.
2. Slide fingers distally onto the smaller radial head while passively pronating and supinating the forearm, making it pivot under your fingers.

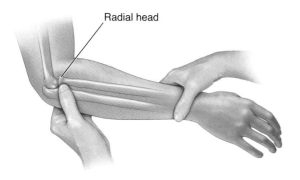

5-3E. **Radial Head.**

Palpating the Ulnar Ridge

Positioning: client supine with elbow flexed and forearm neutral.

1. Locate the olecranon process of the ulna.
2. Slide fingers distally following the sharp edge of the ulnar ridge toward the wrist.

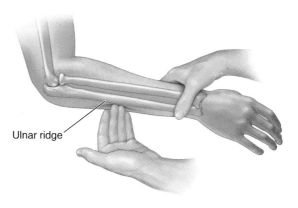

5-3F. **Ulnar Shaft.**

Palpating the Ulnar Styloid Process

Positioning: client supine with elbow relaxed and forearm pronated.

1. Locate the lateral edge of the wrist.
2. Slide fingers anteriorly onto the prominent bump of the ulnar styloid process.

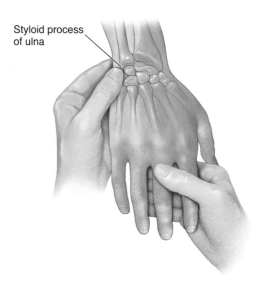

5-3G. **Ulnar Styloid Process.**

Palpating Lister's Tubercle

Positioning: client supine with elbow relaxed and forearm pronated.

1. Locate the ulnar styloid process.
2. Slide fingers medially onto the deeper, smaller bump formed by Lister's tubercle.

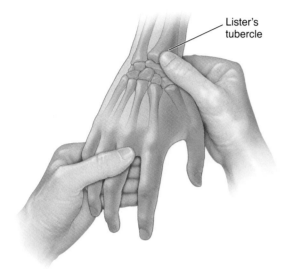

5-3H. **Lister's Tubercle.**

Palpating the Radial Styloid Process

Positioning: client supine with elbow relaxed and forearm pronated.

1. Locate Lister's tubercle of the radius.
2. Slide fingers medially and distally onto the rounded prominence of the radial styloid process.

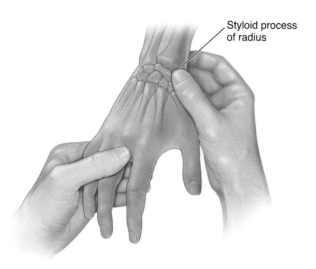

5-3I. **Radial Styloid Process.**

Dorsal Palpation of the Carpals

Positioning: client supine with elbow relaxed and forearm pronated.

1. Using the thumbs of both hands, locate the radial and ulnar styloid processes.
2. Slide thumbs distally onto the dorsal surfaces of the carpal bones.

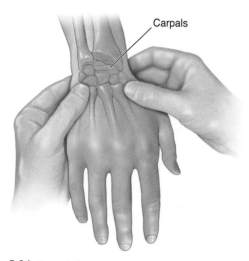

5-3J. **Dorsal Carpals.**

Palpating the Scaphoid

Positioning: client supine with elbow relaxed and forearm pronated.

1. Using the thumb of one hand, locate the radial styloid process.
2. Passively ulnar deviate the wrist and slide thumb distally and deep onto the flat surface of the scaphoid.

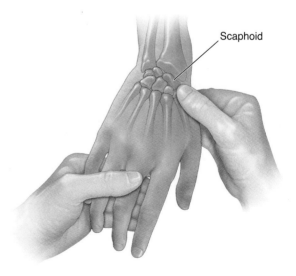

5-3K. **Scaphoid.**

Palpating the Metacarpals

Positioning: client supine with elbow relaxed and forearm pronated.

1. Using the thumbs of both hands locate the knuckles.
2. Slide thumbs proximally along the long, slender shafts of the metacarpals.

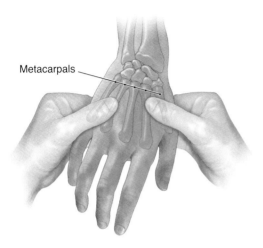

Metacarpals

5-3L. **Metacarpals.**

Palmar Palpation of the Carpals

Positioning: client supine with elbow relaxed and forearm supinated.

1. Using the thumbs of both hands, locate the thenar and hypothenar eminence of the palm.
2. Palpate deeply under and between these two soft structures onto the palmar surfaces of the carpals.

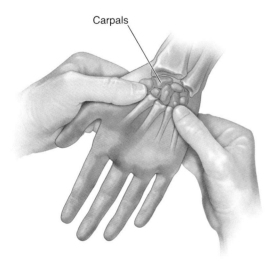

Carpals

5-3M. **Palmar Carpals.**

Palpating the Pisiform

Positioning: client supine with elbow relaxed and forearm supinated.

1. With the thumb of one hand locate the hypothenar eminence.
2. Slide thumb proximally onto the small bump of the pisiform.

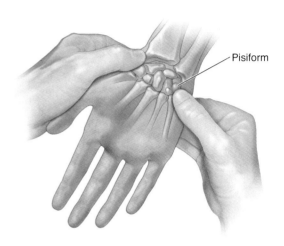

Pisiform

5-3N. **Pisiform.**

Palpating the Hook of the Hamate

Positioning: client supine with elbow relaxed and forearm supinated.

1. With the thumb of one hand locate the pisiform.
2. Slide thumb slightly medial, distal, and deep onto the small hook of the hamate.

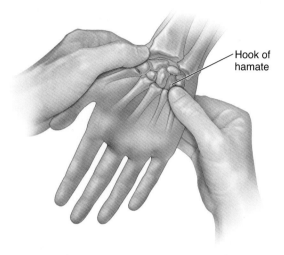

Hook of hamate

5-3O. **Hook of the Hamate.**

Palpating the Phalanges

Positioning: client supine with elbow relaxed and forearm supinated.

1. Using a pincer, grasp with both hands locate the knuckles.
2. Slide grasp distally onto the fingers palpating the phalanges, proximal interphalangeal joints and distal interphalangeal joints.

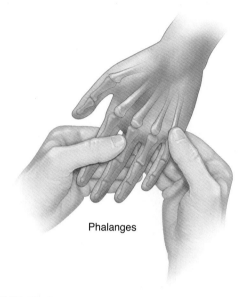

Phalanges

5-3P. **Phalanges.**

▶ MUSCLE ATTACHMENT SITES

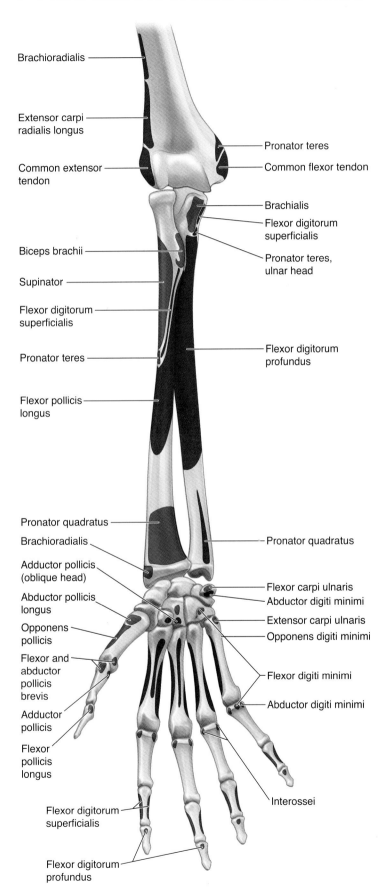

Brachioradialis

Extensor carpi radialis longus

Common extensor tendon

Biceps brachii

Supinator

Flexor digitorum superficialis

Pronator teres

Flexor pollicis longus

Pronator quadratus

Brachioradialis

Adductor pollicis (oblique head)

Abductor pollicis longus

Opponens pollicis

Flexor and abductor pollicis brevis

Adductor pollicis

Flexor pollicis longus

Flexor digitorum superficialis

Flexor digitorum profundus

Pronator teres

Common flexor tendon

Brachialis

Flexor digitorum superficialis

Pronator teres, ulnar head

Flexor digitorum profundus

Pronator quadratus

Flexor carpi ulnaris

Abductor digiti minimi

Extensor carpi ulnaris

Opponens digiti minimi

Flexor digiti minimi

Abductor digiti minimi

Interossei

5-4A. Arm muscle attachments: anterior view. Primarily, muscles of the elbow, forearm, wrist, and hand originate (marked in red) on the humerus and proximal portions of the radius and ulna. Most insert (marked in blue) distally on the carpals, metacarpals, and phalanges. Muscles usually bring their more mobile, distal insertions toward their more stable, proximal origins as they shorten.

MUSCLE ATTACHMENT SITES

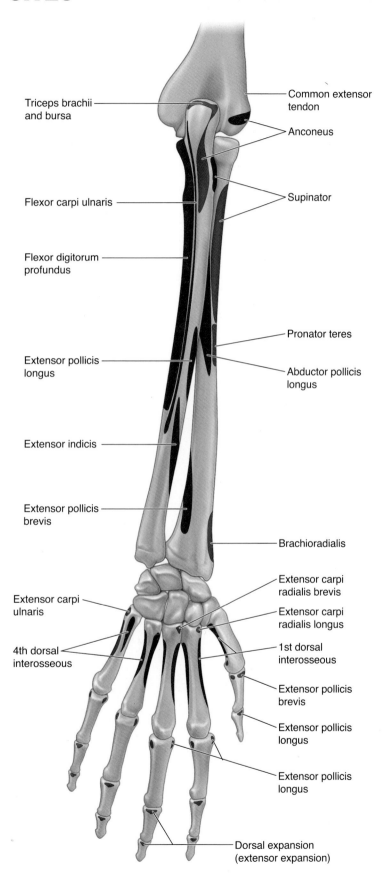

Triceps brachii and bursa

Common extensor tendon

Anconeus

Flexor carpi ulnaris

Supinator

Flexor digitorum profundus

Pronator teres

Extensor pollicis longus

Abductor pollicis longus

Extensor indicis

Extensor pollicis brevis

Brachioradialis

Extensor carpi ulnaris

Extensor carpi radialis brevis

Extensor carpi radialis longus

4th dorsal interosseous

1st dorsal interosseous

Extensor pollicis brevis

Extensor pollicis longus

Extensor pollicis longus

Dorsal expansion (extensor expansion)

5-4B. Arm muscle attachments: posterior view.

▌ LIGAMENTS OF THE ELBOW, FOREARM, WRIST, AND HAND

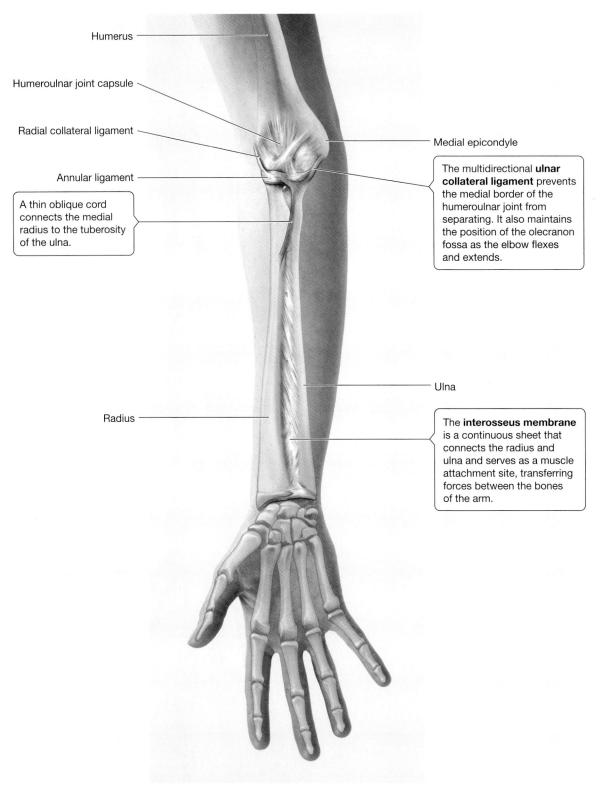

Humerus

Humeroulnar joint capsule

Radial collateral ligament

Annular ligament

A thin oblique cord connects the medial radius to the tuberosity of the ulna.

Medial epicondyle

The multidirectional **ulnar collateral ligament** prevents the medial border of the humeroulnar joint from separating. It also maintains the position of the olecranon fossa as the elbow flexes and extends.

Ulna

Radius

The **interosseus membrane** is a continuous sheet that connects the radius and ulna and serves as a muscle attachment site, transferring forces between the bones of the arm.

5-5A. Elbow ligaments: anterior view.

▶ LIGAMENTS OF THE ELBOW, FOREARM, WRIST, AND HAND

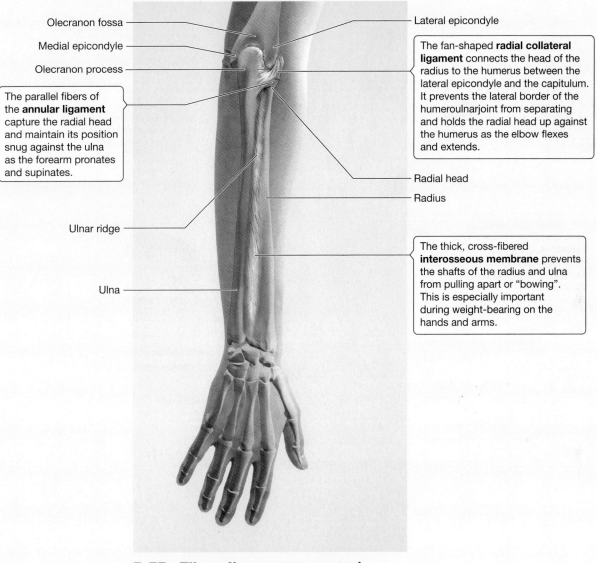

Olecranon fossa

Medial epicondyle

Olecranon process

The parallel fibers of the **annular ligament** capture the radial head and maintain its position snug against the ulna as the forearm pronates and supinates.

Ulnar ridge

Ulna

Lateral epicondyle

The fan-shaped **radial collateral ligament** connects the head of the radius to the humerus between the lateral epicondyle and the capitulum. It prevents the lateral border of the humeroulnarjoint from separating and holds the radial head up against the humerus as the elbow flexes and extends.

Radial head

Radius

The thick, cross-fibered **interosseous membrane** prevents the shafts of the radius and ulna from pulling apart or "bowing". This is especially important during weight-bearing on the hands and arms.

5-5B. Elbow ligaments: posterior view.

▶ LIGAMENTS OF THE ELBOW, FOREARM, WRIST, AND HAND

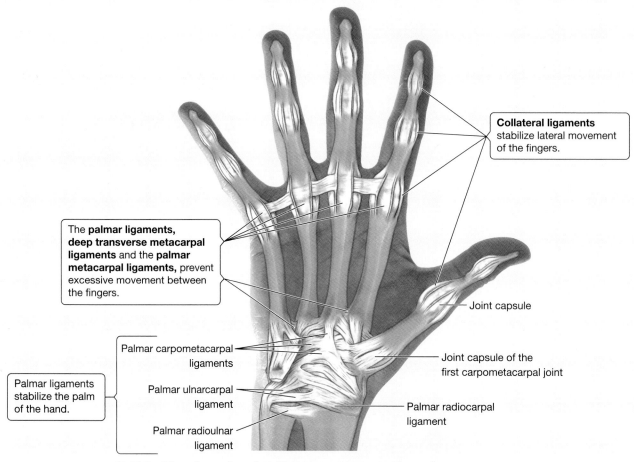

Collateral ligaments stabilize lateral movement of the fingers.

The **palmar ligaments, deep transverse metacarpal ligaments** and the **palmar metacarpal ligaments,** prevent excessive movement between the fingers.

Joint capsule

Palmar ligaments stabilize the palm of the hand.

Palmar carpometacarpal ligaments

Palmar ulnarcarpal ligament

Palmar radioulnar ligament

Joint capsule of the first carpometacarpal joint

Palmar radiocarpal ligament

5-5C. Hand and wrist ligaments: anterior view.

▶ SUPERFICIAL MUSCLES OF THE ELBOW, FOREARM, WRIST, AND HAND

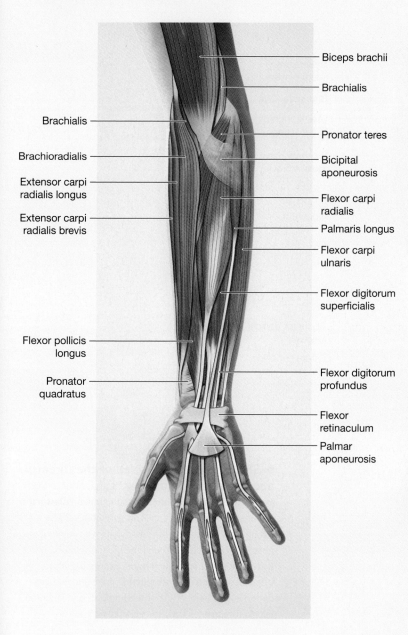

Biceps brachii

Brachialis

Pronator teres

Bicipital aponeurosis

Flexor carpi radialis

Palmaris longus

Flexor carpi ulnaris

Flexor digitorum superficialis

Flexor digitorum profundus

Flexor retinaculum

Palmar aponeurosis

Brachialis

Brachioradialis

Extensor carpi radialis longus

Extensor carpi radialis brevis

Flexor pollicis longus

Pronator quadratus

5-6A. Superficial muscles of the forearm and hand: anterior view. These large muscles have thick bellies near the elbow and taper to tendons in the wrist and hand. **Brachioradialis** and the wrist extensors lie laterally. **Pronator teres** lies superiorly, deep to the insertion of **biceps brachii. Flexor carpi radialis, palmaris longus, and flexor carpi ulnaris** span the medial forearm. Both the **bicipital aponeurosis** and the **palmar aponeurosis** are superficial on the anterior arm, as is the anchoring connective tissue of the **flexor retinaculum**. Superficial muscles tend to be stronger and more complex in their actions than their deeper counterparts (pronator quadratus and flexor digitorum profundus, shown in Figure 5-7A).

▶ SUPERFICIAL MUSCLES OF THE ELBOW, FOREARM, WRIST, AND HAND

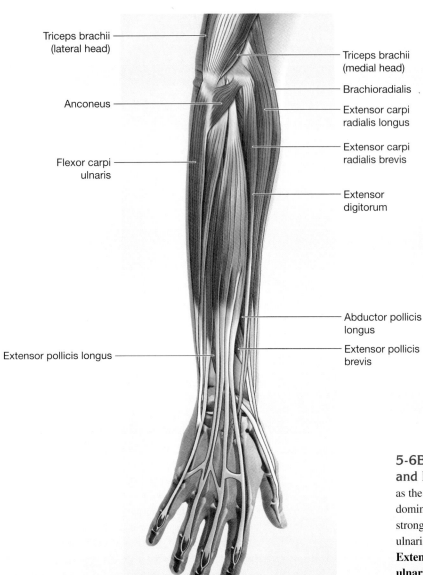

Triceps brachii (lateral head)

Anconeus

Flexor carpi ulnaris

Extensor pollicis longus

Triceps brachii (medial head)

Brachioradialis

Extensor carpi radialis longus

Extensor carpi radialis brevis

Extensor digitorum

Abductor pollicis longus

Extensor pollicis brevis

5-6B. Superficial muscles of the forearm and hand: posterior view. Large muscles such as the **extensor carpi ulnaris** and **extensor digitorum** dominate the posterior forearm. **Anconeus** shares a strong attachement on the ulnar shaft with flexor carpi ulnaris, which wraps around the medial forearm. **Extensor carpi radialis longus, extensor carpi ulnaris,** and **extensor digitorum** share attachments on the lateral epicondyle of the humerus and span the lateral forearm.

▶ DEEP MUSCLES OF THE ELBOW, FOREARM, WRIST, AND HAND

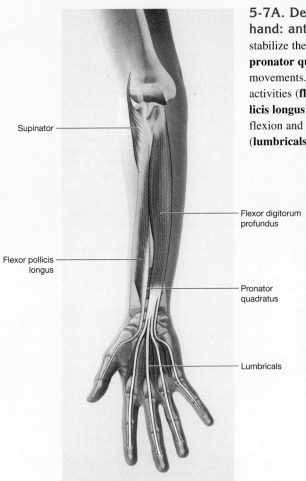

5-7A. Deep muscles of the forearm and hand: anterior view. Deep muscles of this region stabilize the elbow and forearm (**supinator** and **pronator quadratus**). They also create more subtle movements. Deep muscles in the hand control grasping activities (**flexor digitorum profundus** and **flexor pollicis longus**) and fine finger movements like segmented flexion and opening and closing of the hand (**lumbricals**).

Supinator

Flexor digitorum profundus

Flexor pollicis longus

Pronator quadratus

Lumbricals

Anconeus

Supinator

Abductor pollicis brevis

Extensor pollicis brevis

Extensor pollicis longus

Extensor indicis

5-7B. Deep muscles of the forearm and hand: posterior view. The deep muscles of the posterior arm and hand wrap around the forearm and stabilize rotation (**supinator** and **anconeus**). Several deep muscles move the thumb (**abductor pollicis longus, extensor pollicis brevis** and **longus**) and index finger (**extensor indicis**).

▶ SPECIAL STRUCTURES OF THE ELBOW, FOREARM, WRIST, AND HAND

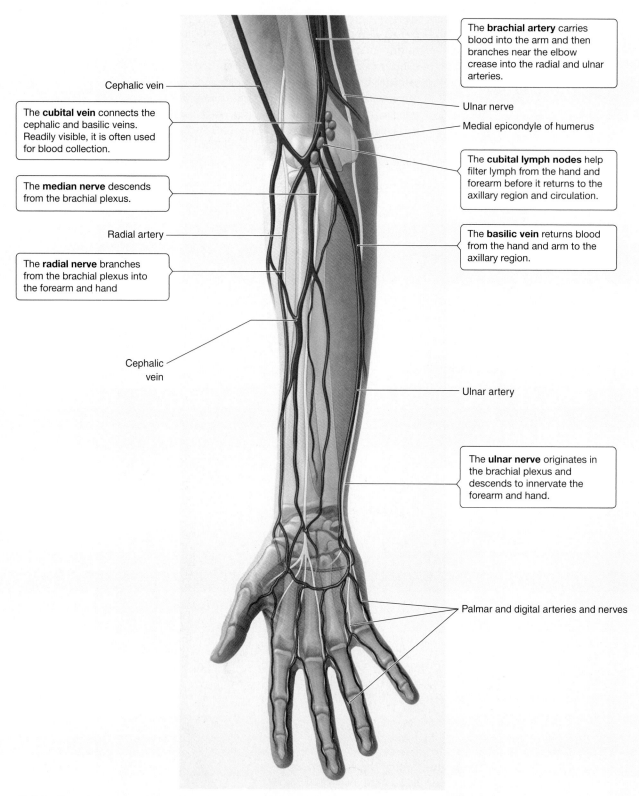

Cephalic vein

The **brachial artery** carries blood into the arm and then branches near the elbow crease into the radial and ulnar arteries.

Ulnar nerve

Medial epicondyle of humerus

The **cubital vein** connects the cephalic and basilic veins. Readily visible, it is often used for blood collection.

The **cubital lymph nodes** help filter lymph from the hand and forearm before it returns to the axillary region and circulation.

The **median nerve** descends from the brachial plexus.

Radial artery

The **basilic vein** returns blood from the hand and arm to the axillary region.

The **radial nerve** branches from the brachial plexus into the forearm and hand

Cephalic vein

Ulnar artery

The **ulnar nerve** originates in the brachial plexus and descends to innervate the forearm and hand.

Palmar and digital arteries and nerves

5-8A. Special structures of the elbow, forearm, wrist, and hand. A. Lymph nodes, nerves, and blood vessels of the forearm and hand: anterior view. *(continued)*

▶ SPECIAL STRUCTURES OF THE ELBOW, FOREARM, WRIST, AND HAND

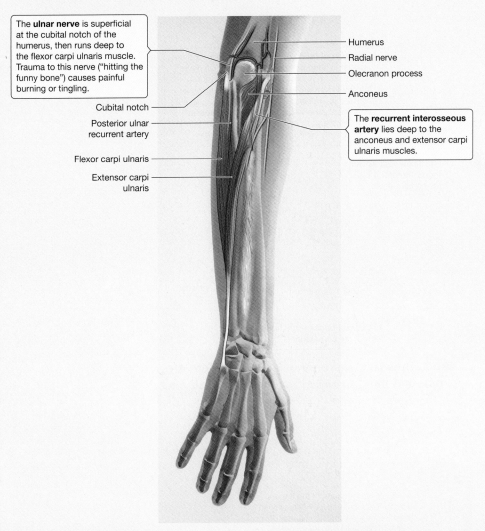

The **ulnar nerve** is superficial at the cubital notch of the humerus, then runs deep to the flexor carpi ulnaris muscle. Trauma to this nerve ("hitting the funny bone") causes painful burning or tingling.

Cubital notch

Posterior ulnar
recurrent artery

Flexor carpi ulnaris

Extensor carpi
ulnaris

Humerus
Radial nerve
Olecranon process
Anconeus

The **recurrent interosseous artery** lies deep to the anconeus and extensor carpi ulnaris muscles.

5-8B. Special structures of the elbow, forearm, wrist, and hand. *(continued)*
B. Special structures of the elbow: posterior view.

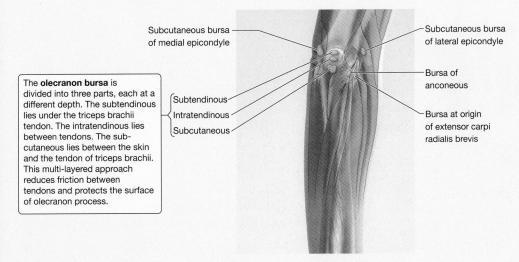

Subcutaneous bursa
of medial epicondyle

Subcutaneous bursa
of lateral epicondyle

Bursa of
anconeous

Bursa at origin
of extensor carpi
radialis brevis

Subtendinous
Intratendinous
Subcutaneous

The **olecranon bursa** is divided into three parts, each at a different depth. The subtendinous lies under the triceps brachii tendon. The intratendinous lies between tendons. The subcutaneous lies between the skin and the tendon of triceps brachii. This multi-layered approach reduces friction between tendons and protects the surface of olecranon process.

5-8C. Special structures of the elbow, forearm, wrist, and hand. *(continued)*
C. Bursae of the elbow: posterior view. *(continued)*

SPECIAL STRUCTURES OF THE ELBOW, FOREARM, WRIST, AND HAND

Palmar side of hand

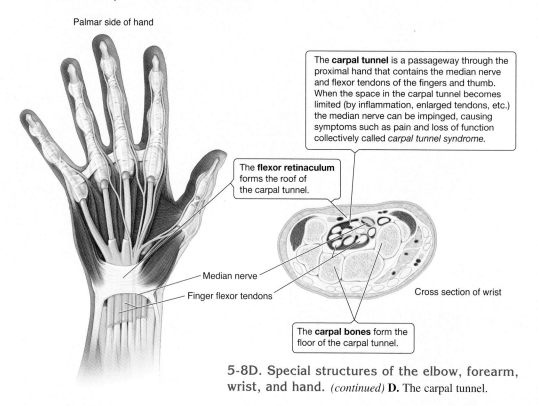

The **carpal tunnel** is a passageway through the proximal hand that contains the median nerve and flexor tendons of the fingers and thumb. When the space in the carpal tunnel becomes limited (by inflammation, enlarged tendons, etc.) the median nerve can be impinged, causing symptoms such as pain and loss of function collectively called *carpal tunnel syndrome.*

The **flexor retinaculum** forms the roof of the carpal tunnel.

Median nerve

Finger flexor tendons

Cross section of wrist

The **carpal bones** form the floor of the carpal tunnel.

5-8D. Special structures of the elbow, forearm, wrist, and hand. *(continued)* **D.** The carpal tunnel.

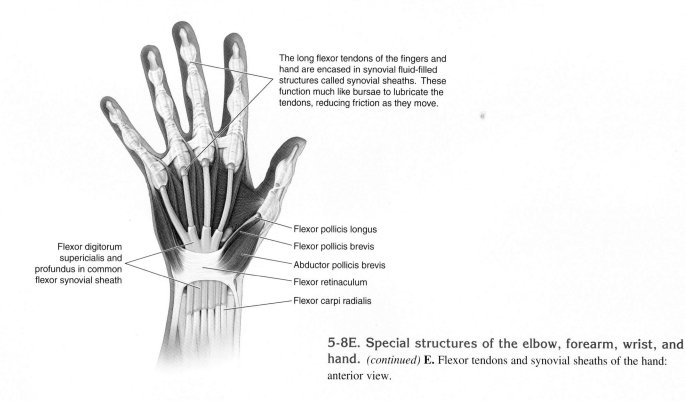

The long flexor tendons of the fingers and hand are encased in synovial fluid-filled structures called synovial sheaths. These function much like bursae to lubricate the tendons, reducing friction as they move.

Flexor digitorum superficialis and profundus in common flexor synovial sheath

Flexor pollicis longus

Flexor pollicis brevis

Abductor pollicis brevis

Flexor retinaculum

Flexor carpi radialis

5-8E. Special structures of the elbow, forearm, wrist, and hand. *(continued)* **E.** Flexor tendons and synovial sheaths of the hand: anterior view.

MOVEMENTS AVAILABLE: ELBOW AND WRIST

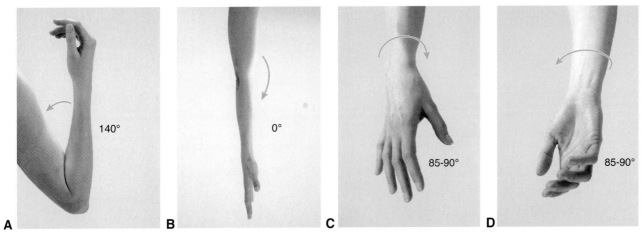

5-9 A. Elbow flexion, B. Elbow extension, C. Supination, D. Pronation

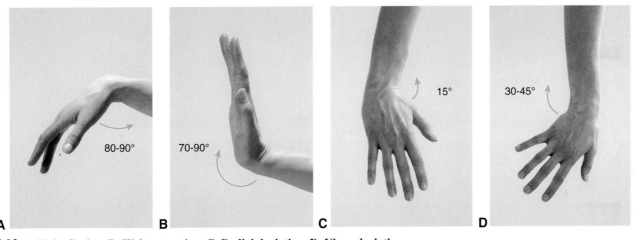

5-10 A. Wrist flexion, B. Wrist extension, C. Radial deviation, D. Ulnar deviation

◗ MOVEMENTS AVAILABLE: HAND

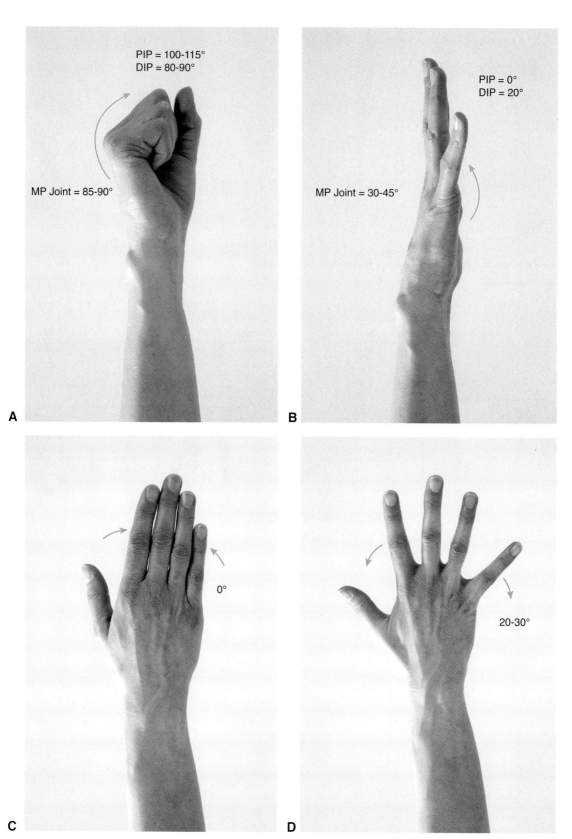

5-11 A. Finger flexion, B. Finger extension, C. Finger adduction, D. Finger abduction

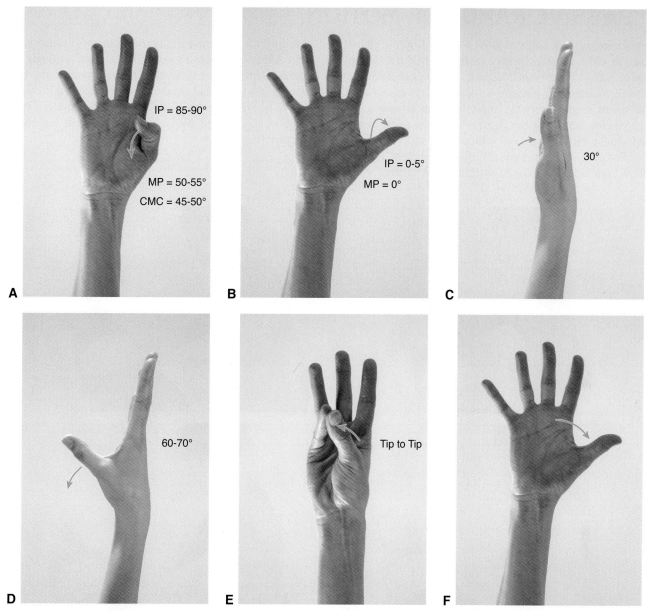

5-12 Movements available: thumb. A. Thumb flexion, B. Thumb extension, C. Thumb adduction, D. Thumb abduction, E. Thumb opposition, F. Thumb reposition

▶ PASSIVE RANGE OF MOTION

Performing passive range of motion (PROM) in the elbow, forearm, wrist, and hand helps establish the health and function of inert structures such as joint capsules and ligaments as well as length of antagonist (opposite) muscle groups. The client should be lying comfortably on a massage or examination table. Ask the client to relax and allow you to perform the PROM exercises without "helping."

For each of the movements illustrated below, take the elbow, forearm, wrist, or hand through to endfeel while watching for compensation (extraneous movement) in the other joints or regions. Some motions, such as finger and thumb adduction, are limited by approximation (the body running into itself) and are therefore not included in evaluation of passive range of motion. Information about passive range of motion and endfeel can be found at the end of Chapter 3.

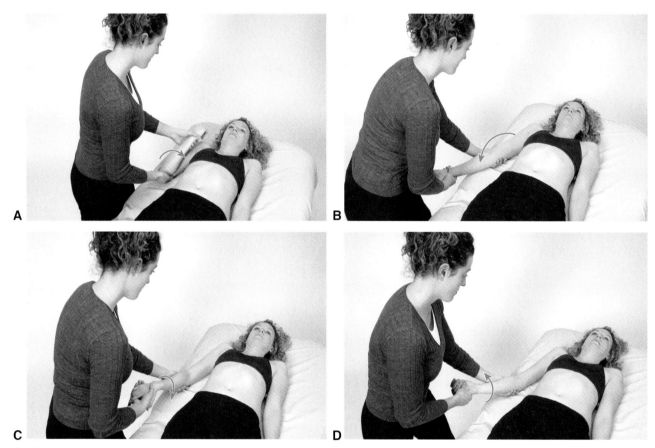

A   B

C   D

5-13 A. Passive elbow flexion. The blue arrow indicates the direction of movement. Stand at the side of the table and face the client's body. Hold the client's wrist with one hand and grasp the elbow with the other hand to stabilize the limb. Supinate the forearm while keeping the elbow extended. Then bend the elbow to move the client's forearm from the side of the body toward the upper arm. Assess the ROM of the joint capsule as well as the muscles that extend the elbow. B. Passive elbow extension. Stand at the client's side and support the wrist and elbow in the same way as for passive elbow flexion. With the client's forearm supinated and starting with the elbow flexed, bring the arm back down to the client's side straightening the elbow as far as is comfortable. Assess the ROM of the joint capsule as well as the muscles that flex the elbow. C. Passive forearm pronation. Stand at the client's side. Hold the client's wrist with one hand and grasp the elbow with the other hand to stabilize the limb. Start with forearm supinated or in palm-up position then gently rotate the client's arm into palm-down position as far as is comfortable. Assess the ROM of the joint capsule as well as the muscles that supinate the forearm. D. Passive forearm supination. Stand at the client's side. Hold the client's wrist with one hand and grasp the elbow with the other hand to stabilize the limb. Start with the client's forearm pronated in palm-down position then gently rotate the arm into palm-up position as far as is comfortable. Assess the ROM of the joint capsule as well as the muscles that pronate the forearm.

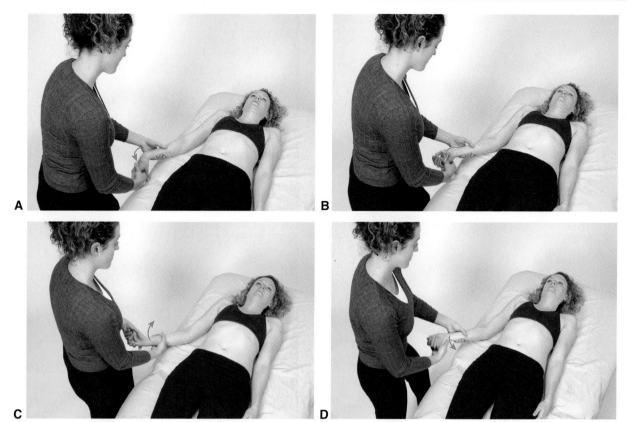

5-14 A. **Passive wrist flexion.** Stand at the client's side. Hold the client's hand with one hand and grasp the forearm with the other hand to stabilize the limb. Start with the client's forearm pronated and gently bend the wrist and move the hand toward the floor as far as is comfortable. Assess the ROM of the joint capsule as well as the muscles that extend the wrist. **B. Passive wrist extension.** Stand at the client's side. Hold the client's hand with one hand and grasp the forearm with the other hand to stabilize the limb. Start with the client's forearm supinated and gently bend the wrist and move the hand toward the floor as far as is comfortable. Assess the ROM of the joint capsule as well as the muscles that flex the wrist. **C. Passive radial deviation.** Stand at the client's side. Hold the client's hand with one hand and grasp the forearm with the other hand to stabilize the limb. Start with the client's forearm supinated, then gently bend the wrist and move the hand laterally as far as is comfortable. Assess the ROM of the joint capsule as well as the muscles that ular deviate the wrist. **D. Passive ulnar deviation.** Stand at the client's side. Hold the client's hand with one hand and grasp the forearm with the other hand to stabilize the limb. Start with the client's forearm supinated, then gently bend the wrist and move the hand medially as far as is comfortable. Assess the ROM of the joint capsule as well as the muscles that radially deviate the wrist.

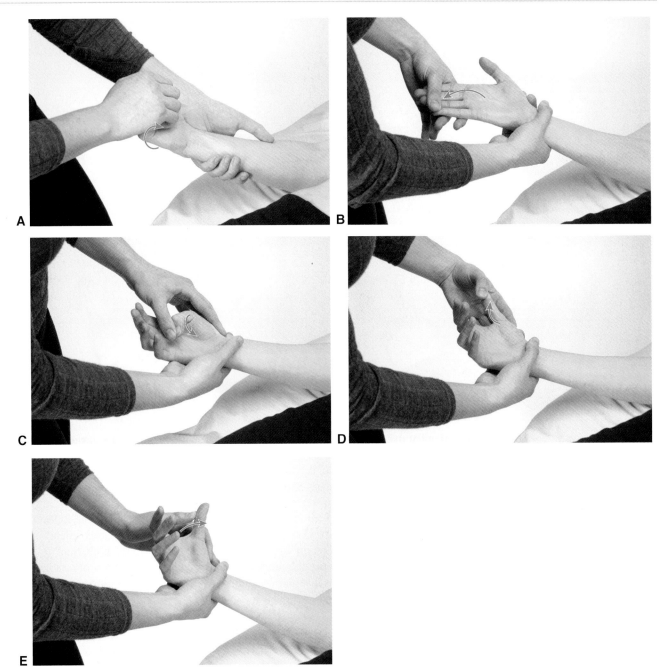

5-15 A. Passive finger flexion. Stand at the client's side. Hold the client's hand with one hand and grasp the forearm with the other hand to stabilize the limb. Start with the client's forearm supinated, then gently bend the fingers into the hand as far as is comfortable. Assess the ROM of the joint capsules as well as the muscles that extend the fingers. **B. Passive finger extension.** Stand at the client's side. Hold the client's hand with one hand and grasp the forearm with the other hand to stabilize the limb. Start with the client's forearm supinated, then gently bend the fingers back as far as is comfortable. Assess the ROM of the joint capsules as well as the muscles that flex the fingers. *Note: passive finger adduction and abduction are not included.* **C. Passive thumb flexion.** Stand at the client's side. Hold the client's thumb with one hand and grasp the wrist with the other hand to stabilize the limb. Start with the client's forearm supinated, then gently bend the thumb and move the tip toward the palm as far as is comfortable. Assess the ROM of the joint capsule as well as the muscles that extend the thumb. **D. Passive thumb extension.** Stand at the client's side. Hold the client's thumb with one hand and grasp the wrist with the other hand to stabilize the limb. Start with the client's forearm supinated, then gently straighten the thumb, moving the tip away from the palm as far as is comfortable. Assess the ROM of the joint capsule as well as the muscles that flex the thumb. **E. Passive thumb abduction.** Stand at the client's side. Hold the client's thumb with one hand and grasp the wrist with the other hand to stabilize the limb. Start with the forearm supinated, then gently move the thumb away from the index finger as far as is comfortable. Assess the ROM of the joint capsule as well as the muscles that adduct the thumb. *Note: passive thumb adduction is limited by approximation and thus not included.*

RESISTED RANGE OF MOTION

Performing resisted range of motion (RROM) helps establish the health and function of the dynamic stabilizers and prime movers in the elbow, forearm, wrist, and hand. Evaluating functional strength and endurance helps identify balance and potential imbalance between the muscles that bend and turn the arm as well as grasp and release objects. The client should be seated comfortably in a chair or on a massage or examination table. For each of the movements illustrated below, resist your client's movement while assessing strength and endurance. Also be sure and watch for compensation (muscle recruitment) in the other joints or regions. Procedures for performing and grading resisted ROM are outlined in Chapter 3.

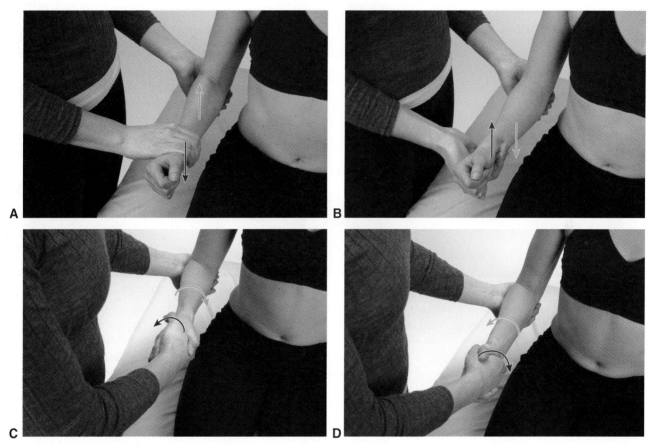

5-16 A. Resisted elbow flexion. The green arrow indicates the direction of movement of the client and the red arrow indicates the direction of resistance from the practitioner. Stand at the client's side. Place one hand under the client's elbow to stabilize the joint and place the other hand on top of the client's forearm. Instruct the client to meet your resistance by pulling the forearm up as you gently but firmly press the forearm down. Assess the strength and endurance of the muscles that flex the elbow. **B. Resisted elbow extension.** Stand at the client's side. Place one hand under client's elbow to stabilize the joint and the other underneath the client's forearm. Instruct the client to meet your resistance by pushing the forearm down as you gently but firmly press the forearm up. Assess the strength and endurance of the muscles that extend the elbow. **C. Resisted pronation.** Stand in front of the client. Place one hand under the client's elbow to stabilize the joint and grasp the client's hand with the other. Instruct the client to meet your resistance by turning the forearm palm down as you gently but firmly turn the forearm palm up. Assess the strength and endurance of the muscles that pronate the forearm. **D. Resisted supination.** Stand in front of the client. Place one hand under the client's elbow to stabilize the joint and grasp the client's hand with the other. Instruct the client to meet your resistance by turning the forearm palm up as you gently but firmly turn the forearm palm down. Assess the strength and endurance of the muscles that supinate the forearm.

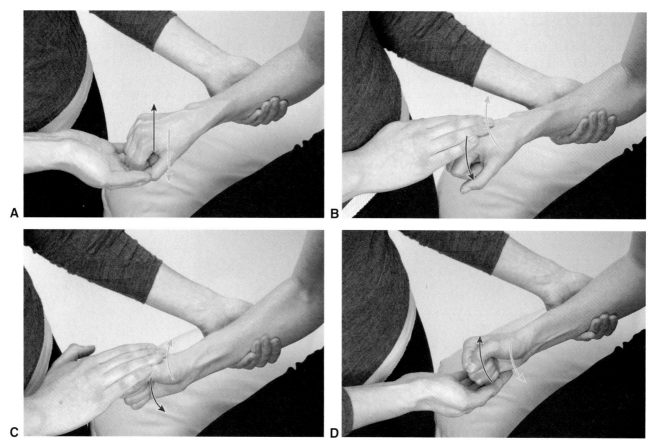

5-17 A. Resisted wrist flexion. Stand in front of the client. Place one hand under the client's forearm to stabilize it and the other on top of the client's pronated, closed hand. Instruct the client to meet your resistance by bending the wrist and pushing the closed hand down toward the floor as you gently but firmly push the hand up. Assess the strength and endurance of the muscles that flex the wrist. **B. Resisted wrist extension.** Stand in front of the client. Place one hand under the client's forearm to stabilize it and the other on top of the client's pronated, closed hand. Instruct the client to meet your resistance by bending the wrist and bringing the closed hand up toward the ceiling as you gently but firmly push the hand down. Assess the strength and endurance of the muscles that extend the wrist. **C. Resisted radial deviation.** Stand in front of the client. Place one hand under the client's forearm to stabilize it and the other on top of the client's neutral (thumb superior) closed hand. Instruct the client to meet your resistance by bending their wrist and bringing the closed hand up as you gently but firmly push it toward the floor. Assess the strength and endurance of the muscles that radially deviate the wrist. **D. Resisted ulnar deviation.** Stand in front of the client. Place one hand under the client's forearm to stabilize it and the other under the client's neutral (thumb superior) closed hand. Instruct the client to meet your resistance by bending their wrist and pushing the closed hand down as you gently but firmly push it toward the ceiling. Assess the strength and endurance of the muscles that ulnar deviate the wrist.

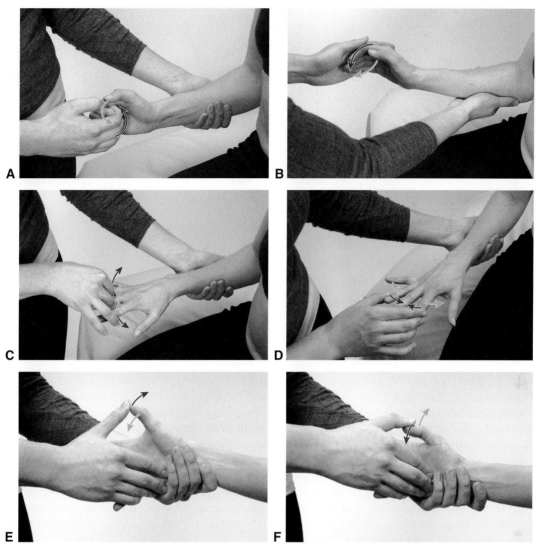

5-18 A. **Resisted finger flexion.** Stand in front of the client. Place one hand under the client's forearm to stabilize it. Place the fingers of your other hand on the pads of the client's fingertips. Instruct the client to meet your resistance by closing the fingers as you gently but firmly open them. Assess the strength and endurance of the muscles that flex the fingers. **B. Resisted finger extension.** Stand in front of the client. Place one hand under the client's forearm to stabilize it. Place the fingers of your other hand on the backs of the client's fingers. Instruct the client to meet your resistance by opening the fingers as you gently but firmly close them. Assess the strength and endurance of the muscles that extend the fingers. **C. Resisted finger adduction.** Stand in front of the client. Place one hand under the client's forearm to stabilize it. Place the fingers of your other hand on the inside edge of the client's fingers. Instruct the client to meet your resistance by bringing the fingers together as you gently but firmly pull them apart. Assess the strength and endurance of the muscles that adduct the fingers. **D. Resisted finger abduction.** Stand in front of the client. Place one hand under the client's forearm to stabilize it. Place the fingers of your other hand on the outside edge of the client's fingers. Instruct the client to meet your resistance by spreading the fingers as you gently but firmly push them together. Assess the strength and endurance of the muscles that abduct the fingers. **E. Resisted thumb flexion.** Stand in front of the client. Place one hand under the client's wrist to stabilize it. Place the pad of your other thumb on the pad of the client's thumb. Instruct the client to meet your resistance by closing the thumb as you gently but firmly open it. Assess the strength and endurance of the muscles that flex the thumb. **F. Resisted thumb extension.** Stand in front of the client. Place one hand under the client's wrist to stabilize it. Place the pad of your other thumb on the top of the client's thumb. Instruct the client to meet your resistance by opening the thumb as you gently but firmly close it. Assess the strength and endurance of the muscles that extend the thumb. *(continues)*

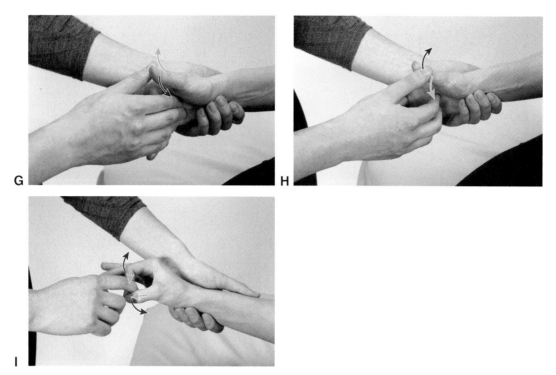

5-18 *(continued)* **G. Resisted thumb adduction.** Stand in front of the client. Place one hand under the client's wrist to stabilize it. Place the pad of your other thumb on the inside edge of the client's thumb. Instruct the client to meet your resistance by bringing the thumb toward the index finger as you gently but firmly push it away. Assess the strength and endurance of the muscles that adduct the thumb. **H. Resisted thumb abduction.** Stand in front of the client. Place one hand under the client's wrist to stabilize it. Place the pad of your other thumb on the outside edge of the client's thumb. Instruct the client to meet your resistance by pushing the thumb away from the index finger as you gently but firmly bring it closer. Assess the strength and endurance of the muscles that abduct the thumb. **I. Resisted thumb opposition.** Stand in front of the client. Place one hand under the client's wrist to stabilize it and instruct the client to make an "ok" sign with the index finger and thumb. Place the pad of your index finger at the joint of the circle and instruct the client to meet your resistance by keeping the fingertips together as you gently but firmly pull them apart. Assess the strength and endurance of the muscles that create opposition in the thumb.

Brachialis • brā-kē-ā'lis • "brachium" Latin *arm*

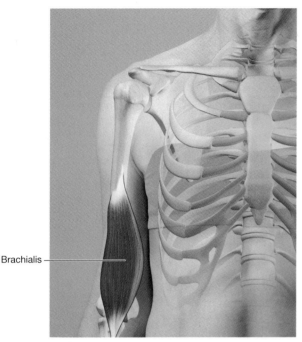

Brachialis

5-19

Palpating Brachialis

Positioning: client supine with forearm pronated.

1. Passively flex elbow to slack tissue.

2. On anterior upper arm find the medial and lateral borders of the elbow flexors in a pincer grasp.

3. Gently slide fingers distally toward the elbow crease, stopping a few inches above.

4. Client gently resists elbow flexion to ensure proper location.

Attachments
O: Humerus, distal one-half of anterior surface
I: Ulna, tuberosity, and coronoid process

Actions
• Flexes the elbow

Innervation
• Musculocutaneous nerve
• C5–C6

Functional Anatomy

Brachialis works primarily with biceps brachii and brachio-radialis to flex the elbow. It differs from biceps brachii in that it attaches to the ulna rather than the radius; thus, it cannot rotate the forearm. Brachialis is unique in that it is a pure elbow flexor and maintains its leverage regardless of forearm position. Both biceps brachii and brachioradialis have varying strength depending upon the rotational position of the forearm.

Brachialis is strongly anchored to a broad section of the anterior humerus. This feature allows it to generate large amounts of force without being damaged. Powerful movements such as lifting, pulling, and performing chin-ups rely on brachialis. This muscle is particularly important when the forearm is pronated (palm down) because both biceps brachii and brachioradialis lose their mechanical advantage in this position. Both brachialis and biceps brachii are rapid flexors; that is, position on the arm generates quick movement through a large range of motion. The forces produced by brachialis and biceps brachii are distributed between the ulna and the radius, maximizing joint function and minimizing injury.

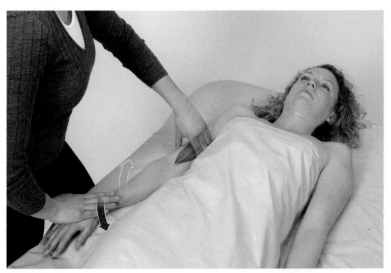

5-20

Brachioradialis
brā'kē ō rā dē ā'lis • "brachium" Latin *arm* "radius" Latin *spoke* or *ray*

Attachments
O: Humerus, proximal two-thirds of lateral supracondylar ridge
I: Radius, lateral side of styloid process

Actions
• Flexes the elbow
• Pronates the forearm from supinated to neutral
• Supinates the forearm from pronated to neutral

Innervation
• Radial nerve
• C5–C6

Functional Anatomy

Brachioradialis is different than its synergists, biceps brachii and brachialis. All three muscles flex the elbow, but brachioradialis has its origin near the joint rather than its insertion like the others. This arrangement makes brachioradialis very strong at the elbow joint and more effective in lifting and carrying heavy loads like buckets of water or grocery bags.

Brachioradialis is strongest when the forearm is in a neutral (thumb up) position. This position aligns its origin on the lateral edge of the humerus with its insertion on the radial styloid process. In fact, brachioradialis will assist with pronation and supination in an effort to return the forearm to that position. So, if you carry groceries or do arm curls with a supinated forearm, your biceps brachii will work the hardest. If you have a pronated forearm, your brachialis will work the hardest. But if you have a neutral (thumb up) forearm, your brachioradialis will work the hardest.

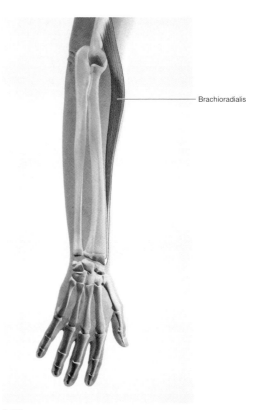

Brachioradialis

5-21

Palpating Brachioradialis

Positioning: client supine with neutral forearm.

1. Passively flex elbow to slack tissue.
2. Palpate the lateral forearm distal to the lateral epicondyle.
3. Pincer grasp muscle belly just distal to lateral epicondyle and follow toward insertion on radial styloid process.
4. Client resists elbow flexion to ensure proper location.

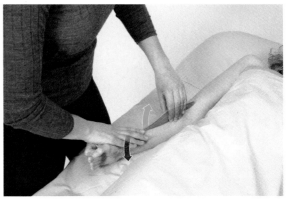

5-22

Flexor Carpi Radialis

fleks'ōr kar'pī rā dē ā'lis • "flexor" Latin *bender* "carpi" Greek *wrist* "radius" Latin *spoke* or *ray*

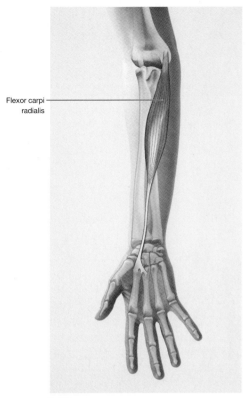

Flexor carpi radialis

5-23

Attachments

O: Humerus, medial epicondyle
I: Metacarpals, base of 2nd and 3rd on palmar side

Actions

* Flexes the wrist
* Radially deviates (abducts) the wrist
* Slightly flexes the elbow
* Slightly pronates the forearm

Innervation

* Median nerve
* C6–C8

Functional Anatomy

Flexor carpi radialis is the most lateral of the three superficial wrist flexors and lies just lateral to the brachioradialis. This muscle serves a dual purpose in the wrist. First, along with several other muscles that originate from the medial epicondyle of the humerus, it flexes the wrist. It is particularly strong in this function when the forearm is supinated; for example, when we carry an object such as a small tray on a flat, upward facing palm. Strong wrist flexion from this supinated position is also necessary when bowling and throwing underhand, as with softball pitching.

The second function of flexor carpi radialis is to radially deviate (abduct) the wrist. Here it works with extensor carpi radialis longus and brevis, as well as several muscles working on the thumb. The final movement when shoveling or throwing a discus activates flexor carpi radialis.

Palpating Flexor Carpi Radialis

Positioning: client supine with forearm supinated.

1. Passively flex elbow and wrist to slack tissue.

2. Locate belly of brachioradialis distal to lateral epicondyle with thumb.

3. Move thumb medially into flexor carpi radialis, staying distal to the elbow crease.

4. Client resists wrist flexion and radial deviation to ensure proper location.

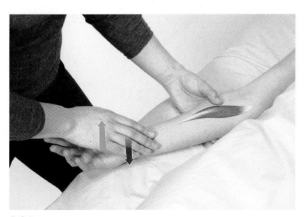

5-24

Palmaris Longus • pahl'măr ēz long'gŭs • "palmaris" Latin *palm* "longus" long

Attachments
O: Humerus, medial epicondyle
I: Flexor retinaculum and palmar aponeurosis

Actions
• Tenses the palmar fascia
• Flexes the wrist
• Slightly flexes the elbow

Innervation
• Median nerve
• C6–C8 and T1

Functional Anatomy

Palmaris longus is centrally located on the anterior forearm between flexor carpi radialis and ulnaris. Because of this location, it does not abduct or adduct the wrist. The efforts of this muscle are focused on flexing the wrist and tensing the *palmar fascia*, a web of connective tissue that attaches to the base of the 2nd–5th metacarpals. When under tension, this fascia helps close the hand. This function contributes to grasping and maintaining grip strength.

Because of its origin on the medial epicondyle of the humerus, palmaris longus contributes to elbow flexion; however, it is weak in this action compared with biceps brachii, brachialis, and brachioradialis. It may contribute to joint stability when the elbow is near full extension. This is a factor when golfing, throwing, and hitting overhead, such as in tennis or volleyball. All of these activities require powerful wrist flexion with the elbow near full extension.

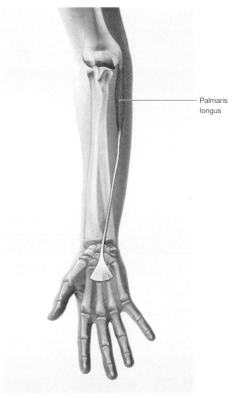

Palmaris longus

5-25

Palpating Palmaris Longus

Positioning: client supine with forearm supinated.

1. Passively flex elbow and wrist to slack tissue.
2. Locate muscle belly of flexor carpi radialis with thumb.
3. Move thumb medially onto muscle belly of palmaris longus.
4. Client makes a fist and resists wrist flexion to ensure proper location.

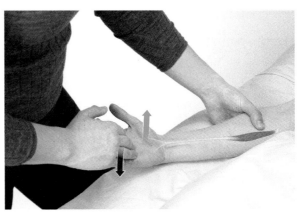

5-26

Flexor Carpi Ulnaris

fleks′ōr kar′pī ūl nā′ris • "flexor" Latin *bender* "carpi" Greek *wrist* "ulna" Latin *elbow*

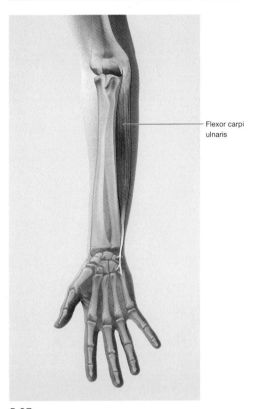

Flexor carpi ulnaris

5-27

Attachments

O: Humeral head: medial epicondyle
O: Ulnar head: medial aspect of olecranon process and proximal two-thirds of posterior border
I: Pisiform, hook of hamate, and base of 5th metacarpal on palmar side

Actions

- Flexes the wrist
- Ulnar deviates (adducts) the wrist
- Slightly flexes the elbow

Innervation

- Ulnar nerve
- C7–C8 and T1

Functional Anatomy

Flexor carpi ulnaris is the most medial of the three superficial wrist flexors lying just medial to palmaris longus. Like flexor carpi radialis, flexor carpi ulnaris has a dual purpose in the wrist. First, it is a strong wrist flexor and, like flexor carpi radialis, is strongest when the forearm is supinated for carrying objects palm up and for underhand activities.

Second, flexor carpi ulnaris ulnar deviates (adducts) the wrist. Here it is an antagonist to flexor carpi radialis. This movement is utilized when hammering, performing a tennis backhand, and throwing overhead when leading with the medial hand. Some baseball pitching and football throwing involve ulnar deviation of the wrist. Flexor carpi ulnaris also is a weak elbow flexor, and more likely contributes to elbow stability during straight-arm activities.

Palpating Flexor Carpi Ulnaris

Positioning: client supine with forearm supinated.

1. Passively flex elbow and wrist to slack tissue.
2. Locate muscle belly of palmaris longus with thumb.
3. Move thumb medially onto muscle belly of flexor carpi ulnaris.
4. Client resists wrist flexion and ulnar deviation to ensure proper location.

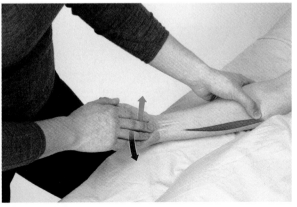

5-28

Flexor Digitorum Superficialis

fleks'ōr dij i tō'rŭm sū'pĕr fish ē āl'is •
"flexor" Latin *bender* "digit" *finger or toe*
"superficialis" *near the surface*

Attachments

O: Humeral head: medial epicondyle and ulnar collateral ligament
O: Ulnar head: medial aspect of coronoid process
O: Radial head: proximal one-half of anterior shaft distal to radial tuberosity
I: Sides of middle phalanges 2–5 by four separate tendons

Actions

- Flexes proximal interphalangeal joints 2–5
- Assists in flexing metacarpophalangeal joints 2–5
- Assists in flexing the wrist

Innervation

- Median nerve
- C7–C8 and T1

Functional Anatomy

The main function of flexor digitorum superficialis is to flex the fingers at the middle joints. The tendons extend only to the middle phalanges, limiting their movement to the metacarpophalangeal and proximal interphalangeal joints. This flexion is utilized in grasping and gripping. All four tendons may be recruited together to make a fist, or individually to play the piano or type.

Flexor digitorum superficialis spreads its origin across the humerus, radius, and ulna. This protects the muscle from damage when generating great force for grasping, holding, and carrying. Because of its origin on the medial epicondyle of the humerus, flexor digitorum superficialis is a weak elbow flexor. It combines efforts with flexor carpi radialis and ulnaris, as well as palmaris longus, to stabilize the elbow and flex the wrist.

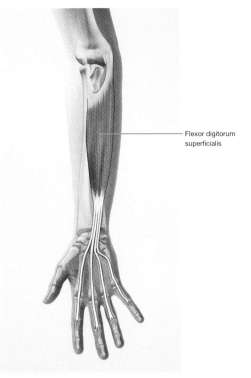

Flexor digitorum superficialis

5-29

Palpating Flexor Digitorum Superficialis

Positioning: client supine with forearm supinated.

1. Passively flex elbow and wrist to slack tissue.

2. Locate muscle belly of palmaris longus and slide thumb distally and deep.

3. Muscle belly of flexor digitorum superficialis is broad and deep to the superficial flexors.

4. Client resists finger flexion and elbow flexion to ensure proper location.

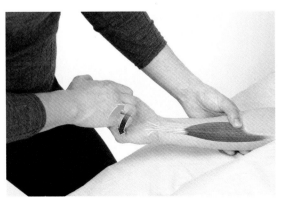

5-30

Flexor Digitorum Profundus

fleks'ōr dij i tō'rŭm prō fŭn'dŭs • "flexor"
Latin *bender* "digit" *finger or toe* "profound"
deep

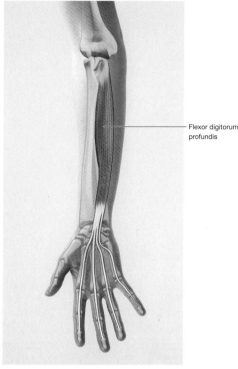

Flexor digitorum
profundis

5-31

Palpating Flexor Digitorum Profundus

Positioning: client supine with forearm supinated.

1. Passively flex wrist to slack tissue.

2. Locate tendons of superficial wrist flexors and slide thumb between and deep.

3. Muscle belly of flexor digitorum profundus is broad and deep to the superficial flexor tendons.

4. Client resists finger flexion to ensure proper location.

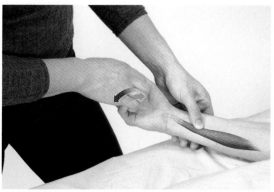

5-32

Attachments

O: Ulna, proximal three-quarters anterior and medial surfaces and interosseous membrane
I: Bases of distal phalanges 2–5, palmar side by four separate tendons

Actions

- Flexes distal interphalangeal joints 2–5
- Assists in flexing proximal interphalangeal joints 2–5
- Assists in flexing metacarpophalangeal joints 2–5
- Assists in flexing the wrist

Innervation

- Median nerve for digits 2 and 3
- Ulnar nerve for digits 4 and 5
- C7–C8 and T1

Functional Anatomy

Flexor digitorum profundus is one of two forearm muscles that flex the fingers. Unlike flexor digitorum superficialis, profundus extends to the distal phalanges. Its tendons dive deep to the split insertions of superficialis and attach to the base of each distal phalange (2–5). This feature makes flexor digitorum profundus the only muscle that flexes all segments of the fingers. Gripping with the fingertips, as when rock climbing or fingering the strings of a guitar, involves activation of this muscle alone.

Flexor digitorum superficialis does not contribute to elbow flexion, but it does assist with wrist flexion. Here it assists flexor carpi radialis and ulnaris, palmaris longus, and flexor digitorum superficialis.

Flexor Pollicis Longus

fleks'ōr pol'i sis long'gŭs • "flexor" Latin *bender* "pollicis" *thumb* "longus" *long*

Attachments

O: Radius, anterior surface of body and interosseous membrane

I: Base of first distal phalange, palmar side

Actions

- Flexes the thumb at carpometacarpal, metacarpophalangeal, and intercarpal joints
- Assists in flexing the wrist

Innervation

- Median nerve
- C6–C8 and T1

Functional Anatomy

The primary function of flexor pollicis longus is to flex the thumb. This function is useful in grasping and gripping activities, since the thumb flexes along with the fingers to make a fist or take hold of an object. Flexor pollicis longus extends to the distal phalange of the thumb, allowing it to act on the carpometacarpal, metacarpophalangeal, and intercarpal joints. Tension of this muscle allows the thumb to wrap around objects such as a tennis racket or baseball.

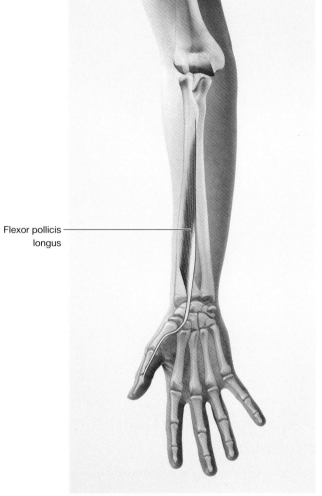

Flexor pollicis longus

5-33

Palpating Flexor Pollicis Longus

Flexor pollicis longus is the deepest of the flexors. It lies underneath the superficial wrist flexors and is thus very difficult to access.

Pronator Teres ● prō nā′tōr tē′res • "pronare" Latin *bend forward* "teres" *round*

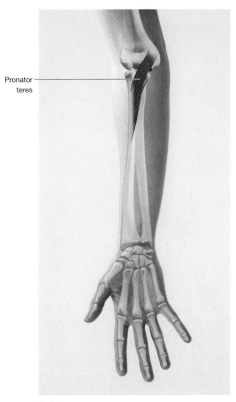

Pronator teres

5-34

Palpating Pronator Teres

Positioning: client seated with forearm supinated.

1. Passively flex elbow and pronate forearm to slack tissue.

2. Locate medial epicondyle with thumb.

3. Slide thumb distally and laterally onto belly of pronator teres.

4. Client resists forearm pronation to ensure proper location.

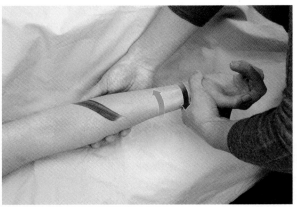

5-35

Attachments

O: Humeral head: medial epicondyle
O: Ulnar head: medial aspect of coronoid process
I: Middle one-third of lateral radius

Actions

• Pronates the forearm
• Assists in flexing the elbow

Innervation

• Median nerve
• C6–C7

Functional Anatomy

Pronator teres crosses the anterior forearm proximal and lateral to flexor carpi radialis. This muscle rotates the forearm to pronate the palm. It also flexes the elbow. It is quite powerful in both of these motions. Using a screwdriver, wrench, or other turning tool requires strong contractions of pronator teres.

Pronator teres is vulnerable to injury during overhead activities such as throwing. The challenge occurs as it turns the forearm over to lead with the palm (pronation). Pronator teres must lengthen as the elbow extends while simultaneously contracting to turn the arm. This can lead to irritation of the medial epicondyle of the humerus where it originates.

Pronator Quadratus

prō nā'tōr kwa drā'tŭs • "pronare" Latin *bend forward* "quadrat" *square*

Attachments

O: Ulna, distal one-fourth on medial side and anterior surface

I: Radius, distal one-fourth on lateral side and anterior surface

Actions

• Pronates the forearm

Innervation

• Median nerve
• C7–C8 and T1

Functional Anatomy

The transverse fibers of pronator quadratus lie distal on the forearm and deep to the flexor tendons. Pronator quadratus works with pronator teres to pronate the forearm. Since two joints (the proximal and distal radioulnar joints) work together to create pronation, muscles are needed at both joints to govern the movement. Pronator quadratus functions more strongly when the elbow is extended as this position decreases the mechanical advantage of pronator teres.

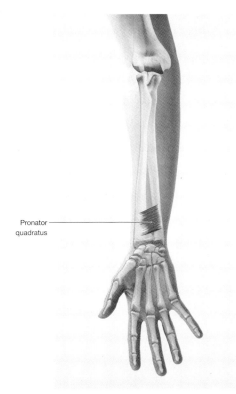

Pronator quadratus

5-36

Palpating Pronator Quadratus

Positioning: client supine with forearm supinated.

1. Passively flex wrist and pronate forearm to slack tissue.

2. Locate radial styloid process with thumb.

3. Slide thumb medially and deep onto lateral edge of pronator quadratus. *(Note: avoid compressing the radial artery, which resides in this location.)*

4. Client resists forearm pronation to ensure proper location.

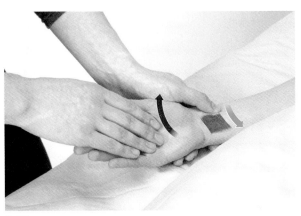

5-37

Supinator • sū pi nā′tōr • "supinare" Latin *place on back*

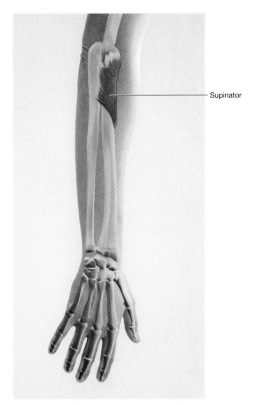

Supinator

5-38

Palpating Supinator

Positioning: client supine with forearm neutral (thumb up).

1. Passively flex elbow to slack tissue.

2. Locate lateral epicondyle with thumb.

3. Follow muscle distally and slightly anteriorly onto radial head. *(Note: avoid compressing the radial nerve, which resides in this location.)*

4. Client resists supination to ensure proper location.

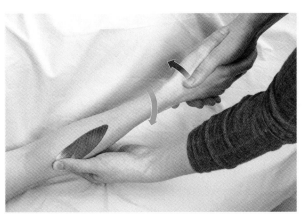

5-39

Attachments

O: Humerus, lateral epicondyle and ulna, supinator crest

I: Radius, proximal one-third of posterior, lateral, and anterior surfaces

Actions

* Supinates the forearm
* Slightly extends the elbow

Innervation

* Radial nerve
* C5–C7

Functional Anatomy

Supinator lies deep to the forearm extensors on the lateral epicondyle of the humerus. It works with biceps brachii and brachioradialis to supinate the forearm. Unlike biceps brachii, supinator is strongest when the elbow is extending or extended. Some of its fibers attach to the lateral epicondyle of the humerus, allowing it to assist with this movement.

The supinator reverses the action of pronator teres and quadratus when turning a screwdriver or wrench. It also is activated when throwing a curve ball in baseball. Here, the elbow extends while the forearm supinates. This generates the characteristic spin of the curve ball.

Anconeus • ang kō'nē ŭs • "ancon" Latin *elbow*

Attachments

O: Humerus, posterior surface of lateral epicondyle
I: Ulna, lateral aspect of olecranon process, and proximal posterior surface of body

Actions

- Extends elbow
- Stabilizes ulna while forearm pronates and supinates

Innervation

- Radial nerve
- C7–C8

Functional Anatomy

The primary function of anconeus is to assist triceps brachii in extending the elbow. It is a comparatively small muscle that resides close to the humeroulnar joint. Anconeus also helps stabilize the ulna while the radius rotates. It anchors the olecranon process to the lateral epicondyle. This tether function prevents the ulna from moving out of the olecranon fossa during pronation and supination of the forearm.

Tensing of anconeus during elbow extension may also protect the joint capsule. Here anconeus pulls the capsule inferiorly and away from the olecranon process as it moves into the olecranon fossa. This prevents the joint capsule from being pinched in the hinge of the humeroulnar joint.

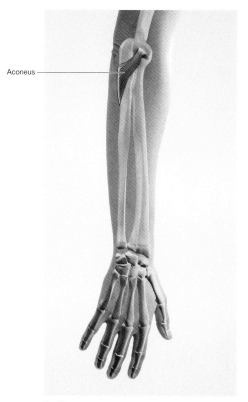

Aconeus

5-40

Palpating Anconeus

Positioning: client supine with forearm neutral (thumb up).

1. Passively flex the elbow to slack tissue.
2. Locate lateral epicondyle of humerus with thumb.
3. Slide thumb posterior and distal toward the olecranon process and onto anconeus.
4. Client resists elbow extension to ensure proper location.

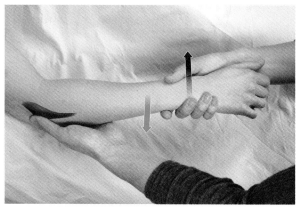

5-41

Extensor Carpi Radialis Longus

eks ten'sōr kar'pī rā dē ā'lis long'gŭs • "extensor" Latin *extender* "carpi" Greek *wrist* "radius" Latin *spoke* or *ray* "longus" *long*

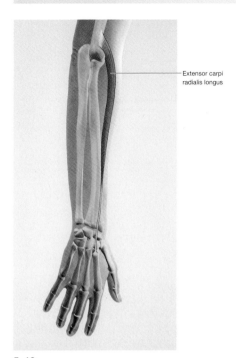

Extensor carpi radialis longus

5-42

Palpating Extensor Carpi Radialis Longus

Positioning: client supine with forearm neutral (thumb up).

1. Passively flex the elbow and radially deviate the wrist to slack tissue.

2. Locate lateral epicondyle of the humerus with thumb.

3. Slide thumb distally onto extensor carpi radialis longus. Be sure and remain lateral to the brachioradialis.

4. Client resists wrist extension and radial deviation to ensure proper location.

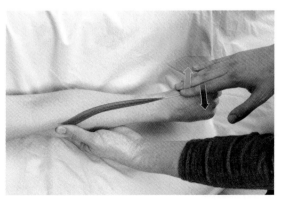

5-43

Attachments

O: Humerus, distal one-third of lateral supracondylar ridge
I: Base of 2nd metacarpal, dorsal side

Actions

• Extends the wrist
• Radially deviates (abducts) the wrist
• Assists in flexing the elbow
• Slightly pronates the forearm

Innervation

• Radial nerve
• C5–C8

Functional Anatomy

Extensor carpi radialis longus has a fairly broad attachment on the lateral supracondylar ridge and epicondyle of the humerus. It is the most lateral of the forearm extensors and lies posterior and medial to brachioradialis. Extensor carpi radialis longus, along with extensor carpi radialis brevis and extensor carpi ulnaris, is a powerful wrist extensor. It helps generate power for a tennis backhand and when lifting with a pronated grip. Overuse of this muscle can result in irritation of the lateral epicondyle, commonly called "tennis elbow."

Extensor carpi radialis also works with extensor carpi radialis brevis and flexor carpi radialis to radially deviate or abduct the wrist. This movement is required for shoveling or throwing a discus.

Some fibers of extensor carpi radialis longus attach anteriorly on the supracondylar ridge of the humerus. This position gives the muscle some function in elbow flexion and forearm supination.

Extensor Carpi Radialis Brevis

eks ten'sōr kar'pī rā dē ā'lis brev'is • "extensor" Latin *extender* "carpi" Greek *wrist* "radius" Latin *spoke* or *ray* "brevis" *short*

Attachments

O: Humerus, lateral epicondyle
I: Base of 3rd metacarpal, dorsal side

Actions

• Extends the wrist
• Radially deviates (abducts) the wrist
• Assists in flexing the elbow

Innervation

• Radial nerve
• C6–C8

Functional Anatomy

Extensor carpi radialis brevis lies just medial to extensor carpi radialis longus and has a more specific origin on the lateral epicondyle of the humerus. It works closely with extensor carpi radialis longus to extend the wrist. Both create the powerful tennis backhand as well as the more subtle "flicking" action of throwing a Frisbee. This muscle also radially deviates (abducts) the wrist along with extensor carpi radialis longus and flexor carpi radialis.

Extensor carpi radialis brevis is one of several muscles that attach to the lateral epicondyle of the humerus. Overuse of these muscles can result in inflammation of this structure, called lateral epicondylitis or "tennis elbow." The extensor muscles are often less developed than the corresponding flexor muscles. This muscle imbalance can contribute to overuse injuries.

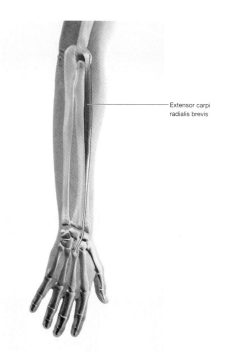

Extensor carpi radialis brevis

5-44

Palpating Extensor Carpi Radialis Brevis

Positioning: client supine with forearm neutral (thumb up).

1. Passively flex the elbow and radially deviate the wrist to slack tissue.

2. Locate lateral epicondyle of the humerus with thumb.

3. Slide thumb distally onto extensor carpi radialis longus. Continue moving distally and slightly laterally onto extensor carpi radialis brevis.

4. Client resists wrist extension and radial deviation to ensure proper location.

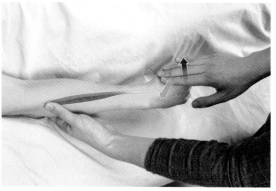

5-45

Extensor Carpi Ulnaris

eks tens'sōr kar'pī ŭl nā'ris • "extensor" Latin *extender* "carpi" Greek *wrist* "ulna" Latin *elbow*

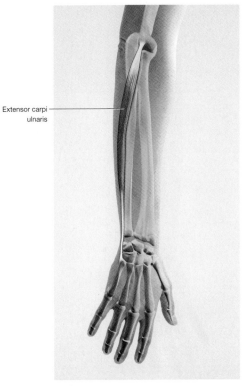

Extensor carpi
ulnaris

5-46

Attachments

O: Humerus, lateral epicondyles and ulna, middle one-third of posterior border
I: Base of 5th metacarpal, dorsal side

Actions

• Extends the wrist
• Ulnar deviates (adducts) the wrist
• Slightly extends the elbow

Innervation

• Radial nerve
• C6–C8

Functional Anatomy

Extensor carpi ulnaris is the most medial of the forearm extensor muscles. It is the medial equivalent to the lateral extensor carpi radialis brevis. It is a powerful wrist extensor as well as ulnar deviator (adductor). This muscle functions synergistically with flexor carpi ulnaris to ulnar deviate the wrist when chopping wood or hammering. Throwing, swinging a baseball bat, and golfing also require ulnar deviation of the wrist and a strong, functional relationship between extensor carpi ulnaris and flexor carpi ulnaris.

Palpating Extensor Carpi Ulnaris

Positioning: client supine with forearm pronated.

1. Passively flex the elbow and ulnar deviate the wrist to slack tissue.
2. Locate the olecranon process with thumb then follow distally along lateral edge of ulna.
3. Slide thumb anteriorly and laterally onto extensor carpi ulnaris.
4. Client resists wrist extension and ulnar deviation to ensure proper location.

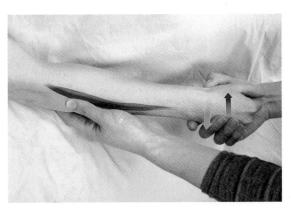

5-47

Extensor Digitorum

eks-ten'sōr dij i tō'rŭm • "extensor" Latin *extender* "digit" *finger or toe*

Attachments

O: Humerus, lateral epicondyle
I: Middle and distal phalanges 2–5, dorsal side

Actions

- Extends digits 2–5 at metacarpophalangeal, proximal interphalangeal, and distal interphalangeal joints
- Extends the wrist
- Slightly extends the elbow

Innervation

- Radial nerve
- C6–C8

Functional Anatomy

Extensor digitorum is the most central of the forearm extensors, lying between extensor carpi radialis brevis and extensor carpi ulnaris. The main function of extensor digitorum is to extend the four fingers. Since less strength is required to open the hand than to close it and grip objects, it's not surprising that this single muscle, as compared to the two flexor muscles, accomplishes extension. Because extensor digitorum crosses the wrist and elbow, it also contributes to wrist extension and slight elbow extension.

The unequal strength between the finger flexors and extensors contributes to the slightly flexed resting hand posture. Caution must be exercised to maintain balanced strength and good ergonomics with repetitive activities like typing. This helps avoid overuse injuries in the elbow, forearm, wrist, and hand.

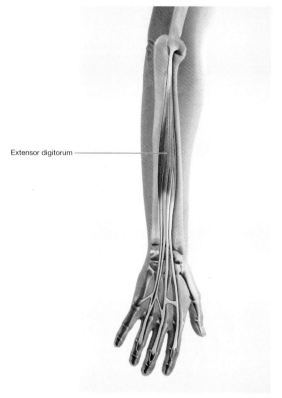

Extensor digitorum

5-48

Palpating Extensor Digitorum

Positioning: client supine with forearm pronated.

1. Passively flex the elbow and extend the wrist to slack tissue.
2. Locate the olecranon process with thumb then follow distally along lateral edge of ulna.
3. Slide thumb anteriorly and laterally onto extensor carpi ulnaris then farther laterally onto extensor digitorum.
4. Client resists finger extension to ensure proper location.

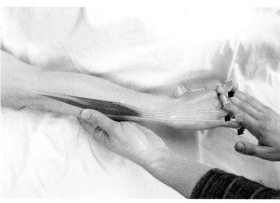

5-49

Extensor Indicis ● eks ten'sōr in'di sis • "extensor" Latin *extender* "indicis" *pointer finger*

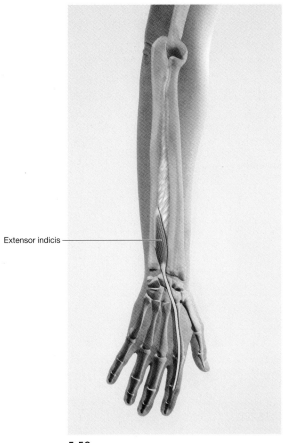

Extensor indicis

5-50

Palpating Extensor Indicis

Positioning: client supine with forearm pronated.

1. Passively extend wrist to slack tissue.

2. Locate the ulnar styloid process with thumb then slide proximally and medially onto extensor indicis.

3. Client resists extension of the index finger to ensure proper location.

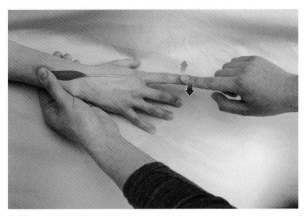

5-51

Attachments

O: Ulna, posterior surface of body, and interosseous membrane

I: Base of 2nd proximal phalange and into tendon of extensor digitorum

Actions

• Extends 2nd digit at metacarpophalangeal joint and interphalangeal joints
• Extends the wrist
• Assists in adducting the index finger
• Slightly supinates the forearm

Innervation

• Radial nerve
• C6–C8

Functional Anatomy

The hand is capable of many fine movements through synchronization or isolation of muscle contractions. Extensor indicis allows the index finger to function independently from the other three fingers. Pointing, clicking a computer mouse, and writing all require individualized movement of the index finger.

Because extensor indicis originates on the ulna and traverses the posterior forearm and wrist, it is able to extend the wrist and supinate the forearm. These actions are slight compared to supinator, extensor carpi radialis longus and brevis, and extensor carpi ulnaris.

Extensor Digiti Minimi

eks ten'sōr dij'i tī min'i mī • "extensor" Latin extender "digiti" finger "minimi" smallest

Attachments

O: Humerus, lateral epicondyle
I: Base of 5th proximal phalange, dorsal side

Actions

* Extends 5th digit at metacarpophalangeal and interphalangeal joints
* Extends wrist
* Assists in abducting little finger
* Slightly extends the elbow

Innervation

* Radial nerve
* C6–C8

Functional Anatomy

Extensor digiti minimi lies between extensor digitorum and extensor carpi ulnaris. It is primarily responsible for extending the pinky finger. Extensor digiti minimi assists extensor digitorum in this function, but allows individualized movement of this digit in much the same way as extensor indicis does for the index finger. This individualized movement allows us to play musical instruments such as the guitar, violin, piano, and flute. It also contributes to fine motor skills such as typing.

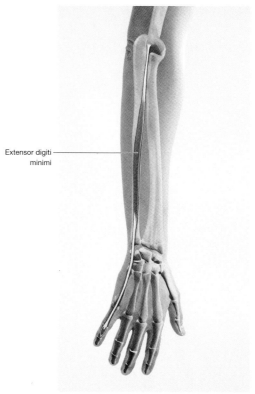

Extensor digiti minimi

5-52

Palpating Extensor Digiti Minimi

Positioning: client supine with forearm pronated.

1. Passively flex elbow and extend wrist to slack tissue.

2. Locate the olecranon process with thumb then slide distally along lateral edge of ulna.

3. Slide thumb laterally past the extensor carpi ulnaris onto extensor digiti minimi.

4. Client resists extension of the little finger to ensure proper location.

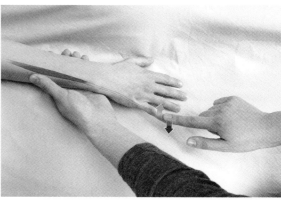

5-53

Abductor Pollicis Longus

ab dŭk′tōr pŏl′ĭ sis lŏn′gus • "abduct" Latin *lead away* "pollicis" *thumb* "longus" *long*

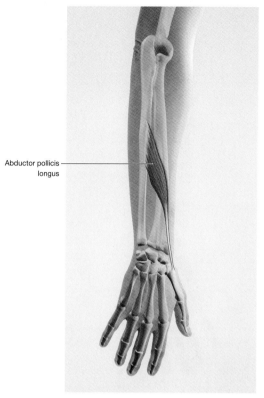

Abductor pollicis longus

5-54

Attachments

O: Ulna, radius, and interosseous membrane, middle one-third of posterior surface
I: Base of first metacarpal, dorsal side

Actions

- Abducts the first carpometacarpal joint
- Extends the first carpometacarpal joint
- Radially deviates (abducts) the wrist
- Slightly flexes the wrist

Innervation

- Radial nerve
- C6–C8

Functional Anatomy

Abductor pollicis longus, which is just distal to supinator, crosses diagonally from the ulna to the radius before inserting on the first metacarpal. This muscle, along with extensor pollicis longus and brevis (discussed next), creates the borders of a structure known as the *anatomical snuffbox*, which is located just distal and posterior to the radial styloid process. Its name comes from its use for holding finely ground tobacco (called *snuff*) prior to inhaling or snorting. Abductor pollicis longus, along with extensor pollicis brevis, forms the lateral border of this structure.

When contracted, abductor pollicis longus pulls the thumb away from the palm of the hand. This motion is a combination of abduction and extension and occurs at the first carpometacarpal joint. Abduction and adduction of the thumb are unique in that they take place on the sagittal plane around the frontal axis. Here, flexion and extension occur on the frontal plane around a sagittal axis. Remember, the first carpometacarpal joint is the only saddle joint in the body and allows specialized movements for grasping and gripping. Abduction and extension of the thumb are critical movements for opening the hand and letting go of objects.

Because of its anterior position on the thumb, abductor pollicis longus is in a position to assist with wrist flexion as well as radial deviation. Along with the other anatomical snuffbox muscles, it is active during wrist activities such as shoveling, bowling, and golfing.

Palpating Abductor Pollicis Longus

Positioning: client seated with forearm neutral (thumb up).

1. Passively radially deviate wrist to tension tissue.

2. Locate radial styloid process with thumb and slide distally onto tendon of abductor pollicis longus. Abductor pollicis longus makes up the lateral border of the anatomical snuffbox.

3. Client resists thumb abduction to ensure proper location.

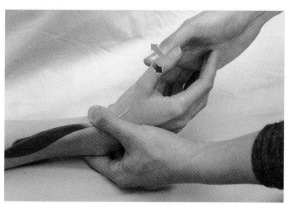

5-55

Extensor Pollicis Brevis

eks ten'sŏr pōle¯'cēs brā'vēs • "extensor" Latin *extender* "pollicis" *thumb* "brevis" *short*

Attachments

O: Radius, distal one-third of posterior surface and interosseous membrane
I: Base of 1st proximal phalange, dorsal side

Actions

- Extends the thumb at the carpometacarpal and metacarpophalangeal joints
- Abducts the thumb at the carpometacarpal joint
- Slightly radially deviates (abducts) the wrist

Innervation

- Radial nerve
- C6–C8

Functional Anatomy

Extensor pollicis brevis crosses the posterior surface of the distal radius. It is one of three muscles that make up the anatomical snuffbox (see abductor pollicis longus) and forms the lateral border along with abductor pollicis longus. Its main function is to extend the thumb at the carpometacarpal and metacarpophalangeal joints. This movement helps the hand open to grasp objects. It is also instrumental in letting those objects go.

Extensor pollicis longus stretches across the back of the wrist and down the thumb, giving it some leverage to radially deviate (abduct) the wrist. This action is utilized in shoveling, bowling, and golfing.

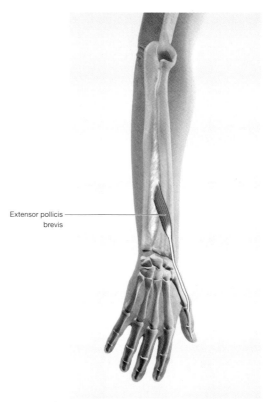

Extensor pollicis brevis

5-56

Palpating Extensor Pollicis Brevis

Positioning: client supine with forearm neutral (thumb up).

1. Passively ulnar deviate wrist to create tension in the tissue.

2. Locate radial styloid process with thumb and slide distally onto tendon of extensor pollicis brevis. Extensor pollicis brevis helps makes up the lateral border of the anatomical snuffbox.

3. Client resists thumb extension to ensure proper location.

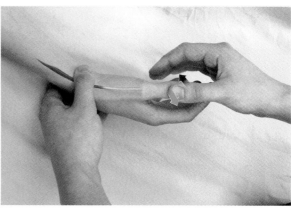

5-57

Extensor Pollicis Longus

eks ten'sŏr pō lē'cēs lŏn gus • "extensor" Latin *extender* "pollicis" *thumb* "longus" *long*

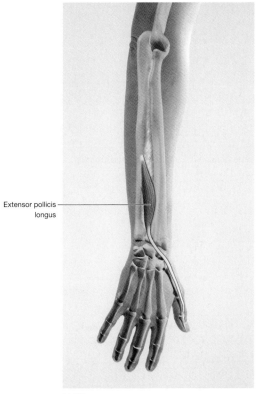

Extensor pollicis longus

5-58

Palpating Extensor Pollicis Longus

Positioning: client supine with forearm neutral (thumb up).

1. Passively ulnar deviate wrist to create tension in the tissue.

2. Locate radial styloid process with thumb and slide laterally onto tendon of extensor pollicis longus. Extensor pollicis longus makes up the lateral border of the anatomical snuffbox (from this position).

3. Client resists thumb extension to ensure proper location.

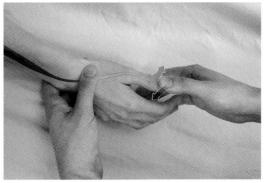

5-59

Attachments

O: Ulna, middle one-third of posterior surface and interosseous membrane
I: Base of 1st distal phalange, dorsal side

Actions

• Extends the thumb at the carpometacarpal, metacarpophalangeal, and interphalangeal joints
• Slightly radially deviates (abducts) the wrist
• Slightly extends the wrist

Innervation

• Radial nerve
• C6–C8

Functional Anatomy

Extensor pollicis longus spans the distal radioulnar joint and lies medial to extensor pollicis brevis. It is the third muscle of the anatomical snuffbox (see abductor pollicis longus) and forms its medial border. Extensor pollicis longus is a synergist to extensor pollicis brevis in extending the thumb and radially deviating the wrist. Together, these two muscles extend the thumb as the hand opens and releases objects, and bend the wrist toward the thumb. This movement is part of household activities such as shoveling and sports activities such as bowling and the volleyball bump.

Because extensor pollicis longus attaches more proximally on the forearm than brevis, it is stronger in radial deviation and able to extend the wrist. This function is of particular importance in finely controlled movements such as at the end of a golf swing.

▶ INTRINSIC MUSCLES OF THE HAND

Muscle	Location	Action	Function
Opponens digiti minimi	Hypothenar eminance	Opposition of pinky finger	Grasping and pinching
Flexor digiti minimi brevis	Hypothenar eminance	Flexes pinky finger at metacarpo-phalangeal joint	Grasps round objects
Abductor digiti minimi	Hypothenar eminance	Abducts pinky finger	Wraps hand around round objects
Opponens pollicis	Thenar eminance	Opposition, flexion, and adduction of thumb	Grasping round objects and fine gripping like a pencil
Flexor pollicis brevis	Thenar eminance	Flexes and abducts first carpometacarpal joint and flexes first metacarpophalangeal joint, opposition	Pincer gripping and lateral gripping to hold a key or a card

▶ INTRINSIC MUSCLES OF THE HAND (continued)

Muscle	Location	Action	Function
Abductor pollicis brevis 	Thenar eminence	Abducts thumb, opposition	Grasping round or cylindrical objects
Adductor pollicis 	Central hand	Adducts the first carpometacarpal joint and flexes the first metacarpophalangeal joint	Grasping and making a fist
Interossei 	Central hand *Palmar:* between 2nd and 3rd, 3rd and 4th, and 4th and 5th metacarpals and proximal phalanges *Dorsal:* Between all five metacarpals and proximal phalanges	*Palmar:* Flex MP joints, extend PIP joints, adduct fingers *Dorsal:* Flex MP joints, extend PIP joints, abduct fingers	Staggered finger flexing and closing (palmar) and spreading (dorsal) of fingers
Lumbricals 	Central hand from tendons of flexor digitorum profundus to 2nd, 3rd, 4th, and 5th MP joints	Flex MP joints, extend PIP and DIP joints	Staggered finger flexion

▶ SYNERGISTS/ANTAGONISTS: ELBOW AND WRIST

Motion		Muscles Involved	Motion		Muscles Involved
Elbow Flexion	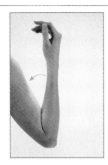	*Biceps brachii (Ch 4) *Brachialis *Brachioradialis Flexor carpi radialis Palmaris longus Flexor carpi ulnaris Pronator teres Extensor carpi radialis longus Extensor carpi radialis brevis	Elbow Extension	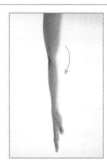	*Triceps brachii (Ch 4) Anconeus Supinator Extensor carpi ulnaris Extensor digitorum Extensor digiti minimi
Pronation	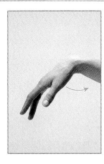	Brachioradialis *Flexor carpi radialis *Pronator teres *Pronator quadratus Extensor carpi radialis longus	Supination	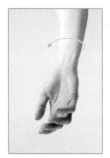	*Biceps brachii (Ch 4) Brachioradialis *Supinator Extensor indicis
Wrist Flexion	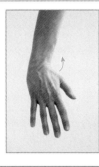	*Flexor carpi radialis Palmaris longus *Flexor carpi ulnaris Flexor digitorum superficialis Flexor digitorum profundus Flexor pollicis longus Abductor pollicis longus	Wrist Extension	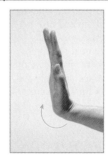	*Extensor carpi radialis longus *Extensor carpi radialis brevis *Extensor carpi ulnaris Extensor digitorum Extensor indicis Extensor digiti minimi Extensor pollicis longus
Radial Deviation	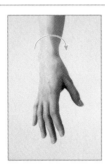	*Flexor carpi radialis *Extensor carpi radialis longus Extensor carpi radialis brevis *Abductor pollicis longus *Extensor pollicis brevis Extensor pollicis longus	Ulnar Deviation	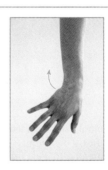	*Flexor carpi ulnaris *Extensor carpi ulnaris

*Indicates prime movers.

▶ SYNERGISTS/ANTAGONISTS: HAND

Motion		Muscles Involved	Motion		Muscles Involved
Finger flexion		*Flexor digitorum superficialis (MP's and PIP's) *Flexor digitorum profundus (MP's, PIP's, and DIP's) *Flexor digiti minimi brevis (5th MP joint) *Lumbricals (MP joints) *Interossei (MP joints)	Finger extension		*Extensor digitorum (MP's, PIP's, and DIP's) *Extensor indicis (2nd MP, PIP, and DIP) *Extensor digiti minimi (5th MP, PIP, and DIP) Interossei (PIP joints) Lumbricals (PIP and DIP joints)
Finger adduction		Extensor indicis (2nd digit) *Palmar interossei	Finger abduction		Extensor digiti minimi (5th digit) *Abductor digiti minimi *Dorsal interossei
Thumb flexion		*Flexor pollicis longus (CM, MP, and IC joints) *Flexor pollicis brevis (CM and MP joints) *Opponens pollicis Adductor pollicis (MP joint)	Thumb extension		*Abductor pollicis longus (CM joint) *Extensor pollicis brevis (CM and MC joints) *Extensor pollicis longus (CM, MC, and IP joints)
Thumb adduction		Opponens pollicis *Adductor pollicis (CM joint)	Thumb abduction		*Abductor pollicis longus (CM joint) Extensor pollicis brevis (CM joint) Flexor pollicis brevis *Abductor pollicis brevis
Thumb opposition		*Opponens digiti minimi *Opponens pollicis *Flexor pollicis brevis *Abductor pollicis brevis			

*Indicates prime movers.

▶ PUTTING IT IN MOTION

Muscles of the elbow, forearm, wrist, and hand work together to perform common movements such as lifting, grasping, twisting, and throwing. Coordinated effort is required for these complex movements to occur smoothly and efficiently. Proper balance between agonist and antagonist groups maintains proper alignment of joints as well as adequate control of powerful movements.

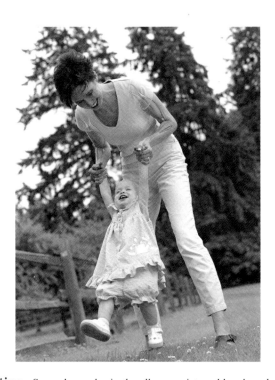

Lifting. Several muscles in the elbow, wrist, and hand work together to help us lift and carry objects. When the forearm is pronated, the wrist extensors and elbow flexors work together. When the forearm is supinated, the wrist flexors are working. In either case, the finger flexors and intrinsic hand muscles are responsible for grasping and holding the object.

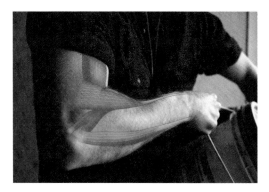

Twisting. Movements such as turning a screwdriver, opening a bottle with a corkscrew, or rolling the hands in golf or baseball activates the pronators and supinators of the forearm. The biceps brachii and supinator turn the forearm from palm down to palm up. The pronator teres, pronator quadratus, and flexor carpi radialis turn the forearm from palm up to palm down.

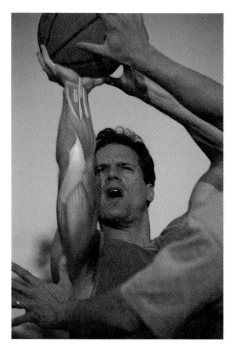

Shooting. The majority of force for shooting a basketball is produced in the lower body, trunk, and shoulders. The position of the arm and hand fine-tune the shot and help determine the motion and direction of the ball. Here, the pronator teres, pronator quadratus, and flexor carpi radialis pronate the forearm as the triceps brachii and anconeus extend the elbow. The finger flexors are helping to grip the ball, but the extensors must be activated for release. All of the wrist flexors remain active propelling the ball forward until it rolls off of the fingertips.

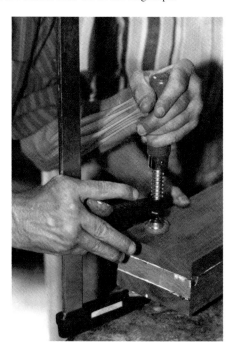

Grasping. A closer view of grasping reveals the coordinated efforts of muscles such as the palmaris longus, flexor digitorum superficialis, flexor digitorum profundus, flexor pollicis longus, flexor pollicis brevis, and opponens pollicis. Complex hand movements require activation of multiple muscle groups.

SUMMARY

- The elbow is composed of three bones (humerus, radius, and ulna) and two joints (humeroulnar and proximal radioulnar), which allow it to hinge (flexion and extension) and rotate (pronation and supination).
- The wrist and hand contain several bones and joints including the radius, ulna, carpals, metacarpals, and phalanges. This complex architecture allows various movements in this region.
- Powerful muscles such as the brachialis and brachioradialis create strength for lifting and carrying objects.
- Many muscles that control movement in the wrist and hand reside close to the elbow, including the flexors and extensors of the wrist and fingers.
- Specialized muscles like the pronator teres, pronator quadratus, and supinator pivot the forearm, helping to position the hand and perform twisting motions.
- The thumb is unique and has a separate muscle group to control its movements including pressing, grasping, and releasing.
- Muscles of the elbow, forearm, wrist, and hand work in harmony to create movements such as lifting, twisting, shooting, and grasping.

FOR REVIEW

Answers to review questions can be found in Appendix A.

Multiple Choice

1. The two joints that allow the forearm to rotate are:
   A. the humeroulnar and the radiocarpal
   B. the humeroulnar and the proximal radioulnar
   C. the humeroulnar and distal radioulnar
   D. the proximal and distal radioulnar

2. The ulnar notch is located on the:
   A. humerus
   B. radius
   C. ulna
   D. scaphoid

3. The ligament that maintains the position of the radial head during pronation and supination is called the:
   A. ulnar collateral ligament
   B. radial collateral ligament
   C. anular ligament
   D. transverse carpal ligament

4. The nerve that lies within the carpal tunnel is the:
   A. ulnar nerve
   B. radial nerve
   C. median nerve
   D. brachial plexus

5. The artery that is superficial on the lateral aspect of the wrist and can be used to take a person's pulse is the:
   A. ulnar artery
   B. radial artery
   C. median artery
   D. brachial artery

6. The cubital lymph nodes are located:
   A. in the axilla
   B. in the carpal tunnel
   C. near the medial elbow crease
   D. near the lateral elbow crease

7. The purpose of the synovial sheaths in the hand is:
   A. to lubricate the tendons of fingers
   B. to protect the olecranon process
   C. to reduce friction at the medial and lateral epicondyles
   D. to cushion the bones when grasping or holding objects

8. The ligament that forms the roof of the carpal tunnel is called the:
   A. ulnar collateral ligament
   B. radial collateral ligament
   C. anular ligament
   D. transverse carpal ligament

9. The purpose of the interosseous membrane is to:
   A. prevent medial separation of the humeroulnar joint
   B. prevent lateral separation of the humeroulnar joint
   C. prevent "bowing" or separation of the radius and ulna
   D. maintain the position of the radial head

10. The anatomical term for finger bones is:
    A. carpals
    B. phalanges
    C. metacarpals
    D. tarsals

Matching

Different muscle attachments are listed below. Match the correct muscle with its attachment.

11. _____ Base of 1st distal phalange, dorsal side

12. _____ Pisiform, hook of hamate, and base of 5th metacarpal on palmar side

13. _____ Humerus, distal one-third of lateral supracondylar ridge

14. _____ Middle one-third of lateral radius

15. _____ Metacarpals, base of 2nd and 3rd on palmar side

16. _____ Humerus, distal one-half of anterior surface

17. _____ Radius, lateral side of styloid process

18. _____ Ulna, proximal three-fourths anterior and medial surfaces and interosseous membrane

19. _____ Ulna, lateral aspect of olecranon process and proximal posterior surface of body

20. _____ Middle and distal phalanges 2–5, dorsal side

A. Anconeus
B. Brachialis
C. Extensor carpi radialis longus
D. Pronator teres
E. Flexor digitorum profundus
F. Brachioradialis
G. Abductor pollicis longus
H. Flexor carpi radialis
I. Extensor digitorum
J. Flexor carpi ulnaris

Different muscle actions are listed below. Match the correct muscle with its action. Answers may be used more that once.

21. _____ flexes the elbow

22. _____ extends the elbow

23. _____ pronates the forearm

24. _____ supinates the forearm

25. _____ flexes the wrist

26. _____ extends the wrist

27. _____ radially deviates the wrist

28. _____ ulnar deviates the wrist

29. _____ flexes the fingers

30. _____ extends the fingers

A. Brachioradialis
B. Extensor digitorum
C. Pronator quadratus
D. Flexor digitorum profundus
E. Extensor carpi ulnaris
F. Brachialis
G. Flexor carpi radialis longus
H. Anconeus
I. Palmaris longus
J. Flexor carpi ulnaris

Short Answer

31. Briefly describe why the elbow is able to flex and extend as well as rotate. What joints make this possible?

32. Make a list of all the muscles that have attachments to the lateral epicondyle of the humerus. Do the same for those attaching to the medial epicondyle of the humerus.

33. Briefly contrast the thumb with the other digits. What motions are possible here, and which are unique? How are these unique movements possible?

Try This!

Activity: Find a partner and have him or her perform one of the skills identified in the *Putting It in Motion* segment. Identify the specific actions of the elbow, forearm, wrist and hand that make up this skill. Write them down. Use the synergist list to identify which muscles work together to create this movement. Make sure you put the actions in the correct sequence. See if you can discover which muscles are stabilizing or steering the joint into position and which are responsible for powering the movement.

Switch partners and perform a different skill from *Putting It in Motion*. Repeat the steps above. Confirm your findings with the *Putting It in Motion* segment on the student CD included with your textbook. To further your understanding, practice this activity with skills not identified in *Putting It in Motion*.

SUGGESTED READINGS

Bongers PM. The cost of shoulder pain at work: variation in work tasks and good job opportunities are essential for prevention. *BMJ.* 2001;322(7278):64–65.

Cogley RM, Archambault TA, Fiberger JF, et al. Comparison of muscle activation using various hand positions during the push-up exercise. *J. Strength Cond. R.* 2005;19(3):628–633.

Grezios AK, Gissis IT, Sotiropoulos AA, et al. Muscle-contraction properties in overarm throwing movements. *J Strength Cond. R.* 2006;20(1):117–123.

McMullen J, Uhl TL. A kinetic chain approach for shoulder rehabilitation. *J Athl Train.* 2000;35(3):329–337.

Myers JB, Pasquale MR, Laudner KG, et al. On-the-field resistance-tubing exercises for throwers: an electromyographic analysis. *J Athl Train.* 2005;40(1):15–22.

Zimmerman GR. Carpal Tunnel Syndrome. *J Athl Train.* 1994;29(1):22–24,26–28,30.

Head, Neck, and Face

6

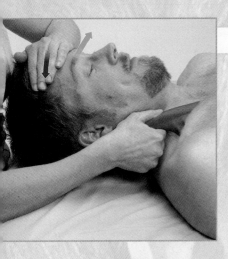

Learning Objectives

After working through the material in this chapter, you should be able to:

- Identify the main structures of the head, neck, and face, including bones, joints, special structures, and deep and superficial muscles.

- Label and palpate the major surface landmarks of the head, neck, and face.

- Identify and demonstrate all actions of the muscles of the head, neck, and jaw.

- Demonstrate passive and resisted range of motion of the neck.

- Draw, label, palpate, and fire the superficial and deep muscles of the head, neck, and face.

- Locate the attachments and nerve supply of the muscles of the head, neck, and face.

- Describe the unique functional anatomy and relationships between each muscle of the head, neck, and face.

- Identify both the synergists and antagonists involved in each movement of the neck and jaw (flexion, extension, etc.).

- Identify muscles used in performing four coordinated movements of the neck: heading in soccer, looking up, cocking to one side, and turning the head.

▶ OVERVIEW OF THE REGION

The head, neck, and face house the most critical organs of the nervous system. The head encases the brain, the organ of cognition and consciousness, as well as the entire length of eleven of the twelve cranial nerves. It also contains the organs of four special senses: sight, sound, smell, and taste. The neck contains the cervical spinal cord, from which nerves branch throughout the upper body including the diaphragm muscle, which is essential for breathing. Complex interactions between this region and all other regions of the body are thus critical to survival and optimal function.

Several bones fit together to form the skull. Some form the round cranium, which contains the brain. Others form the bones of the face and protect underlying structures, such as the openings of the digestive and respiratory systems. A complex union between two bones forms the jaw joint, which allows the movements required for speaking, chewing, and facial expression.

The cervical spine contains seven vertebrae and two types of joints, making it the most mobile region of the spine. Multiple layers of ligaments and muscles maintain alignment between the skull, individual vertebrae, and the cervical spine as a whole. The size, shape, and location of these muscles reflect their function in this complex region. Some muscles that act on the head and neck also act on the entire spine. These will be explored in Chapter 7.

▶ SURFACE ANATOMY OF THE HEAD, NECK, AND FACE

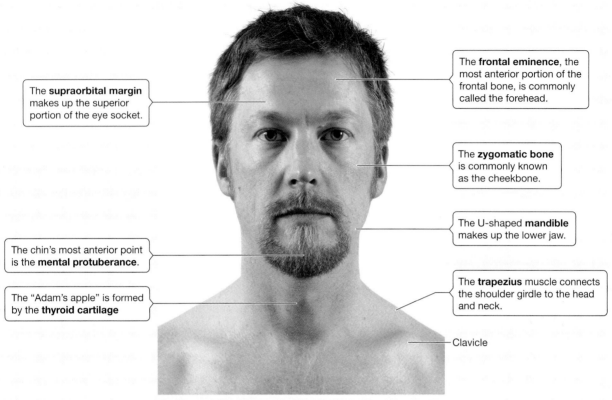

The **supraorbital margin** makes up the superior portion of the eye socket.

The **frontal eminence**, the most anterior portion of the frontal bone, is commonly called the forehead.

The **zygomatic bone** is commonly known as the cheekbone.

The U-shaped **mandible** makes up the lower jaw.

The chin's most anterior point is the **mental protuberance**.

The "Adam's apple" is formed by the **thyroid cartilage**

The **trapezius** muscle connects the shoulder girdle to the head and neck.

Clavicle

6-1A. Anterior view.

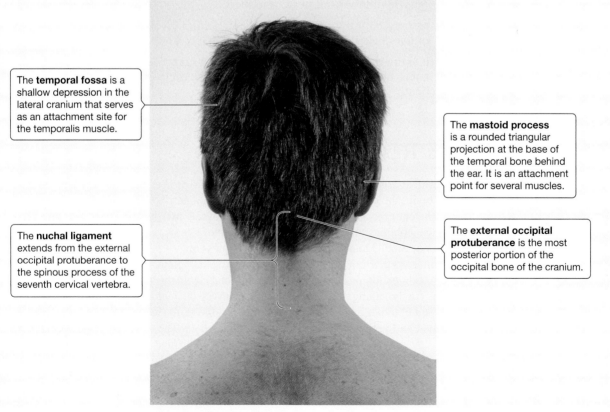

The **temporal fossa** is a shallow depression in the lateral cranium that serves as an attachment site for the temporalis muscle.

The **mastoid process** is a rounded triangular projection at the base of the temporal bone behind the ear. It is an attachment point for several muscles.

The **nuchal ligament** extends from the external occipital protuberance to the spinous process of the seventh cervical vertebra.

The **external occipital protuberance** is the most posterior portion of the occipital bone of the cranium.

6-1B. Posterior view.

▶ SURFACE ANATOMY OF THE HEAD, NECK, AND FACE

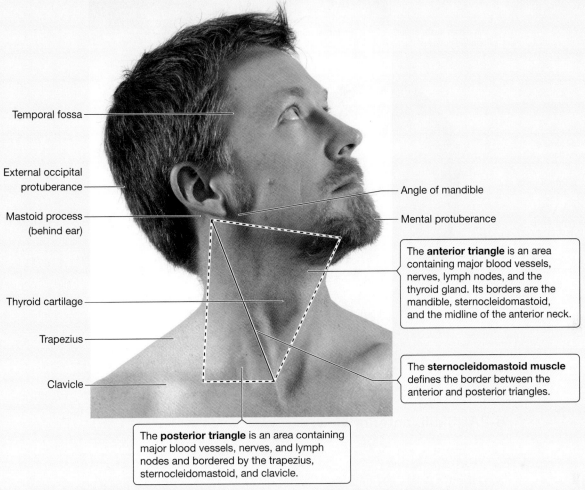

Temporal fossa

External occipital protuberance

Mastoid process (behind ear)

Thyroid cartilage

Trapezius

Clavicle

Angle of mandible

Mental protuberance

The **anterior triangle** is an area containing major blood vessels, nerves, lymph nodes, and the thyroid gland. Its borders are the mandible, sternocleidomastoid, and the midline of the anterior neck.

The **sternocleidomastoid muscle** defines the border between the anterior and posterior triangles.

The **posterior triangle** is an area containing major blood vessels, nerves, and lymph nodes and bordered by the trapezius, sternocleidomastoid, and clavicle.

6-1C. Anterolateral view.

▶ SKELETAL STRUCTURES OF THE HEAD, NECK, AND FACE

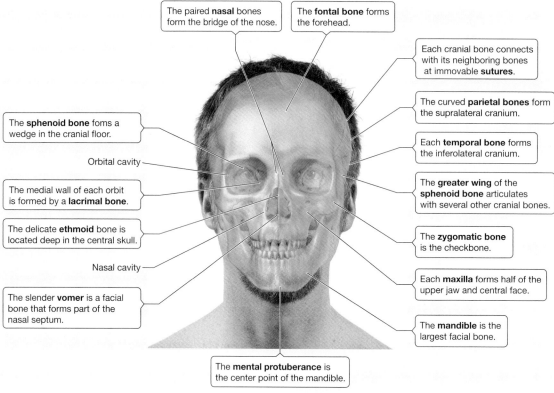

The paired **nasal** bones form the bridge of the nose.

The **fontal bone** forms the forehead.

Each cranial bone connects with its neighboring bones at immovable **sutures**.

The **sphenoid bone** foms a wedge in the cranial floor.

The curved **parietal bones** form the supralateral cranium.

Orbital cavity

Each **temporal bone** forms the inferolateral cranium.

The medial wall of each orbit is formed by a **lacrimal bone**.

The **greater wing** of the **sphenoid bone** articulates with several other cranial bones.

The delicate **ethmoid** bone is located deep in the central skull.

The **zygomatic bone** is the checkbone.

Nasal cavity

Each **maxilla** forms half of the upper jaw and central face.

The slender **vomer** is a facial bone that forms part of the nasal septum.

The **mandible** is the largest facial bone.

The **mental protuberance** is the center point of the mandible.

6-2A. Skull, anterior view.

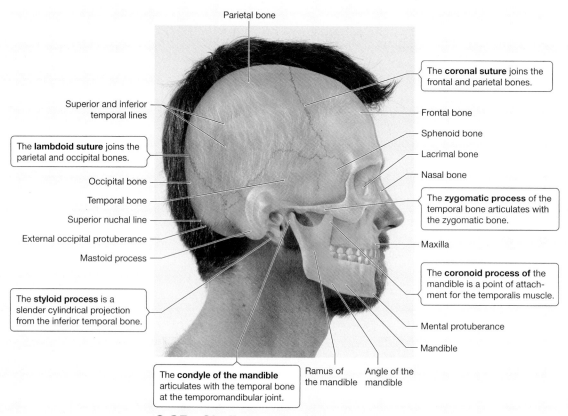

Parietal bone

The **coronal suture** joins the frontal and parietal bones.

Superior and inferior temporal lines

Frontal bone

Sphenoid bone

The **lambdoid suture** joins the parietal and occipital bones.

Lacrimal bone

Nasal bone

Occipital bone

Temporal bone

The **zygomatic process** of the temporal bone articulates with the zygomatic bone.

Superior nuchal line

External occipital protuberance

Maxilla

Mastoid process

The **coronoid process of** the mandible is a point of attach-ment for the temporalis muscle.

The **styloid process** is a slender cylindrical projection from the inferior temporal bone.

Mental protuberance

Mandible

The **condyle of the mandible** articulates with the temporal bone at the temporomandibular joint.

Ramus of the mandible

Angle of the mandible

6-2B. Skull, lateral view.

▶ SKELETAL STRUCTURES OF THE HEAD, NECK, AND FACE

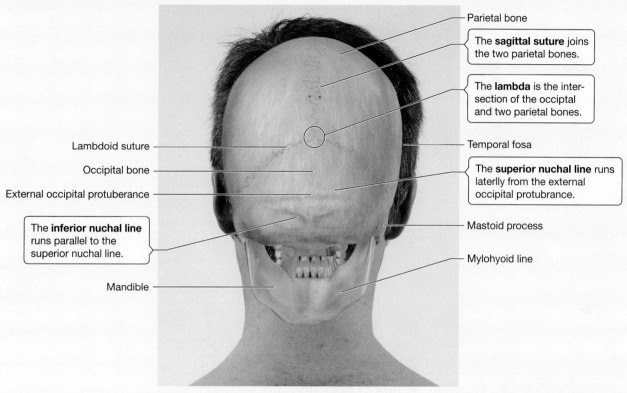

Parietal bone

The **sagittal suture** joins the two parietal bones.

The **lambda** is the inter-section of the occipital and two parietal bones.

Lambdoid suture

Occipital bone

External occipital protuberance

Temporal fosa

The **superior nuchal line** runs laterlly from the external occipital protubrance.

The **inferior nuchal line** runs parallel to the superior nuchal line.

Mastoid process

Mylohyoid line

Mandible

6-2C. Skull, posterior view.

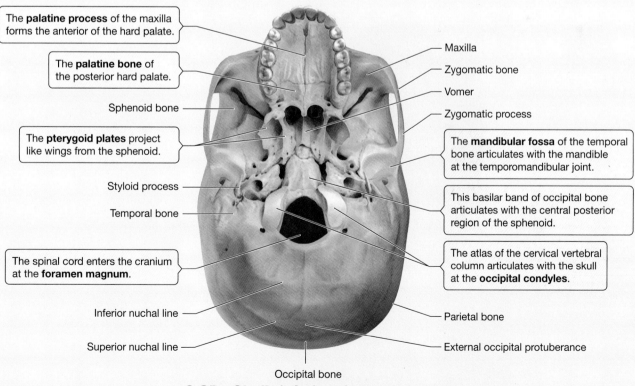

The **palatine process** of the maxilla forms the anterior of the hard palate.

The **palatine bone** of the posterior hard palate.

Sphenoid bone

The **pterygoid plates** project like wings from the sphenoid.

Styloid process

Temporal bone

The spinal cord enters the cranium at the **foramen magnum**.

Inferior nuchal line

Superior nuchal line

Maxilla

Zygomatic bone

Vomer

Zygomatic process

The **mandibular fossa** of the temporal bone articulates with the mandible at the temporomandibular joint.

This basilar band of occipital bone articulates with the central posterior region of the sphenoid.

The atlas of the cervical vertebral column articulates with the skull at the **occipital condyles**.

Parietal bone

External occipital protuberance

Occipital bone

6-2D. Skull, inferior view. (The mandible is not shown.)

▶ SKELETAL STRUCTURES OF THE HEAD, NECK, AND FACE

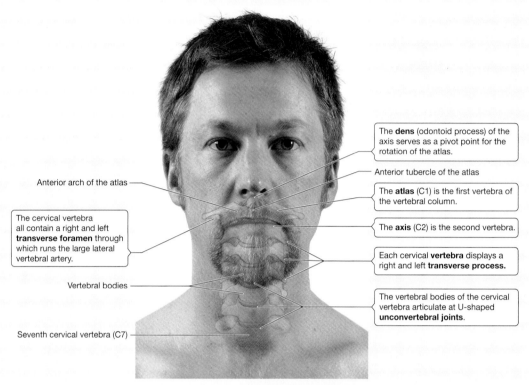

The **dens** (odontoid process) of the axis serves as a pivot point for the rotation of the atlas.

Anterior tubercle of the atlas

The **atlas** (C1) is the first vertebra of the vertebral column.

Anterior arch of the atlas

The **axis** (C2) is the second vertebra.

The cervical vertebra all contain a right and left **transverse foramen** through which runs the large lateral vertebral artery.

Each cervical **vertebra** displays a right and left **transverse process.**

Vertebral bodies

The vertebral bodies of the cervical vertebra articulate at U-shaped **unconvertebral joints**.

Seventh cervical vertebra (C7)

6-2E. Cervical vertebral column: anterior view.

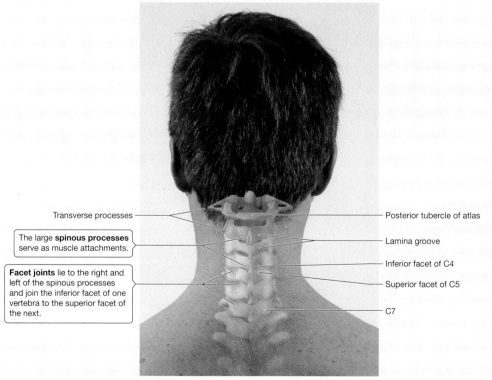

Transverse processes

Posterior tubercle of atlas

The large **spinous processes** serve as muscle attachments.

Lamina groove

Inferior facet of C4

Facet joints lie to the right and left of the spinous processes and join the inferior facet of one vertebra to the superior facet of the next.

Superior facet of C5

C7

6-2F. Cervical vertebral column: lateral view.

▶ SKELETAL STRUCTURES OF THE HEAD, NECK, AND FACE

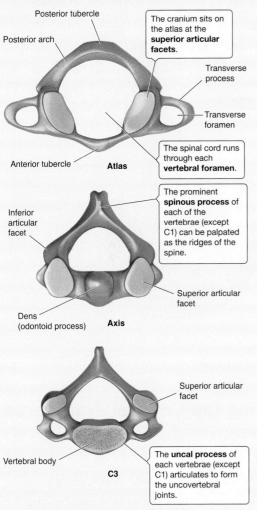

Posterior tubercle

Posterior arch

Transverse process

Transverse foramen

The cranium sits on the atlas at the **superior articular facets**.

Anterior tubercle **Atlas**

The spinal cord runs through each **vertebral foramen**.

Inferior articular facet

The prominent **spinous process** of each of the vertebrae (except C1) can be palpated as the ridges of the spine.

Superior articular facet

Dens (odontoid process) **Axis**

Superior articular facet

Vertebral body **C3**

The **uncal process** of each vertebrae (except C1) articulates to form the uncovertebral joints.

6-2G. Cervical vertebrae: Superior view.

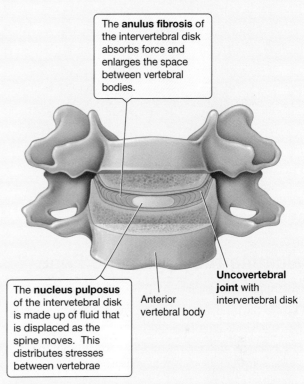

The **anulus fibrosis** of the intervertebral disk absorbs force and enlarges the space between vertebral bodies.

The **nucleus pulposus** of the intervetebral disk is made up of fluid that is displaced as the spine moves. This distributes stresses between vertebrae

Anterior vertebral body

Uncovertebral joint with intervertebral disk

6-2H. Cervical vertebrae: anterior view.

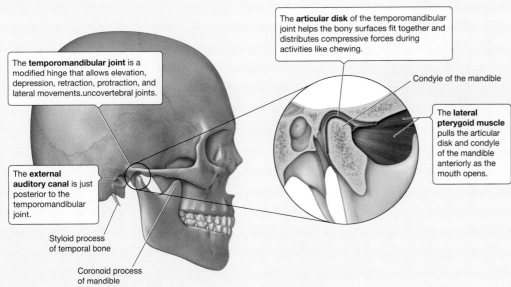

The **articular disk** of the temporomandibular joint helps the bony surfaces fit together and distributes compressive forces during activities like chewing.

Condyle of the mandible

The **lateral pterygoid muscle** pulls the articular disk and condyle of the mandible anteriorly as the mouth opens.

The **temporomandibular joint** is a modified hinge that allows elevation, depression, retraction, protraction, and lateral movements.uncovertebral joints.

The **external auditory canal** is just posterior to the temporomandibular joint.

Styloid process of temporal bone

Coronoid process of mandible

6-2I. Temperomandibular joint: lateral view.

▶ BONY LANDMARKS OF THE HEAD, NECK, AND FACE

Palpating the Temporal Fossa

Positioning: client supine.

1. Locate the junction of your client's head and the top of their ear with your four fingertips.
2. Slide your fingertips superiorly into the broad, shallow temporal fossa.

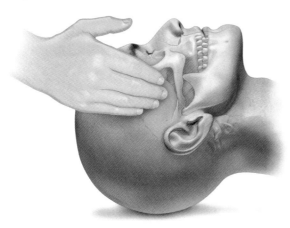

6-3A. **Temporal fossa**

Palpating the Zygomatic Bone

Positioning: client supine.

1. Locate the prominent ridge just anterior to your client's ear canal with your fingertips.
2. Slide fingers anteriorly across the cheek toward the nose, palpating the narrow zygomatic bone.

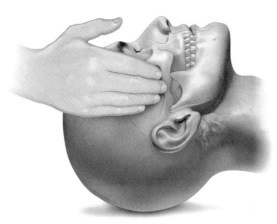

6-3B. **Zygomatic bone**

Palpating the Mastoid Process

Positioning: client supine.

1. Place the pad of one of your fingertips directly behind your client's ear.
2. Sweep the pad of your finger around the large, rounded mastoid process.

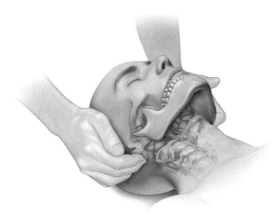

6-3C. **Mastoid process**

Palpating the Cervical Transverse Processes

Positioning: client supine.

1. Locate the mastoid process with your fingertips.
2. Slide fingers inferiorly and anteriorly onto the small, laterally protruding transverse process of C1.
3. Continue palpating inferiorly to find the vertically aligned transverse processes of C2–C7.

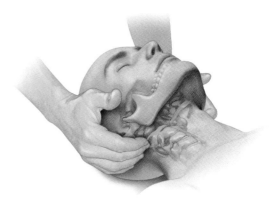

6-3D. **Cervical Transverse Processes**

Palpating the Cervical Spinous Processes

Positioning: client supine.

1. Cup your fingertips around the side of your client's head and palpate the midline of the cervical spine.

2. Gently probe the indented midline locating the posteriorly protruding spinous processes of C2–C7 (C1 spinous process is too small to palpate).

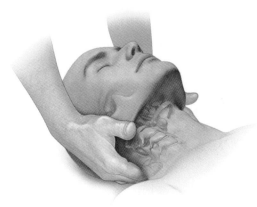

6-3E. **Cervical Spinous Processes**

Palpating the External Occipital Protuberance

Positioning: client supine.

1. Cup your fingertips under your client's head and onto the occiput.

2. Palpate the midline of the occiput, locating the bump marking the center of the superior nuchal line.

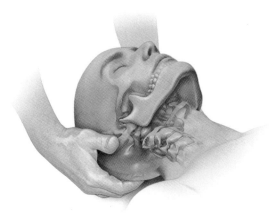

6-3F. **External Occipital Protuberance**

Palpating the Ramus and Angle of the Mandible

Positioning: client supine with jaw relaxed.

1. Locate the inferior edge of your client's zygomatic bone with your fingertips.

2. Slide your fingertips inferiorly onto the broad, flat ramus of the mandible and follow its surface where it curves anteriorly at the angle.

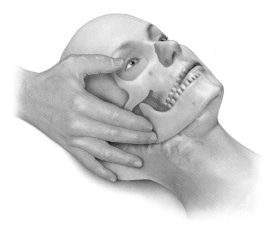

6-3G. **Ramus and Angle of Mandible**

Palpating the Coronoid Process of the Mandible

Positioning: client supine with jaw slightly depressed.

1. Locate the center of the zygomatic bone with the pad of one finger.

2. Slide your finger inferiorly as client depresses the mandible palpating the anteriorly protruding coronoid process.

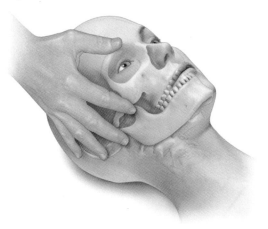

6-3H. **Coronoid Process of Mandible**

Palpating the Condyle of the Mandible

Positioning: client supine with mandible slightly depressed.

1. Locate the posterior edge of the zygomatic bone just anterior to the ear canal.
2. Instruct your client to depress the mandible as you slide your fingertips inferiorly. Palpate the condyle as it moves anterior and inferior.

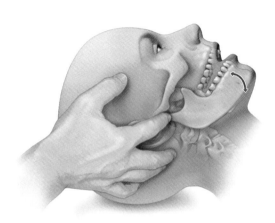

6-3I. **Condyle of Mandible**

Palpating the Submandibular Fossa

Positioning: client supine.

1. Locate the posterior edge of angle of the mandible with your fingertip.
2. Slide your fingertip deep behind the inferior edge of the mandible into the submandibular fossa.

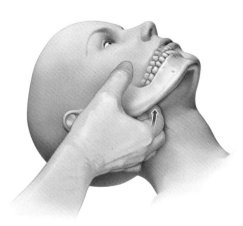

6-3J. **Submandibular Fossa**

Palpating the Hyoid Bone

Positioning: client supine.

1. Cup your index finger and thumb around the anterior neck just above the thyroid cartilage.
2. Gently pincer your thumb and finger, palpating the lateral edges of the slender hyoid bone.

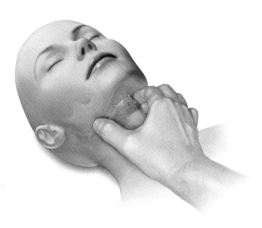

6-3K. **Hyoid Bone**

Palpating the Cervical Anterior Vertebral Bodies

Positioning: client supine.

1. Locate the depression between the thyroid cartilage and sternocleidomastoid muscle with your fingertips.
2. Palpate deeply between these two structures onto the flat, firm anterior vertebral bodies.

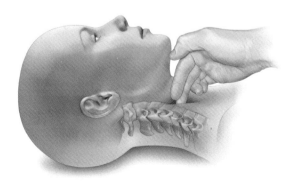

6-3L. **Cervical Anterior Vertebral Bodies**

❱ MUSCLE ATTACHMENT SITES

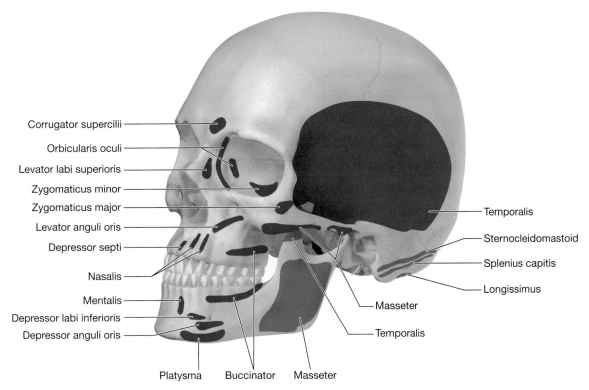

Corrugator supercilii
Orbicularis oculi
Levator labi superioris
Zygomaticus minor
Zygomaticus major
Levator anguli oris
Depressor septi
Nasalis
Mentalis
Depressor labi inferioris
Depressor anguli oris

Temporalis
Sternocleidomastoid
Splenius capitis
Longissimus
Masseter
Temporalis

Platysma   Buccinator   Masseter

6-4A. Skull muscle attachments: anterolateral view. When a muscle shortens, the insertion point (blue) tends to move toward the origin point (red). Shown here are the facial, cranial, and cervical muscles that attach to the front and side of the skull.

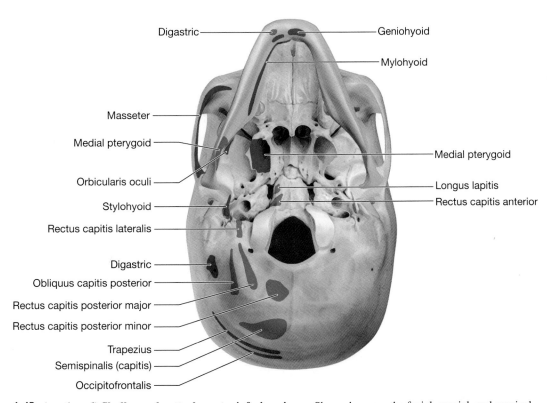

Digastric
Geniohyoid
Mylohyoid
Masseter
Medial pterygoid
Medial pterygoid
Orbicularis oculi
Longus lapitis
Rectus capitis anterior
Stylohyoid
Rectus capitis lateralis
Digastric
Obliquus capitis posterior
Rectus capitis posterior major
Rectus capitis posterior minor
Trapezius
Semispinalis (capitis)
Occipitofrontalis

6-4B. *(continued)* Skull muscle attachments: inferior view. Shown here are the facial, cranial, and cervical muscles that attach to the bottom of the skull. *(continues)*

❱ MUSCLE ATTACHMENT SITES

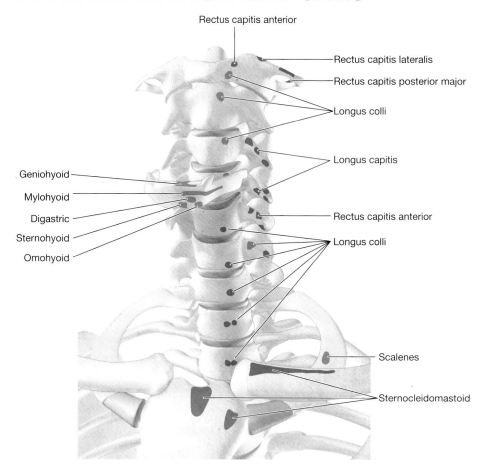

6-4C. *(continued)* **Cervical spine muscle attachments: anterior view.** Shown here are the facial, cranial, and cervical muscles that attach to the front of the spine, hyoid, and shoulder girdle.

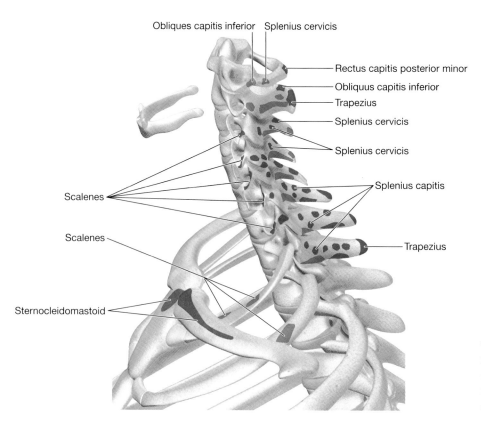

6-4D. *(continued)* **Cervical spine muscle attachments: lateral view.** Shown here are cranial and cervical muscles that attach to the side of the spine, hyoid, and shoulder girdle.

▶ MUSCLE ATTACHMENT SITES

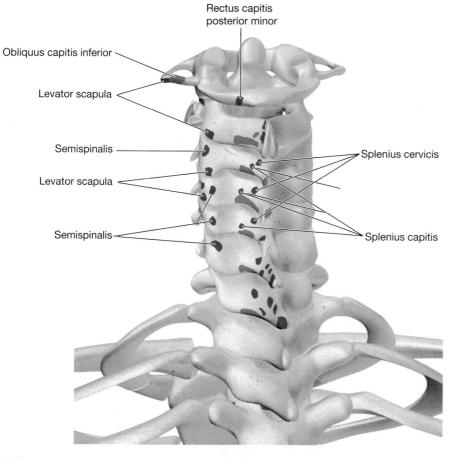

Rectus capitis
posterior minor

Obliquus capitis inferior

Levator scapula

Semispinalis

Splenius cervicis

Levator scapula

Semispinalis

Splenius capitis

6-4E. *(continued)* **Cervical spine muscle attachments: posterior view.**   Shown here are cranial and cervical muscles that attach to the back of the neck.

▶ LIGAMENTS OF THE HEAD, NECK, AND FACE

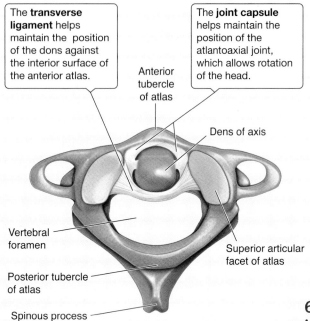

The **transverse ligament** helps maintain the position of the dons against the interior surface of the anterior atlas.

The **joint capsule** helps maintain the position of the atlantoaxial joint, which allows rotation of the head.

Anterior tubercle of atlas

Dens of axis

Vertebral foramen

Superior articular facet of atlas

Posterior tubercle of atlas

Spinous process of axis

6-5A. Transverse ligament of the atlantoaxial joint: superior view.

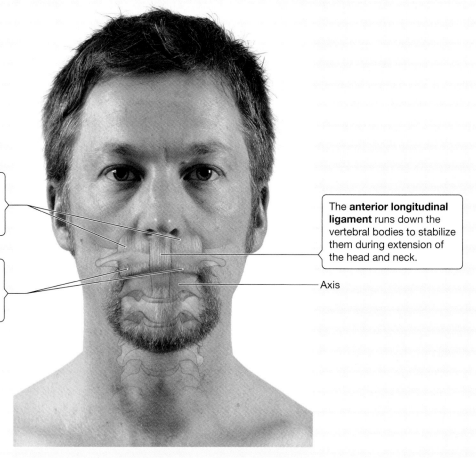

The **anterior atlanto-occipital membrane** and articular capsules connect and stablize the atlanto-occipital joint.

The **anterior atlantoaxial membrane** and articular capsules connect and stabilize the atlantoaxial joint.

The **anterior longitudinal ligament** runs down the vertebral bodies to stabilize them during extension of the head and neck.

Axis

6-5B. Cervical ligaments: anterior view.

▶ LIGAMENTS OF THE HEAD, NECK, AND FACE

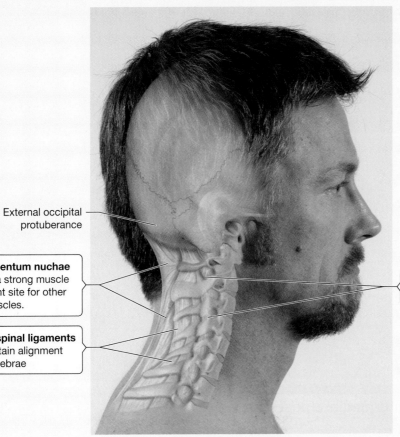

External occipital protuberance

The **ligamentum nuchae** provides a strong muscle attachment site for other spinal muscles.

The **ligamenta flava** help stabilize the neck.

The **interspinal ligaments** help maintain alignment of the vertebrae

6-5C. Cervical ligaments: lateral view.

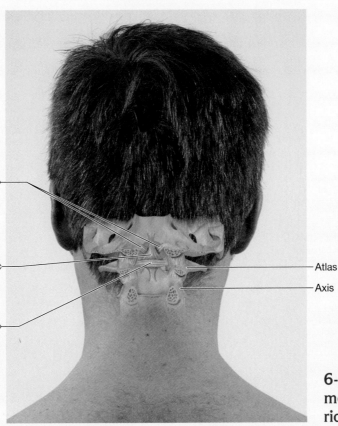

The deep, oblique, **alar ligaments** connect the occiput and atlas and prevent excessive rotation at the atlanto-occipital joint.

The **apical ligament** is a deep vertical ligament that limits vertical movement between the occiput, atlas, and axis.

The **cruciform ligament** is a deep ligament that helps the transverse ligament maintain the position of the dens against the interior surface of the anterior atlas.

Atlas

Axis

6-5D. Cervical ligaments: deep posterior view.

▶ LIGAMENTS OF THE HEAD, NECK, AND FACE

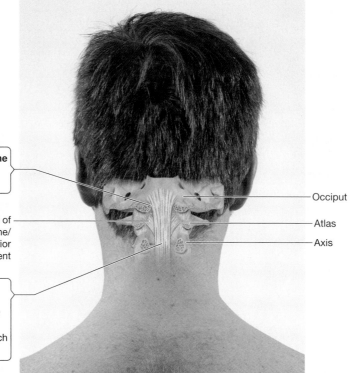

The broad, **tectorial membrane** attaches above the anterior edge of the foramen magnum.

Deep portions of tectorial membrane/ longitudinal posterior ligament

Occiput

Atlas

Axis

The tectorial membrane descends to form the **posterior longitudinal ligament** that connects the posterior vertebral bodies. This strong vertical ligament has deep portions that attach to the intervertebral disks.

6-5E. Cervical ligaments: intermediate posterior view.

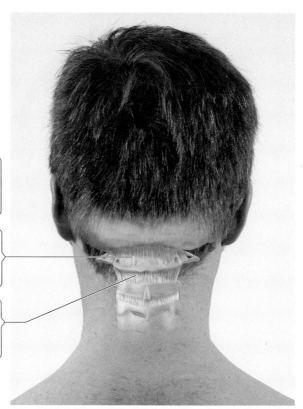

As with the front, two membranes stabilize the back of the upper neck. These structures are pulled taught during the flexion of the upper cervicals.

The **posterior atlanto-occipital membrane** and articular capsules connect and stablize the atlanto-occipital joint.

The **posterier atlantoaxial membrane** and the articular capsules connect and stabilize the atlantoaxial joint.

6-5F. Cervical ligaments: superficial posterior view.

LIGAMENTS OF THE HEAD, NECK, AND FACE

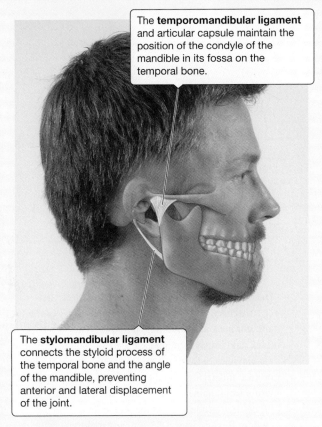

The **temporomandibular ligament** and articular capsule maintain the position of the condyle of the mandible in its fossa on the temporal bone.

The **stylomandibular ligament** connects the styloid process of the temporal bone and the angle of the mandible, preventing anterior and lateral displacement of the joint.

6-5G. Temporomandibular ligaments: lateral view.

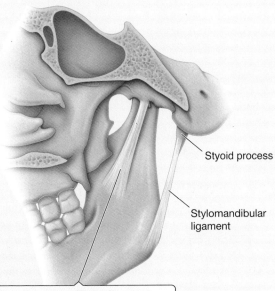

Styoid process

Stylomandibular ligament

The **sphenomandibular ligament**, along with the stylomandibular ligament, limits protraction and lateral movement of the mandible.

6-5H. Temporomandibular ligaments: medial view.

▶ SUPERFICIAL MUSCLES OF THE HEAD AND NECK

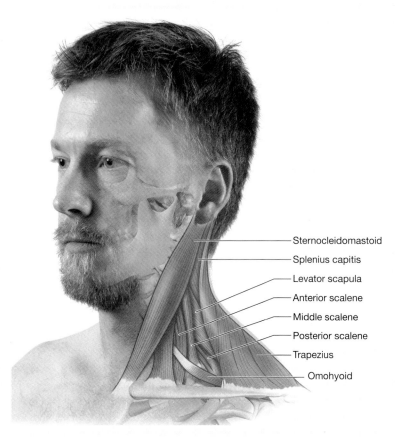

- Sternocleidomastoid
- Splenius capitis
- Levator scapula
- Anterior scalene
- Middle scalene
- Posterior scalene
- Trapezius
- Omohyoid

6-6A. Superficial cervical muscles: anterolateral view. The superficial muscles of the anterior neck serve multiple purposes. They are large, thick, and broad forming a cape-like structure spanning the clavicles, base of the skull, and upper spine. They protect underlying structures and suspend the shoulder girdle from the head. These large muscles on the front of the neck produce gross movement in this region including flexion, lateral flexion, and rotation.

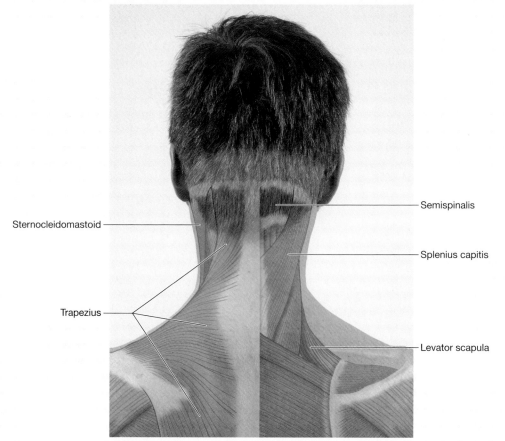

- Sternocleidomastoid
- Trapezius
- Semispinalis
- Splenius capitis
- Levator scapula

6-6B. Superficial cervical muscles: posterior view. The kite-shaped trapezius muscle dominates the posterior neck and can move the head, neck, and scapula. The sternocleidomastoid can be seen from the side and tips the head back, juts the head forward, laterally bends the head, and rotates the head away from the shoulder. Directly underneath the trapezius is the splenius capitis and splenius cervicis. These muscles extend, laterally bend, and rotate the head toward the shoulder.

▶ INTERMEDIATE MUSCLES OF THE HEAD AND NECK

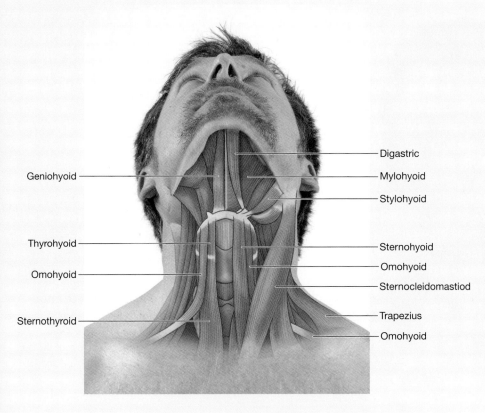

Geniohyoid

Thyrohyoid

Omohyoid

Sternothyroid

Digastric

Mylohyoid

Stylohyoid

Sternohyoid

Omohyoid

Sternocleidomastiod

Trapezius

Omohyoid

6-7A. Intermediate cervical muscles: anterior view. The muscles of swallowing dominate the central layer of muscle in the front of the neck. These include the suprahyoid and infrahyoid muscles, named for their relative location to the hyoid bone. This group of muscles assists during chewing, swallowing, and speaking.

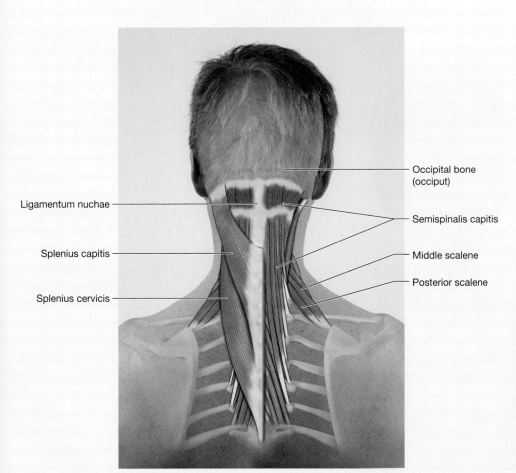

Ligamentum nuchae

Splenius capitis

Splenius cervicis

Occipital bone (occiput)

Semispinalis capitis

Middle scalene

Posterior scalene

6-7B. Intermediate cervical muscles: posterior view. The central layer of muscles in the back of the neck contains longer and broader muscles. These span multiple joints and produce gross movements in this region including extension, lateral flexion, and rotation.

▶ DEEP MUSCLES OF THE HEAD AND NECK

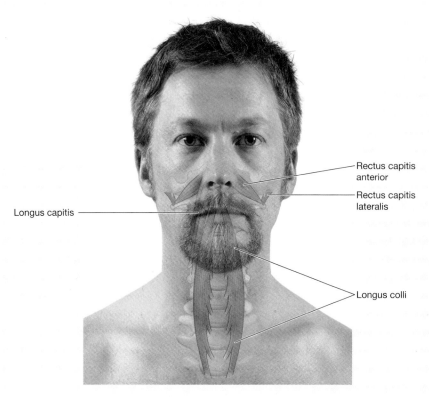

Rectus capitis anterior

Rectus capitis lateralis

Longus capitis

Longus colli

6-8A. Deep cervical muscles: anterior view. Several deep muscles connect the anterior surfaces of the skull and vertebrae. These muscles maintain the alignment of the cervical vertebrae and perform fine flexion and lateral flexion movements in this region.

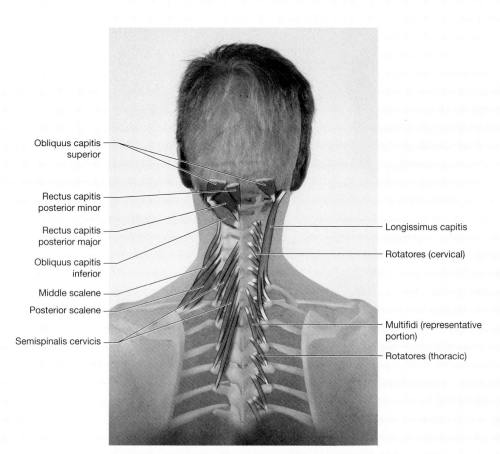

Obliquus capitis superior

Rectus capitis posterior minor

Rectus capitis posterior major

Obliquus capitis inferior

Middle scalene

Posterior scalene

Semispinalis cervicis

Longissimus capitis

Rotatores (cervical)

Multifidi (representative portion)

Rotatores (thoracic)

6-8B. Deep cervical muscles: posterior view. The suboccipital and semispinalis muscles of the neck work with the rotatores and multifidi, other deep spinal muscles (see Chapter 7), to stabilize the head and neck posteriorly. These small, specialized muscles maintain the alignment of the skull and cervical vertebrae. They also perform fine extension, lateral flexion, and rotational movements in this region.

MUSCLES OF THE FACE

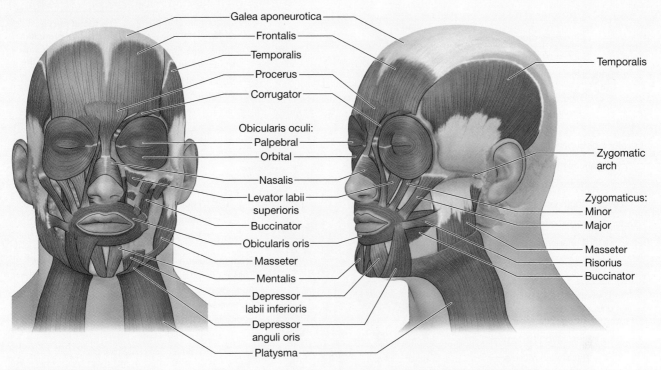

Galea aponeurotica
Frontalis
Temporalis
Procerus
Corrugator

Obicularis oculi:
Palpebral
Orbital

Nasalis
Levator labii superioris
Buccinator
Obicularis oris
Masseter
Mentalis
Depressor labii inferioris
Depressor anguli oris
Platysma

Temporalis

Zygomatic arch

Zygomaticus:
Minor
Major

Masseter
Risorius
Buccinator

6-9. Facial muscles. Several muscles produce facial expressions. Some are rounded or circular for closing the mouth or eyes. Others move the forehead, eyebrows, lips, cheeks, ears, and lips. There are even specialized muscles for moving the nostrils.

▶ SPECIAL STRUCTURES OF THE HEAD, NECK, AND FACE

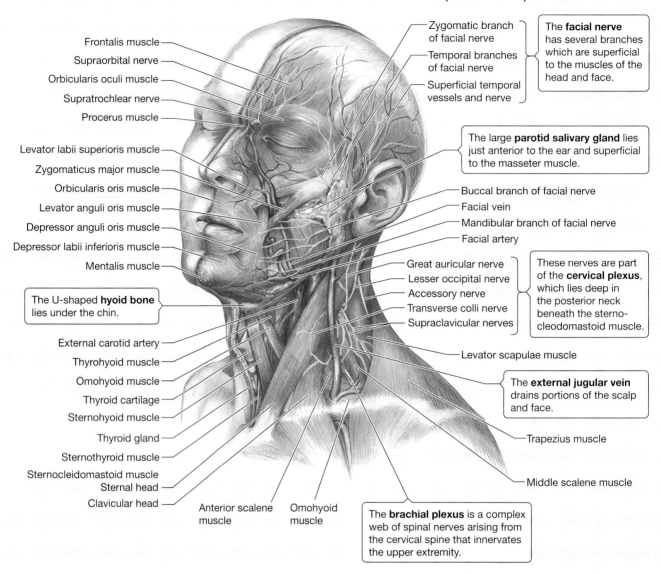

Frontalis muscle

Supraorbital nerve

Orbicularis oculi muscle

Supratrochlear nerve

Procerus muscle

Levator labii superioris muscle

Zygomaticus major muscle

Orbicularis oris muscle

Levator anguli oris muscle

Depressor anguli oris muscle

Depressor labii inferioris muscle

Mentalis muscle

Zygomatic branch of facial nerve

Temporal branches of facial nerve

Superficial temporal vessels and nerve

The **facial nerve** has several branches which are superficial to the muscles of the head and face.

The large **parotid salivary gland** lies just anterior to the ear and superficial to the masseter muscle.

Buccal branch of facial nerve

Facial vein

Mandibular branch of facial nerve

Facial artery

Great auricular nerve

Lesser occipital nerve

Accessory nerve

Transverse colli nerve

Supraclavicular nerves

These nerves are part of the **cervical plexus**, which lies deep in the posterior neck beneath the sterno-cleodomastoid muscle.

The U-shaped **hyoid bone** lies under the chin.

External carotid artery

Thyrohyoid muscle

Omohyoid muscle

Thyroid cartilage

Sternohyoid muscle

Thyroid gland

Sternothyroid muscle

Sternocleidomastoid muscle
Sternal head
Clavicular head

Anterior scalene muscle

Omohyoid muscle

Levator scapulae muscle

The **external jugular vein** drains portions of the scalp and face.

Trapezius muscle

Middle scalene muscle

The **brachial plexus** is a complex web of spinal nerves arising from the cervical spine that innervates the upper extremity.

6-10A. Blood vessels, glands, and other structures of the face and neck: superficial anterolateral view.

▶ SPECIAL STRUCTURES OF THE HEAD, NECK, AND FACE

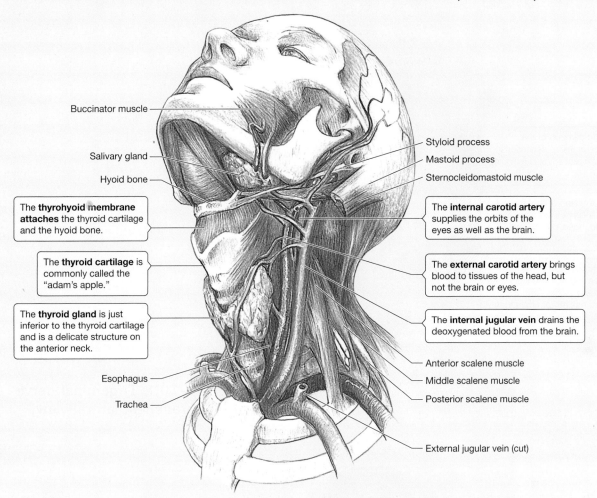

Buccinator muscle

Salivary gland

Hyoid bone

The **thyrohyoid membrane attaches** the thyroid cartilage and the hyoid bone.

The **thyroid cartilage** is commonly called the "adam's apple."

The **thyroid gland** is just inferior to the thyroid cartilage and is a delicate structure on the anterior neck.

Esophagus

Trachea

Styloid process

Mastoid process

Sternocleidomastoid muscle

The **internal carotid artery** supplies the orbits of the eyes as well as the brain.

The **external carotid artery** brings blood to tissues of the head, but not the brain or eyes.

The **internal jugular vein** drains the deoxygenated blood from the brain.

Anterior scalene muscle

Middle scalene muscle

Posterior scalene muscle

External jugular vein (cut)

6-10B. Blood vessels, glands, and other structures of the neck: deep antero-lateral view.

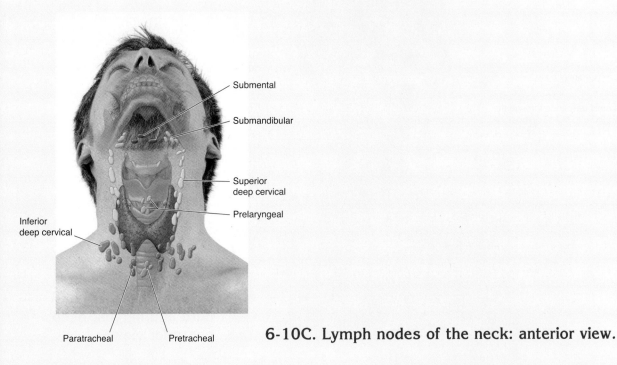

Submental

Submandibular

Superior deep cervical

Prelaryngeal

Inferior deep cervical

Paratracheal   Pretracheal

6-10C. Lymph nodes of the neck: anterior view.

▶ SPECIAL STRUCTURES OF THE HEAD, NECK, AND FACE

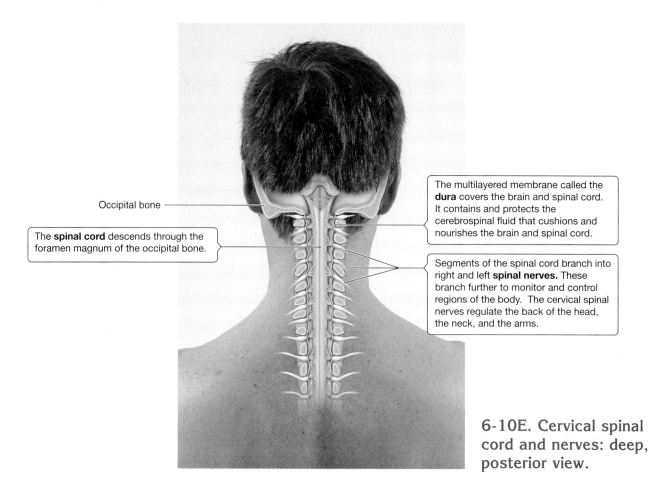

The **ophthalmic division** of the trigeminal nerve picks up sensations from the scalp, forehead, upper eyelid, and nose.

The **maxillary division** of the trigeminal nerve senses impulses from the lower eyelid, nose, mouth, and cheek.

The **mandibular division** of the trigeminal nerve transmits sensory data from the lower teeth, chin , and the temples. It also has motor fibers that help regulate chewing and swallowing.

Trigeminal nerve

6-10D. Trigeminal nerve branches: lateral view.

Occipital bone

The **spinal cord** descends through the foramen magnum of the occipital bone.

The multilayered membrane called the **dura** covers the brain and spinal cord. It contains and protects the cerebrospinal fluid that cushions and nourishes the brain and spinal cord.

Segments of the spinal cord branch into right and left **spinal nerves.** These branch further to monitor and control regions of the body. The cervical spinal nerves regulate the back of the head, the neck, and the arms.

6-10E. Cervical spinal cord and nerves: deep, posterior view.

▶ SPECIAL STRUCTURES OF THE HEAD, NECK, AND FACE

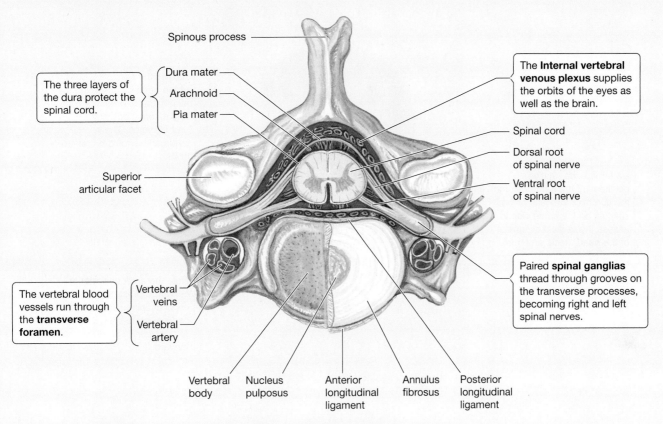

Spinous process

Dura mater

Arachnoid

Pia mater

The three layers of the dura protect the spinal cord.

The **Internal vertebral venous plexus** supplies the orbits of the eyes as well as the brain.

Spinal cord

Dorsal root of spinal nerve

Ventral root of spinal nerve

Superior articular facet

Paired **spinal ganglias** thread through grooves on the transverse processes, becoming right and left spinal nerves.

The vertebral blood vessels run through the **transverse foramen**.

Vertebral veins

Vertebral artery

Vertebral body

Nucleus pulposus

Anterior longitudinal ligament

Annulus fibrosus

Posterior longitudinal ligament

6-10F. Integrated cervical structures: superior view.

▶ POSTURE OF THE HEAD AND NECK

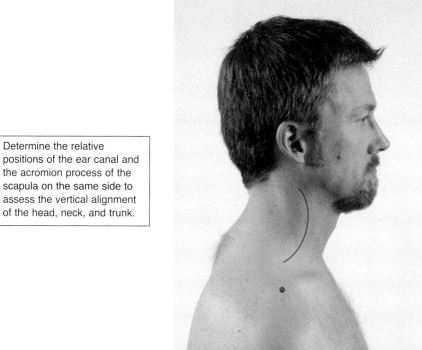

Determine the relative positions of the ear canal and the acromion process of the scapula on the same side to assess the vertical alignment of the head, neck, and trunk.

Assess the horizontal position of the head by observing the alignment between the eyes and external occipital protuberance. These landmarks should be relatively level.

Note the anterior/posterior curvature present in the cervical spine. Normally, the cervical spine should have a *lordotic curve*, or round forward.

A

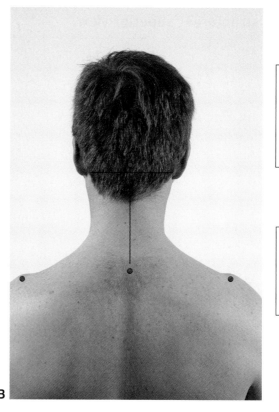

Assess the horizontal position of the head by comparing the position of the right and left earlobes. This helps determine if the head is level, laterally flexed to one side, or rotated.

Assess the vertical alignment of the head and neck by observing whether the external occipital protuberance is centered over the spinous processes of the cervical vertebrae.

Observe the distance between each earlobe and the acromion process of the scapula to further establish horizontal alignment of the head and neck.

B

6-11A. **Lateral view.** Use the lateral view to assess posture in the sagittal plane. **B. Posterior view.** Use the posterior view to assess posture in the frontal and transverse planes.

▶ MOVEMENTS AVAILABLE: NECK

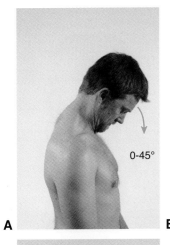

A

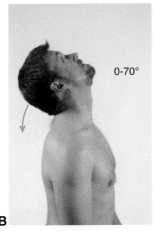

B

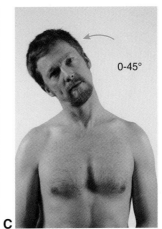

C

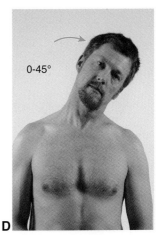

D

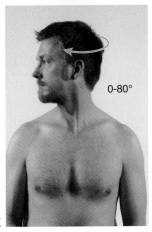

E

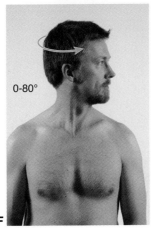

F

6-12 **A.** Cervical flexion. **B.** Cervical extension. **C.** Cervical lateral flexion: right. **D.** Cervical lateral flexion: left.
E. Cervical rotation: right. **F.** Cervical rotation: left.

▶ MOVEMENTS AVAILABLE: JAW

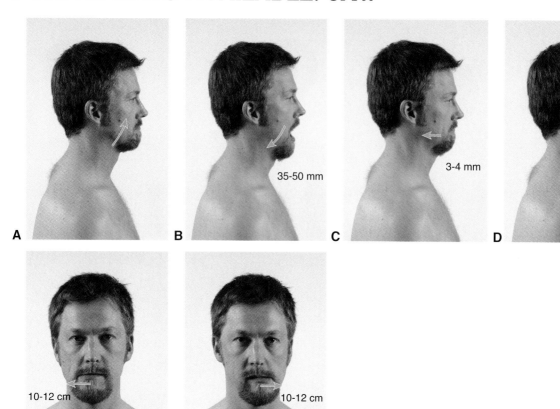

6-13 **A.** Temporomandibular elevation. **B.** Temporomandibular depression. **C.** Temporomandibular retraction.
D. Temporomandibular protraction. **E.** Temporomandibular lateral deviation: right. **F.** Temporomandibular lateral deviation: left.

FACIAL EXPRESSION

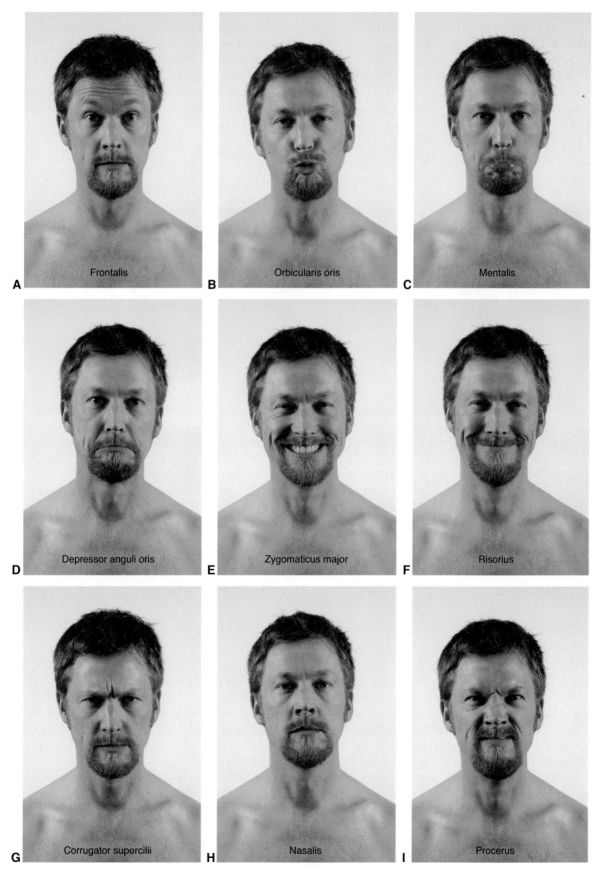

6-14 A–I. **Muscles of facial expression.**

❯ PASSIVE RANGE OF MOTION

Performing passive range of motion in the cervical spine helps establish the health and function of the inert structures, such as the intervertebral ligaments and joint capsules, as well as the larger ligaments, such as the nuchal ligament. It also allows you to evaluate the relative movements between the individual vertebral joints.

The client should be lying supine on a massage or examination table. Ask the client to relax and allow you to perform the ROM exercises without the client "helping." This can be particularly challenging in the cervical spine. Be sure to support the head with both hands to assure the client that passive movements are safe.

For each of the movements illustrated below, take the head and neck through to endfeel while watching for compensation (extraneous movement) in the shoulder or trunk. Procedures for performing passive ROM are described toward the end of Chapter 3.

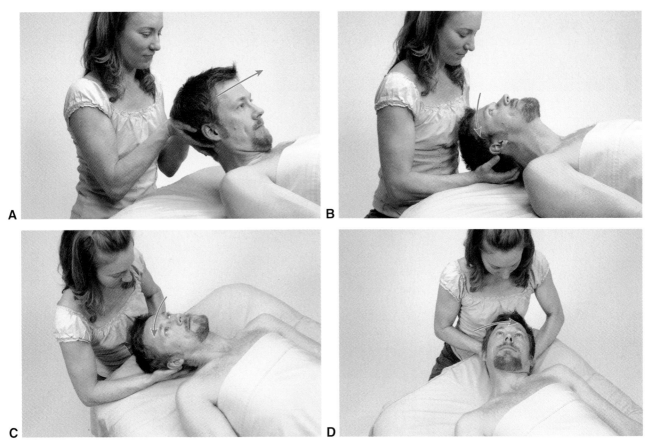

6-15 A. Passive cervical flexion. The arrow indicates the direction of movement. Sit at the head of the table. Hold the back of the client's head with the palms of both hands. Instruct the client to remain relaxed as you lift their head off the table and bring their chin toward their chest. Assess the ROM of the posterior cervical ligaments, joint capsules, and muscles that extend the head and neck. B. Passive cervical extension. Sit at the head of the table. Hold the back of the client's head with the palms of both hands. Instruct the client to remain relaxed as you tip their head back. Assess the ROM of the anterior cervical ligaments, joint capsules, and muscles that flex the head and neck. C. Passive cervical lateral flexion: right. Sit at the head of the table. Hold the back of the client's head with the palms of both hands. Instruct the client to remain relaxed as you gently tip their head toward their right shoulder. Maintain client's face up to avoid rotating the head. Assess the ROM of the left lateral cervical ligaments, joint capsules, and muscles that laterally flex the head and neck to the left. D. Passive cervical lateral flexion: left. Sit at the head of the table. Hold the back of the client's head with the palms of both hands. Instruct the client to remain relaxed as you gently tip their head toward their left shoulder. Their head remains supported by the table as you move it. Maintain client's face up to avoid rotating the head. Assess the ROM of the right lateral cervical ligaments, joint capsules, and muscles that laterally flex the head and neck to the right. *(continues)*

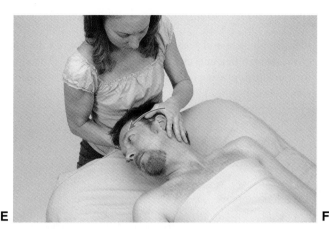

E

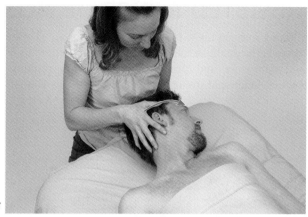

F

6-15 *(continued)* E. **Passive cervical rotation: right.** Sit at the head of the table. Hold the back of the client's head with the palms of both hands. Instruct the client to remain relaxed as you gently rotate their head toward their right shoulder. Their head remains supported by the table as you move it. Maintain client's head straight up and down to avoid laterally flexing the head. Assess the ROM of the alar, cruciform, and transverse ligaments, joint capsules, and muscles that rotate the head and neck to the left. F. **Passive cervical rotation: left.** Sit at the head of the table. Hold the back of the client's head with the palms of both hands. Instruct the client to remain relaxed as you gently rotate their head toward their left shoulder. Their head remains supported by the table as you move it. Maintain client's head straight up and down to avoid laterally flexing the head. Assess the ROM of the alar, cruciform, and transverse ligaments, joint capsules, and muscles that rotate the head and neck to the right.

▶ RESISTED RANGE OF MOTION

Performing resisted range of motion (ROM) for the cervical spine helps establish the health and function of the dynamic stabilizers and prime movers in this region. Evaluating functional strength and endurance helps you to identify balance and potential imbalance between the muscles that stabilize and move the head and neck. Procedures for performing and grading resisted ROM are outlined in Chapter 3.

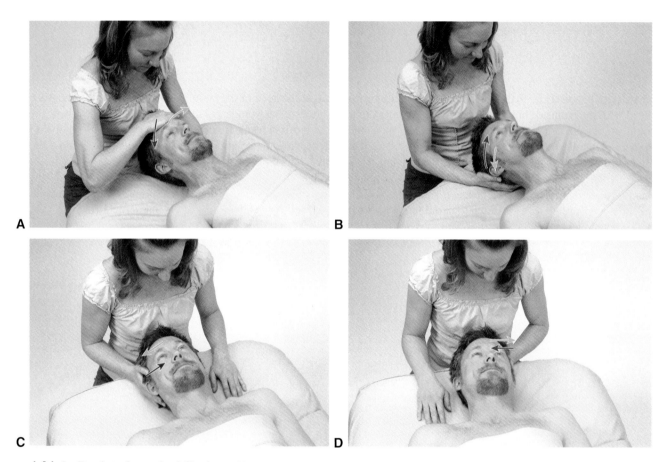

A

B

C

D

6-16 A. Resisted cervical flexion. Sit at client's side facing them. Place one hand on the client's forehead as the table stabilizes their body. Instruct the client to meet your resistance by pushing their forehead up and tuck their chin as you gently but firmly press the forehead down. Assess the strength and endurance of the muscles that flex the head and neck. B. Resisted cervical extension. Sit at client's side facing them. Place one hand on the back of the client's head as the table stabilizes their body. Instruct the client to meet your resistance by pushing their forehead back and looking up as you gently but firmly press the head down. Assess the strength and endurance of the muscles that extend the head and neck. C. Resisted cervical lateral flexion: right. Sit at client's head facing them. Place one hand on the right side of the client's head as the table stabilizes their body. Instruct the client to meet your resistance by pushing their head to the right (keeping their face forward) as you gently but firmly press their head to the left. Assess the strength and endurance of the muscles that laterally flex the head and neck to the right. D. Resisted cervical lateral flexion: left. Sit at client's head facing them. Place one hand on the left side of the client's head as the table stabilizes their body. Instruct the client to meet your resistance by pushing their head to the left (keeping their face forward) as you gently but firmly press their head to the right. Assess the strength and endurance of the muscles that laterally flex the head and neck to the left. *(continues)*

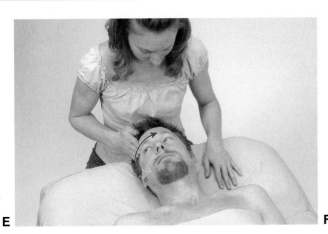

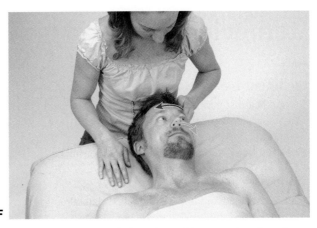

E   F

6-16 *(continued)* **E. Resisted cervical rotation: right.** Sit at client's head facing them. Place one hand on the right side of the client's head as the table stabilizes their body. Instruct the client to meet your resistance by turning their head to the right (keeping their head and neck straight up and down) as you gently but firmly turn their head to the left. Assess the strength and endurance of the muscles that rotate the head and neck to the right. **F. Resisted cervical rotation: left.** Sit at the client's head facing them. Place one hand on the left side of the client's head as the table stabilizes their body. Instruct the client to meet your resistance by turning their head to the left (keeping their head and neck straight up and down) as you gently but firmly turn their head to the right. Assess the strength and endurance of the muscles that rotate the head and neck to the left.

Sternocleidomastoid

ster'no klı do mas'toyd • Greek "**sternon**" *chest* "**kleis**" *clavicle* "**mastos**" *breast* "**eidos**" *resemblance*

Attachments

O: Sternal head: superior manubrium
O: Clavicular head: medial one-third
I: Temporal bone, lateral mastoid process
I: Occipital bone, lateral one-half of superior nuchal line

Actions

- Extends the head and upper cervicals (bilateral action)
- Flexes the neck (bilateral action)
- Laterally flexes the head and neck (unilateral action)
- Rotates the head and neck toward opposite side (unilateral action)

Innervation

- Accesory nerve
- C1 and C2

Functional Anatomy

The sternocleidomastoid is one of the largest and most superficial muscles in the neck. It has two heads and connects the mastoid process of the temporal bone to the manubrium of the sternum and medial clavicle. The sternocleidomastoid runs parallel to the ramus of the mandible and forms an inverted "v" with the splenius capitis. Together, these two muscles center the head front-to-back over the shoulder girdle.

Sternocleidomastoid's strong attachment to the mastoid process of the temporal bone and oblique position on the neck make it a powerful prime mover for flexion, lateral flexion, and rotation of the head and neck. Because it attaches to the back of the skull, it is able to extend the head and upper cervicals. This combination of flexion of the neck and extension of the head creates head movement forward, leading with the chin. Tightness in this muscle, if bilateral, can lead to a forward head posture and, if unilateral, to a condition called *torticollis* (a laterally flexed and rotated neck).

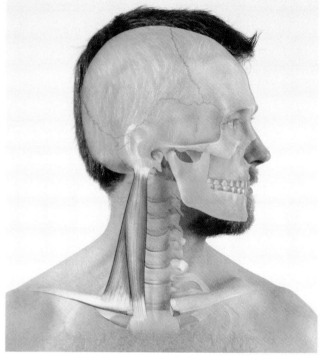

6-17

Palpating Sternocleidomastoid

Positioning: client supine.

1. Sitting at the client's head, slightly rotate the head to the opposite side to slack tissue.

2. Locate the mastoid process with the thumb and slide anteriorly and caudally onto the thick sternocleidomastoid muscle.

3. Gently pincer-grasp the muscle belly and follow it caudally toward the sternum, differentiating between the medial sternal head and lateral clavicular head.

4. Client gently resists flexion to ensure proper location.

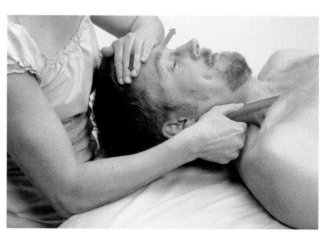

6-18

Scalenes ● *ska len'* • Greek "**skalenos**" *uneven*

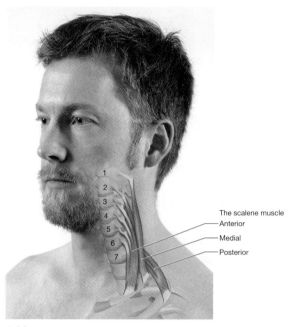

The scalene muscle
- Anterior
- Medial
- Posterior

6-19

Palpating Scalenes

Positioning: client supine.

1. Sitting at your client's head, locate with your fingertips the cervical transverse processes in the space between the trapezius and sternocleidomastoid.

2. Slide your fingertips caudally, following the slender, stringy fibers of the scalenes. *(Caution: the brachial plexus is located in this region. To avoid nerve damage or client discomfort, don't press too firmly on the ropey nerves.)*

3. Follow the fibers of the scalenes toward their attachments on the 1st and 2nd ribs.

4. Client gently resists lateral flexion of the neck to ensure proper location.

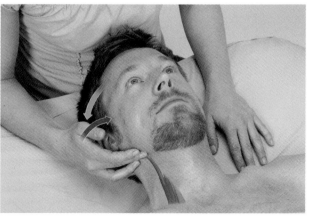

6-20

Attachments

O: C3–C6, anterior tubercles of transverse processes *(anterior)*

O: C2–C7, posterior tubercles of transverse processes *(middle)*

O: C5–C7, posterior tubercles of transverse processes *(posterior)*

I: 1st rib, inner upper edge *(anterior)*

I: 1st rib, outer upper edge *(middle)*

I: 2nd rib, lateral surface *(posterior)*

Actions

- Flexes the head and neck (bilateral action) *anterior only*
- Laterally flexes the head and neck (unilateral action)
- Rotates the head and neck toward opposite side (unilateral action)
- Elevates 1st and 2nd rib during forced inhalation (see Chapter 7)

Innervation

- Cervical spinal nerves C6–8

Functional Anatomy

The scalenes consist of three parts: the anterior, middle, and posterior scalenes. They are located laterally on the neck. A "window" to the scalenes is found between the anterior edge of the upper trapezius and the posterior border of the sternocleidomastoid. All of these large muscles work together to laterally flex and stabilize the head and neck. They also form a protective cape surrounding deeper structures such as the vertebral artery, jugular vein, and brachial plexus.

The scalenes branch to attach to the second rib laterally and the first rib laterally and anteriorly. This dispersion of insertions allows the anterior scalene to flex and rotate the head and neck while the other portions laterally flex.

When the head and neck are fixed, the scalenes can elevate the first and second rib during inhalation. This elevation increases the space in the thoracic cavity, prompting greater inflow of air to the lungs. This occurs more often during labored breathing, as the diaphragm (see Chapter 7) is responsible for normal, relaxed breathing. Labored breathing is common during heavy exercise or with pulmonary pathology such as asthma.

Excessive tightness, hypertrophy (e.g., from overuse), trauma, or structural abnormality of the scalenes can lead to compression of the structures it protects, such as the brachial plexus or subclavian artery. This general pathology is called *thoracic outlet syndrome.*

Platysma · *pla tiz'ma* · Greek "**platy**" *flat*

Attachments
O: Fascia of superior pectoralis major and deltoid muscles
I: Mandible, inferior border

Actions
• Flexes the head and neck (bilateral action)

Innervation
• Facial nerve

Functional Anatomy

Platysma functions primarily in facial expression. It is the most superficial muscle of the anterior neck and extends from the mandible and fascia of the face. Its insertion is not bony; rather, it is attached to the fascia of the chest and the anterior shoulder girdle.

Platysma is a flat, continuous sheet of muscle (generally termed a *panniculus muscle*). Panniculus muscles are found in many animals and perform functions like flicking flies or raising hair. In humans, platysma draws the lower lip downward and laterally while creating ridges or wrinkles in the skin of the neck and chest. This action characterizes facial expressions of stress or anger.

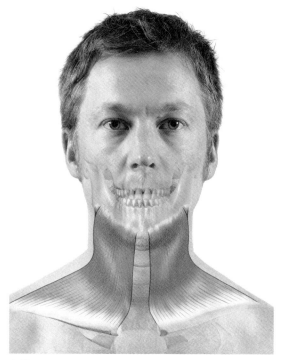

6-21

Palpating Platysma

Positioning: client supine.

1. Sitting at the client's head, locate the superficial flesh on the front of the neck with your fingertips.

2. Have the client draw the lower lip down and make a big frown.

3. Gently palpate the ridges formed between the mandible and chest by the platysma muscle.

4. Client gently resists flexion to further ensure proper location.

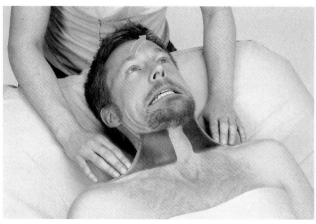

6-22

Longus Colli   • long'gus kol'ı • Latin "**longus**" *long* "**colli**" *neck*

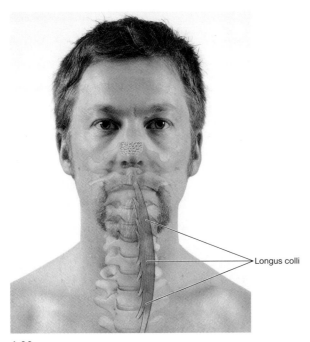

Longus colli

6-23

Palpating Longus Colli

Positioning: client supine.

1. Sitting at client's head, locate the sternocleidomastoid with the fingertips of one hand.

2. Slide fingertips medially into the space between the sternocleidomastoid and the trachea. *(Caution: the thyroid gland and carotid arteries are located in this region. To avoid causing the client discomfort or damaging these structures, be careful to palpate just medial to the muscle.)*

3. Curl fingertips and palpate deep against the vertebral body to find the vertical fibers of longus colli (between C1 and T3).

4. Client gently resists flexion of the neck to ensure proper location.

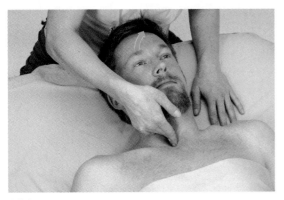

6-24

Attachments

O: C3–C5, anterior tubercles of transverse processes and C5–T3, anterior surface of bodies

I: C2–C6, anterior surfaces

Actions

• Flexes the head and neck (bilateral action)
• Laterally flexes the head and neck (unilateral action)
• Rotates the head and neck toward same side (unilateral action)

Innervation

• C2–C7

Functional Anatomy

The deepest of the anterior neck muscles, the longus colli is long and primarily vertical with multiple segments. It creates an interconnecting network between the anterior surfaces of the cervical and upper thoracic vertebrae. This muscle is a strong flexor of the head and neck when both sides fire, as it spans all of the cervical vertebrae and is segmented.

The longus colli is often associated with the rectus capitis anterior and rectus capitis lateralis as the *paravertebral group*. This group helps stabilize the anterior neck during high-intensity activities like sneezing and rapid arm movements like throwing. It also actively stabilizes the front of the curve of the neck, keeping the head from falling back.

Longus colli is clearly divided into right and left sides with a gap at the midline of the vertebral bodies. This creates some leverage for lateral flexion. Slight horizontal fiber orientation in its superior and inferior segments generates slight rotation to the opposite side when longus colli fires unilaterally.

Longus Capitis • *long'gus* kap'i tis • Latin "**longus**" *long* "**capitis**" *head*

Attachments

O: C3–C6, anterior tubercles of transverse processes
I: Occipital bone, inferior surface of basilar part

Actions

- Flexes the head and neck (bilateral action)
- Rotates the head and neck toward same side (unilateral action)

Innervation

- C1–C3

Functional Anatomy

Like longus colli, the longus capitis is deep to the hyoid bone, suprahyoid muscles, trachea, and esophagus. Its fibers lie more superiorly and run more obliquely than those of longus colli and connect the occiput to the transverse processes of the middle cervical vertebrae. This oblique fiber orientation gives longus capitis better leverage for rotation when firing one side at a time. Longus capitis also is one of several muscles that attaches to the occiput and affects positioning and movement at the atlanto-occipital joint.

    Like longus colli, longus capitis is part of the paravertebral group. This group helps stabilize the anterior neck and keep the head from falling back.

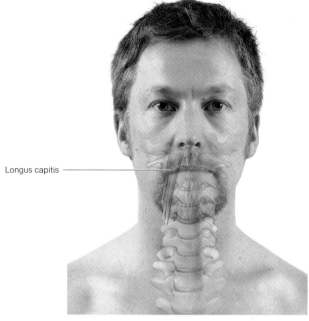

Longus capitis

6-25

Palpating Longus Capitis

Positioning: client supine.

1. Sitting at client's head, locate the sternocleidomastoid with the fingertips of one hand.

2. Slide fingertips medially into the space between sternocleidomastoid and the trachea. *(Caution: the thyroid gland and carotid arteries are located in this region, so be sure to palpate just medial to the muscle.)*

3. Curl fingertips and palpate deep against the vertebral body to find the vertical fibers of longus capitis (superiorly from C5).

4. Client gently resists flexion of the neck to ensure proper location.

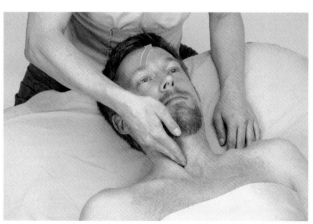

6-26

Suprahyoids ● *su pra hı oyds* • Greek "**supra**" *above* "**hyoeides**" *u-shaped*

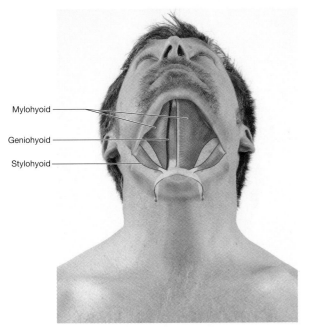

Mylohyoid

Geniohyoid

Stylohyoid

6-27

Palpating Suprahyoids

Positioning: client supine.

1. Sitting at the client's head, locate the underside of the mandible with fingertips. (Client's jaw should be closed, but relaxed.)

2. Slide fingertips posteriorly as client presses their tongue onto the roof of their mouth. *(Caution: the submandibular salivary gland is located in this region. It has a lumpy texture. Avoid pressing firmly on it because doing so could damage this structure.)*

3. Curl fingertips and palpate deeply, following the suprahyoids caudally and posteriorly toward the hyoid bone.

4. Client swallows to ensure proper location.

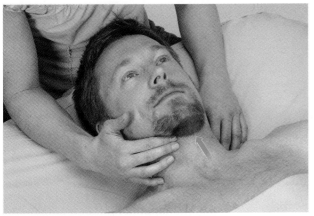

6-28

Attachments

O: Mandible, underside *(geniohyoid and mylohyoid)*
O: Temporal bone, styloid process *(stylohyoid)*
I: Hyoid bone

Actions

• Depress the mandible
• Elevate the hyoid bone and tongue

Innervation

• Hypoglossal nerve *(geniohyoid)*
• Mylohyoid nerve *(mylohyoid)*
• Facial nerve *(stylohyoid)*

Functional Anatomy

The suprahyoid muscle group is composed of the mylohyoid, geniohyoid, and stylohyoid muscles. Each has an attachment to the hyoid bone, a small, u-shaped bone suspended between the mandible and larynx. Together with the digastric, these muscles elevate the hyoid bone and thyroid cartilage during swallowing. They also cocontract with their antagonists, the infrahyoids, to fix the hyoid during chewing.

Besides functioning during chewing and swallowing, the suprahyoids play an important role in speech. The position of the larynx affects the frequency (pitch) and tonal quality of sounds generated by the vocal cords. The suprahyoids help position the larynx, influencing sound production.

Finally, the suprahyoids serve as a weak flexor of the neck when the hyoid bone is fixed. Compared with larger muscles like the sternocleidomastoid, platysma, scalenes, and longus colli, the contribution of the suprahyoids to flexion is minimal.

Digastric • *dɪ gas'trɪk* • Greek "**di**" *two* "**gaster**" *belly*

Attachments

O: Mandible, inferior border near symphysis *(anterior belly)*
O: Temporal bone, mastoid process *(posterior belly)*
I: Hyoid bone

Actions

• Depresses the mandible
• Elevates and pulls the hyoid anteriorly *(anterior belly)*
• Elevates and pulls the hyoid posteriorly *(posterior belly)*

Innervation

• Trigeminal nerve *(anterior belly)*
• Facial nerve *(posterior belly)*

Functional Anatomy

The digastric is unusual in that it descends from the mastoid process of the temporal bone to the hyoid bone posteriorly. From here it bends at the hyoid and ascends to the inner surface of the mandible anteriorly. There is no actual attachment to the hyoid bone; rather, its central tendon runs under a ligamentous sling superiorly on the hyoid. This tethering action allows the digastric to elevate the hyoid when contracted.

Fixation of the different attachments of the digastric also influences its function. If the temporal bone is fixed, the posterior belly of the digastric pulls the hyoid posteriorly. If the mandible is fixed, the anterior belly of the digastric pulls the hyoid anteriorly. These movements of the hyoid are utilized in chewing, swallowing, and speech.

When the hyoid bone is fixed, the digastric depresses and retracts the mandible. These fine mandibular movements also contribute to chewing, swallowing, and speech and can be utilized to establish location during palpation.

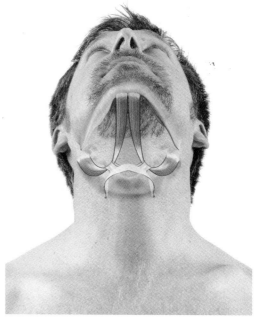

6-29

Palpating the Digastric

Positioning: client supine.

1. Sitting at the client's head, locate the space between the mastoid process and the ramus of the mandible with fingertips.
2. Slide fingertips deep to locate the narrow fibers of the posterior digastric.
3. Follow the fibers of digastric toward the hyoid bone, then pick up the anterior fibers as they traverse the underside of the chin.
4. Client gently resists mandibular depression to ensure proper location.

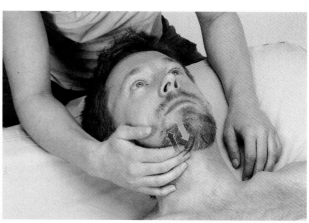

6-30

Infrahyoids
in *fra* hɪ oyds • Greek "**infra**" *below* "**hyoeides**" *u-shaped*

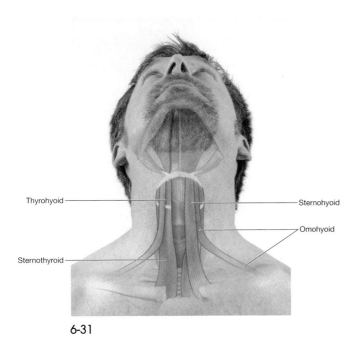

Thyrohyoid

Sternohyoid

Omohyoid

Sternothyroid

6-31

Palpating Infrahyoids

Positioning: client supine.

1. Sitting at the client's head, locate the lateral edge of the trachea, just below the thyroid cartilage (Adam's apple) with fingertips.

2. Slide fingertips caudally and laterally toward the sternocleidomastoid while remaining superficial. *(Caution: the thyroid gland is located in this region. To avoid damaging this structure, don't press too firmly on this lumpy-textured gland.)*

3. Follow the different infrahyoid muscle fibers between the hyoid bone and their attachments on the sternum, clavicle, and scapula.

4. Client swallows to ensure proper location.

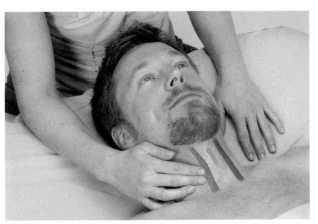

6-32

Attachments
O: Sternum, manubrium (*sternohyoid and sternothyroid*)
O: Thyroid cartilage (*thyrohyoid*)
O: Scapula, superior border (*omohyoid*)
I: Hyoid bone (*sternohyoid, thyrohyoid, and omohyoid*)
I: Thyroid cartilage (*sternothyroid*)

Actions
• Depress hyoid bone and thyroid cartilage

Innervation
• Upper cervical spinal nerves

Functional Anatomy

The infrahyoid muscle group is composed of the thyrohyoid, sternohyoid, sternothyroid, and omohyoid muscles. Each (except the sternothyroid) has an attachment to the hyoid bone. Together, these muscles depress the hyoid bone and thyroid cartilage during swallowing. They also cocontract with their antagonists, the suprahyoids, to fix the hyoid during chewing.

Like the suprahyoids, the infrahyoids also help position the larynx, influencing the pitch and quality of sounds produced by the vocal cords. They also serve as a weak flexor of the neck when the hyoid bone is fixed.

Splenius Capitis • *sple'ne us* kap'i tis • Latin "**splenius**" *bandage* "**capitus**" *head*

Attachments

O: Ligamentum nuchae and C7–T3, spinous processes
I: Temporal bone, mastoid process and occiput, lateral portion of superior nuchal line

Actions

- Extends head and neck (bilateral action)
- Laterally flexes head and neck (unilateral action)
- Rotates head and neck toward same side (unilateral action)

Innervation

- Cervical spinal nerves

Functional Anatomy

Splenius capitus is deep to the trapezius and has a broad origin on the nuchal ligament and spinous processes of the lower cervical and upper thoracic vertebrae. It narrows and thickens to form a strong attachment on the mastoid process and lateral occiput. This muscle forms a strong counterbalance to the large sternocleidomastoid on the front of the neck. Laterally, these two muscles form an inverted "v" and center the head front-to-back over the shoulder girdle when balanced.

Compared to the deeper suboccipitals, the splenius capitus is large and broad, making it a more effective prime mover for extension, lateral flexion, and rotation of the head and neck. It is a direct synergist to the splenius cervicis but has better leverage for lateral flexion and rotation as it attaches more laterally and superiorly than cervicis.

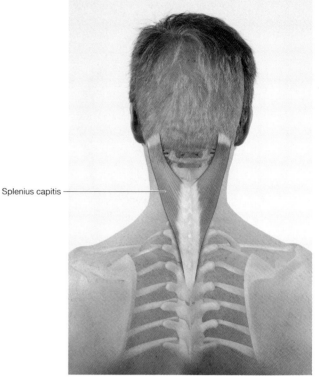

Splenius capitis

6-33

Palpating Splenius Capitis

Positioning: client supine.

1. Sitting at the client's head, place both hands palm-up under client's neck. Find the spinous processes of upper thoracic and lower cervicals with fingertips.
2. Slide fingertips laterally into the lamina groove.
3. Follow oblique muscle fibers on same side toward the mastoid processes.
4. Client gently resists looking up and rotating head to ensure proper location.

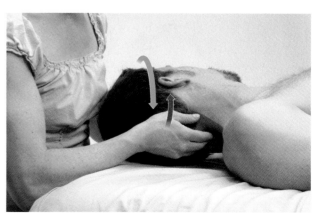

6-34

Splenius Cervicis ● *sple'ne us ser'vi* sis • Latin "**splenius**" *bandage* "**cervicis**" *neck*

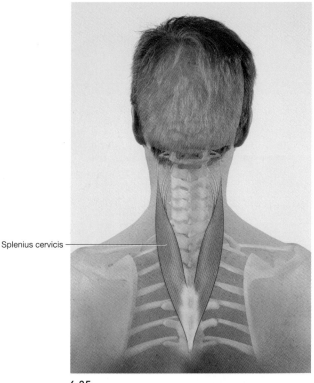

Splenius cervicis

6-35

Palpating Splenius Cervicis

Positioning: client supine.

1. Sitting at client's head, place both hands palm-up under client's neck. Find the spinous processes of T3–T6 with fingertips.

2. Slide fingertips laterally into the lamina groove.

3. Follow oblique muscle fibers on same side toward the cervical transverse processes.

4. Client gently resists looking up and rotating neck to ensure proper location.

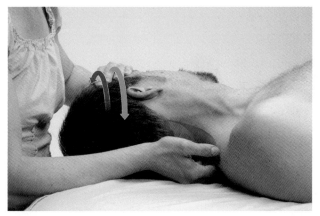

6-36

Attachments
O: T3–T6, spinous processes
I: C2–C3, posterior tubercles of transverse processes

Actions
- Extends the head and neck (bilateral action)
- Laterally flexes the head and neck (unilateral action)
- Rotates the head and neck toward same side (unilateral action)

Innervation
- Cervical spinal nerves

Functional Anatomy

Splenius cervicis connects the spinous processes of the upper thoracic vertebrae to the transverse processes of the upper cervical vertebrae. Its fiber orientation—vertical, slightly oblique—make it a powerful extensor and weak rotator of the cervical spine. It shares its attachments on the cervical transverse processes with the levator scapula (see Chapter 4) posteriorly and the scalenes anteriorly. Proper balance in strength and flexibility in these three muscles maximizes cervical alignment and function.

The splenius cervicis is a direct synergist to the splenius capitis but has less leverage for rotation than its more obliquely oriented counterpart. It also lies just superficial to splenius capitis and levator scapula.

Semispinalis ● *sem'e spi na'lis* • Latin **"semi"** *half* **"spinalis"** *spinous process*

Attachments

O: C4–C6, articular processes and C7–T10, transverse
   processes
I: Occiput, between superior and inferior nuchal lines and
    C2–T4, spinous process

Actions

• Extends the head and neck (bilateral action)
• Laterally flexes the head and neck (unilateral action)
• Rotates the head and neck toward opposite side
  (unilateral action)

Innervation

• Cervical and thoracic spinal nerves

Functional Anatomy

The semispinalis lies deep to the trapezius and just superficial to the deep, stabilizing suboccipital muscles. Its several
divisions include the capitis (attaching to the occiput), cervicis (attaching to the cervical vertebrae), and thoracis (attaching to the thoracic vertebrae). Each segment spans five
or six vertebrae attaching inferiorly to the transverse
processes and superiorly to the spinous processes or occiput
(in the case of capitis). The vertical fibers of semispinalis
make it a strong extensor of the head and neck and a weak
rotator.

   While the suboccipital muscles function to position the
head, the semispinalis is one of several postural muscles that
hold the head upright against gravity. Tightness in this muscle or imbalances in strength between it and its antagonist
flexors can compress the associated occipital nerve, creating
headaches felt in the back of the head.

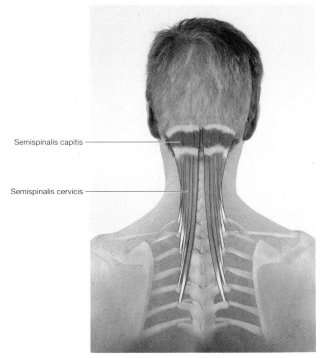

Semispinalis capitis

Semispinalis cervicis

6-37

Palpating Semispinalis

Positioning: client supine.

1. Sitting at the client's head, place both hands palm-up
   under client's head. Find the external occipital protuberance with fingertips.

2. Slide fingertips caudally and laterally into the suboccipital region and lamina groove.

3. Follow vertical muscles fibers caudally within the
   lamina groove as the client tucks the chin to slack
   superficial structures.

4. Client gently resists looking up to ensure proper
   location.

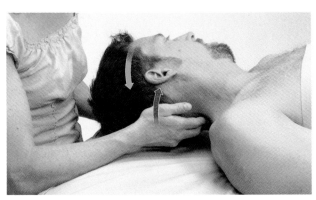

6-38

Rectus Capitis Posterior Major

rek′tus kap′i tis pos te′re or ma′jor • Latin "**rectus**" *straight* "**capitis**" *head* "**posterior**" *toward the back* "**major**" *larger*

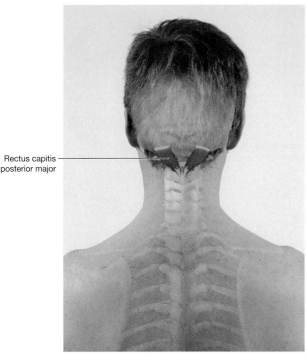

Rectus capitis posterior major

6-39

Palpating Rectus Capitis Posterior Major

Positioning: client supine.

1. Sitting at client's head, place both hands palm-up under client's head. Find external occipital protuberance with fingertips.

2. Slide fingertips caudally and laterally into the suboccipital region and lamina groove.

3. Curl fingertips upward as client tucks chin to slack superficial structures.

4. Client gently looks up to ensure proper location.

Attachments

O: Axis (C2), spinous process
I: Occiput, lateral part of inferior nuchal line

Actions

• Extends the head (bilateral action)
• Rotates the head toward same side (unilateral action)

Innervation

• Suboccipital nerve

Functional Anatomy

The rectus capitus posterior major is one of four muscles that make up the suboccipitial group (sub = *below* occipital = *the occipital bone*). The other three suboccipital muscles include the rectus capitus posterior minor, obliquus capitis superior, and obliquus capitis inferior. Together, these muscles maintain alignment between the skull and the upper cervical vertebrae. They also generate fine movements of the head, for instance, when you read or scan the road as you walk. These movements are especially important in maintaining spatial orientation while the body is in motion.

Rectus capitis posterior major lies at an oblique angle between the second cervical vertebra and the occiput. This muscle is mainly postural and helps stabilize the atlanto-occipital and atlantoaxial joints. It also helps maintain the relative position of the upper vertebral foramen to the foramen magnum. Proper alignment in this region supports the flow of blood and cerebrospinal fluid (fluid that cushions and nourishes the brain and spinal cord) to and from the skull. Imbalances in flexibility and strength of the suboccipital muscles can lead to headaches, cognitive difficulties, and pain.

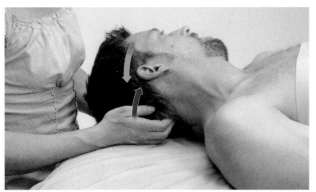

6-40

Rectus Capitus Posterior Minor

rek'tus kap'i tis pos *te're or mi'nor* • Latin "**rectus**" *straight* "**capitis**" *head* "**posterior**" *toward the back* "**minor**" *smaller*

Attachments

O: Atlas (C2), tubercle on posterior arch
I: Occiput, medial part of inferior nuchal line

Actions

• Extends the head (bilateral action)

Innervation

• Suboccipital nerve

Functional Anatomy

The rectus capitus posterior minor is one of four muscles that make up the suboccipitial group. Together, these muscles maintain alignment between the skull and the upper cervical vertebrae and generate fine movements of the head. These movements help maintain spatial orientation while the body is in motion.

Rectus capitis posterior minor, like rectus capitis posterior major, lies at an oblique angle. However, this muscle is more medial and extends between the first cervical vertebra and the occiput. Like the other suboccipital muscles, it is mainly postural and helps stabilize the atlanto-occipital joint.

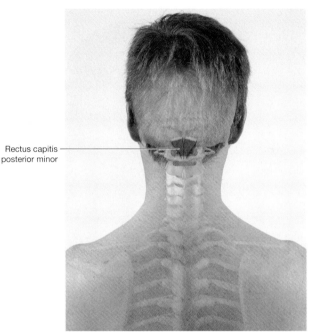

Rectus capitis posterior minor

6-41

Palpating Rectus Capitus Posterior Minor

Positioning: client supine.

1. Sitting at the client's head, place both hands palm-up under client's head. Find the external occipital protuberance with your fingertips.
2. Slide fingertips caudally and laterally into the suboccipital region and lamina groove, slightly medial to rectus capitis posterior major.
3. Curl fingertips upward as the client tucks the chin to slack superficial structures.
4. Client gently looks up to ensure proper location.

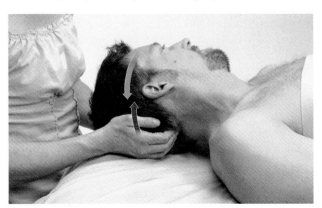

6-42

Obliquus Capitis Superior

ob li´kwus kap´i tes su per e or • Latin "**obliquus**" *oblique* "**capitus**" *head* "**superior**" *higher*

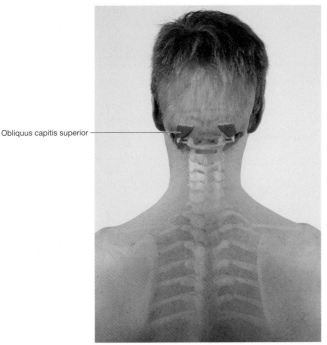

Obliquus capitis superior

6-43

Palpating Obliquus Capitis Superior

Positioning: client supine.

1. Sitting at the client's head, place both hands palm up under client's head. Find the external occipital protuberance with your fingertips.

2. Slide fingertips laterally halfway to the mastoid process and slightly caudal.

3. Curl fingertips upward as your client tucks the chin to slack superficial structures.

4. Client gently looks up to ensure proper location.

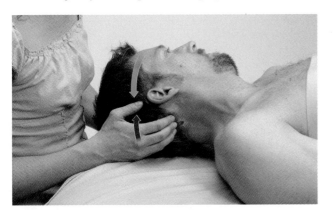

6-44

Attachments

O: Atlas, superior surface of transverse process
I: Occiput, between superior and inferior nuchal lines

Actions

• Extends the head (bilateral action)
• Laterally flexes the head (unilateral action)

Innervation

• Suboccipital nerve

Functional Anatomy

The obliquus capitis superior is one of four muscles that make up the suboccipital group, which maintains alignment between the skull and the upper cervical vertebrae. This muscle group also generates fine movements of the head that are important in maintaining spatial orientation.

Obliquus capitus superior lies more vertically than the other suboccipital muscles. This location makes it a more effective extensor and lateral flexor than rotator. It is also the most superficial of the suboccipital muscles. The rectus capitis posterior major (medial), obliquus capitis inferior (inferolateral), and obliquus capitis superior (superolateral) form a deep stabilizing triangle at the base of the skull.

Obliquus Capitis Inferior

ob li'kwus kap'i tes in fer'e or • Latin "**obliquus**" oblique "**capitus**" head "**inferior**" lower

Attachments

O: Axis (C1), apex of spinous process
I: Atlas (C2), inferior and posterior portion of transverse process

Actions

• Rotates the head toward same side (unilateral action)

Innervation

• Suboccipital nerve

Functional Anatomy

The obliquus capitis inferior is one of four muscles that make up the suboccipitial group. Together, these muscles maintain alignment between the skull and the upper cervical vertebrae. They also generate fine movements of the head that are important in maintaining spatial orientation.

Unlike the other suboccipital muscles, the obliquus capitis inferior does not attach to the occiput. It connects the spinous process of the second cervical vertebra to the transverse process of the first. It lies at a flatter oblique angle, an orientation that makes this suboccipital muscle a more effective rotator. As the transverse process of C1 is pulled toward the spinous process of C2, the head and neck turn (as when you shake your head "no"). The rectus capitis posterior major (medial), obliquus capitis inferior (inferolateral), and obliquus capitis superior (superolateral) form a deep stabilizing triangle at the base of the skull.

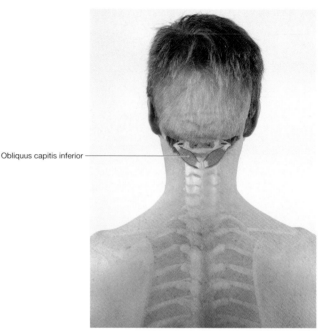

Obliquus capitis inferior

6-45

Palpating Obliquus Capitis Inferior

Positioning: client supine.

1. Sitting at the client's head, place both hands palm-up under client's head. Find the external occipital protuberance with your fingertips.

2. Slide fingertips caudally and laterally into the suboccipital region and lamina groove, slightly caudal to rectus capitis posterior major.

3. Curl fingertips upward as the client tucks the chin to slack superficial structures.

4. Client gently rotates head to ensure proper location.

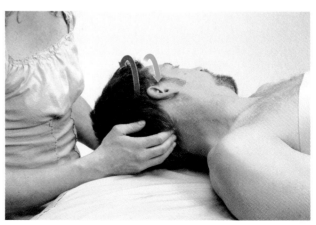

6-46

Rectus Capitis Anterior

rek'tus kap'i tis an *te're or* • Latin "**rectus**" *straight* "**capitis**" *head* "**anterior**" *toward the front*

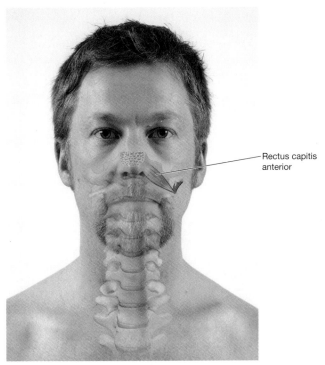

Rectus capitis anterior

6-47

Palpating Rectus Capitis Anterior

Rectus capitis anterior is a deep suboccipital muscle that is too deep to palpate.

Attachments

O: Atlas (C2), anterior surface of transverse process
I: Occipital bone, inferior surface of basilar part

Actions

• Flexes the head and neck (bilateral action)
• Rotates the head and neck toward same side (unilateral action)

Innervation

• C1 and C2

Functional Anatomy

Rectus capitis anterior is very small and deep in the anterior neck. It runs obliquely between the inferior surface of the occiput and the transverse process of the atlas. Its form and function are similar to rectus capitis posterior minor, but rectus capitis anterior flexes rather than extends. Fine bending of the head, such as when you look down, is initiated by rectus capitis anterior.

Rectus capitis anterior also works with the suboccipital muscles to stabilize the atlanto-occipital joint. The antagonist actions of the rectus capitis anterior and the rectus capitis posterior major and minor maintain alignment between the vertebral foramen of the atlas and the foramen magnum of the occiput. Proper alignment in this region supports the flow of blood and cerebrospinal fluid (fluid that cushions and nourishes the brain and spinal cord) to and from the skull. Imbalances in flexibility and strength of the rectus capitis anterior and the suboccipital muscles can lead to headaches, cognitive difficulties, and pain.

Rectus Capitis Lateralis

rek'tus kap'i tis la *ter a'lis* • Latin "**rectus**" *straight* "**capitis**" *head* "**lateralis**" *toward the side*

Attachments

O: Atlas (C2), superior surface of transverse process
I: Occipital bone, inferior surface of jugular process

Actions

• Laterally flexes the head and neck (unilateral action)

Innervation

• C1 and C2

Functional Anatomy

Rectus capitis lateralis runs vertically between the inferior surface of the occiput and the transverse process of the atlas. It has size, orientation, and function similar to the obliquus capitis superior, found in the suboccipital group. Together, these small, deep muscles perform fine lateral flexion of the head. Rectus capitis lateralis is activated when you cock your ear to listen. It also functions to fix your head when you're talking or eating, keeping your eyes level with the horizon.

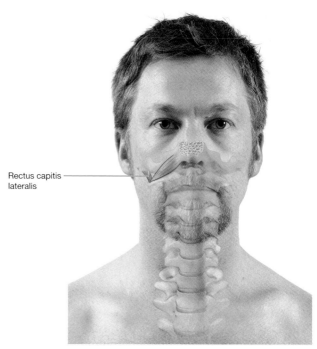

Rectus capitis lateralis

6-48

Palpating Rectus Capitis Lateralis

Positioning: client supine.

1. Sitting at the client's head, locate the mastoid processes just behind the ears with fingertips.

2. Slide fingertips caudally and laterally onto the transverse processes of the atlas.

3. Curl fingertips and palpate superior and deep to find the vertical fibers of rectus capitis lateralis. *(Caution: the styloid process of the temporal bone is a delicate structure located in this region, so don't palpate too deeply).*

4. Client gently resists lateral flexion to ensure proper location.

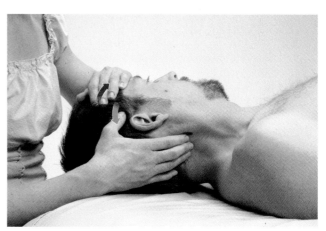

6-49

Temporalis ● tem *por ra'lis* • Latin "**temporal**" *temple*

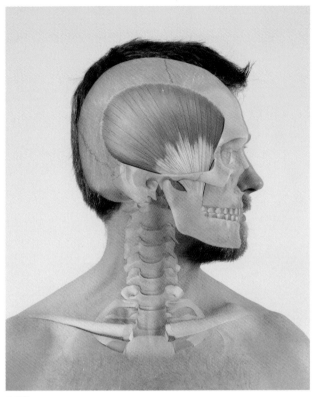

6-50

Attachments
O: Temporal, parietal, sphenoid, and frontal bones, temporal fossa and fascia
I: Mandible, coronoid process and anterior border of ramus

Actions
• Elevates the mandible
• Retracts the mandible

Innervation
• Trigeminal nerve

Functional Anatomy

The temporalis is a broad, fan-shaped muscle that covers the temple. Its fibers connect the parietal, temporal, and frontal bones then converge and run deep to the zygomatic arch. The temporalis connects to the mandible at the pointed coronoid process, which is slightly anterior. This attachment gives the temporalis leverage to retract the mandible as well as elevate it.

The temporalis works with the pterygoids and masseter during chewing. Together, they create the movements necessary for manipulating food.

Palpating Temporalis

Positioning: client supine.

1. Sitting at the client's head, locate the superior edge of the zygomatic arch with your fingertips.

2. Slide your fingertips superiorly toward the temple and onto the fibers of temporalis.

3. Follow the fibers of temporalis as they fan out across the frontal, parietal, and temporal bones.

4. Client gently opens and closes the mouth and/or clenches the jaw to ensure proper location.

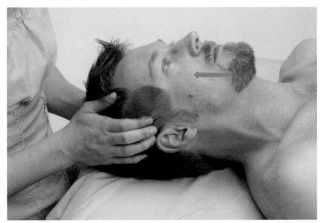

6-51

Masseter •   *mas'e ter* • Greek "**masseter**" *masticator*

Attachments
O: Temporal and zygoma bones, zygomatic arch
I: Mandible, angle, ramus, and lateral surface of coronoid
     process

Actions
• Elevates the mandible

Innervation
• Trigeminal nerve

Functional Anatomy

Masseter is a thick, strong muscle that extends between the zygomatic arch and the mandible. It has two parts, one deep and the other superficial. Their fibers oppose each other: the superficial portion pulls the mandible anteriorly, protracting it, whereas the deep portion pulls the mandible posteriorly, retracting it.

Pound for pound, masseter is the strongest muscle in the body and generates most of the force for biting and chewing. The medial and lateral pterygoid and temporalis muscles also contribute to this complex task.

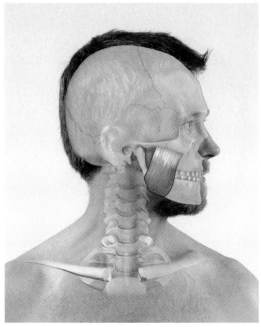

6-52

Palpating Masseter

Positioning: client supine.

1. Sitting at the client's head, locate the inferior edge of the zygomatic arch with your fingertips.

2. Slide fingertips inferiorly toward the angle of the mandible and onto the fibers of masseter. *(Caution: both the trigeminal nerve and the parotid gland are located in this region. To avoid them, carefully feel for the fibers of the masseter muscle when palpating.)*

3. Follow the fibers of masseter to its insertion on the inferior edge of the mandible.

4. Client gently opens and closes the mouth and/or clenches the jaw to ensure proper location.

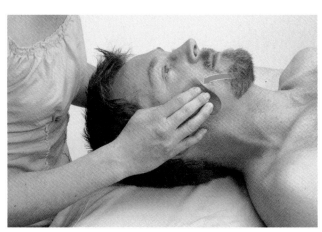

6-53

Medial Pterygoid

me'de al ter'i goyd • Greek "**medialis**" *middle* "**pteryx**" *wing* "**eidos**" *resemblance*

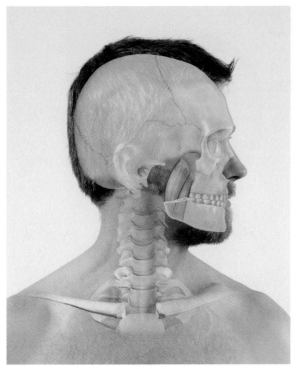

6-54

Palpating Medial Pterygoid

Positioning: client supine.

1. Sitting at the client's head, locate the inner surface of the angle of the mandible with your fingertips.

2. Hook your fingertips deeply onto the inner surface of the mandible.

3. Follow the oblique fibers of the medial pterygoid medially toward the sphenoid.

4. Have the client clench the teeth, elevating the mandible to ensure proper location.

Attachments

O: Sphenoid, pterygoid process, palatine bone, and maxilla bone, tuberosity

I: Mandible, interior surface of angle and ramus

Actions

• Elevates the mandible (bilateral action)
• Protracts the mandible (bilateral action)
• Moves the mandible laterally (unilateral action)

Innervation

• Trigeminal nerve

Functional Anatomy

The medial pterygoid is one of many muscles that move the mandible. It is deep to the masseter and temporalis and medial to its counterpart, the lateral pterygoid. The medial pterygoid connects the sphenoid, maxilla, and palatine bones to the inner surface of the mandible. When contracted, it assists the large, external masseter in elevating the mandible.

The medial pterygoid works with the lateral pterygoid, masseter, and temporalis during chewing. Together, they create the retraction, protraction, and lateral movements necessary for grinding food between the teeth and moving it around the mouth.

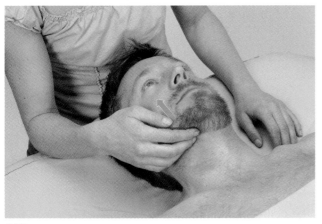

6-55

Lateral Pterygoid

lat'er al ter'i goyd • Greek "**lateralis**" *side* "**pteryx**" *wing* "**eidos**" *resemblance*

Attachments

O: Sphenoid, lateral surface of greater wing and infratemporal crest
I: Mandible, anterior portion of condyle and articular disk

Actions

- Depresses the mandible (bilateral action)
- Protracts the mandible (bilateral action)
- Moves the mandible laterally (unilateral action)

Innervation

- Trigeminal nerve

Functional Anatomy

The lateral pterygoid is one of many muscles that move the mandible. It is deep to the masseter and temporalis and lateral to its counterpart, the medial pterygoid. The lateral pterygoid connects the sphenoid to the neck of the mandible. It also has a direct connection to the capsule and articular disk of the temporomandibular joint, a modified hinge joint that relies on the articular disk to maintain joint alignment during gliding movements. The lateral pterygoid helps position the articular disk during complex movements of the temporomandibular joint, such as chewing and speaking.

The lateral pterygoid works with the medial pterygoid, masseter, and temporalis during chewing. Together, they create the retraction, protraction, and lateral movements necessary for grinding food between the teeth and moving it around the mouth.

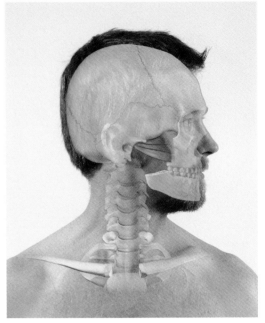

6-56

Palpating Lateral Pterygoid

Positioning: client supine.

1. Sitting at the client's head, locate the inferior surface of the zygomatic arch with your fingertips. *(Caution: the mandibular branch of the trigeminal nerve is located in this region. To avoid causing discomfort or damaging this structure, instruct the client to keep the jaw relaxed during palpation.)*
2. Slide your fingertips slightly inferiorly between the condyle and coronoid process of the mandible onto horizontal fibers of lateral pterygoid.
3. Client gently moves jaw side to side to ensure proper location.

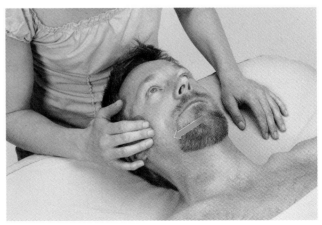

▶ SYNERGISTS/ANTAGONISTS: HEAD AND NECK

Head and Neck Motion	Muscles Involved	Head and Neck Motion	Muscles Involved
Flexion 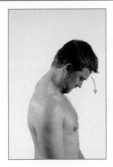	Sternocleidomastoid Platysma Longus colli Longus capitis Scalenes (anterior fibers) Rectus capitis anterior	Extension 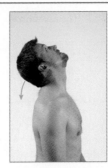	Sternocleidomastoid (upper cervicals only) Splenius capitis Splenius cervicis Semispinalis Rectus capitis posterior major Rectus capitis posterior minor Obliquus capitis superior Levator scapula (see Chapter 4) Trapezius (see Chapter 4) Rotatores (see Chapter 7) Multifidi (see Chapter 7) Semispinalis (see Chapter 7) Interspinalis (see Chapter 7) Iliocostalis (see Chapter 7) Longissimus (see Chapter 7) Spinalis (see Chapter 7)
Lateral Flexion (Right) 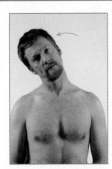	Right sternocleidomastoid Right scalenes Right longus colli Right splenius capitis Right splenius cervicis Right semispinalis Right obliquus capitis superior Right rectus capitis lateralis Right levator scapula (see Chapter 4) Right trapezius (see Chapter 4) Right intertransversarii (see Chapter 7) Right longissimus (see Chapter 7)	Lateral Flexion (Left) 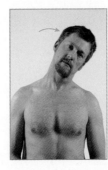	Left sternocleidomastoid Left scalenes Left longus colli Left splenius capitis Left splenius cervicis Left semispinalis Left obliquus capitis superior Left rectus capitis lateralis Left levator scapula (see Chapter 4) Left trapezius (see Chapter 4) Left intertransversarii (see Chapter 7) Left longissimus (see Chapter 7)
Rotation (Right) 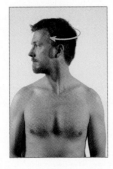	Left sternocleidomastoid Left scalene Right longus colli Right longus capitis Right splenius capitis Right splenius cervicis Left semispinalis Right rectus capitis posterior major Right obliquus capitis inferior Right rectus capitis anterior Right levator scapula (see Chapter 4) Left trapezius (see Chapter 4) Left rotatores (see Chapter 7) Left multifidi (see Chapter 7) Left semispinalis (see Chapter 7)	Rotation (Left) 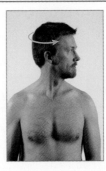	Right sternocleidomastoid Right scalene Left longus colli Left longus capitis Left splenius capitis Left splenius cervicis Right semispinalis Left rectus capitis posterior major Left obliquus capitis inferior Left rectus capitis anterior Left levator scapula (see Chapter 4) Right trapezius (see Chapter 4) Right rotatores (see Chapter 7) Right multifidi (see Chapter 7) Right semispinalis (see Chapter 7)

◗ SYNERGISTS/ANTAGONISTS: JAW

Jaw Motion		Muscles Involved	Jaw Motion		Muscles Involved
Elevation	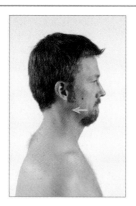	Temporalis Masseter Medial pterygoid	Depression	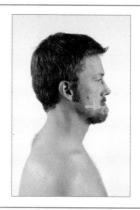	Suprahyoids Digastric Lateral pterygoid
Retraction	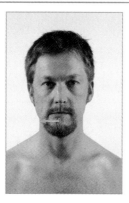	Temporalis	Protraction	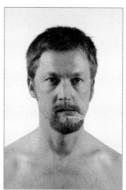	Medial pterygoid Lateral pterygoid
Lateral Motion (Right)		Right medial pterygoid Right lateral pterygoid	Lateral Motion (Left)		Left medial pterygoid Left lateral pterygoid

◗ PUTTING IT IN MOTION

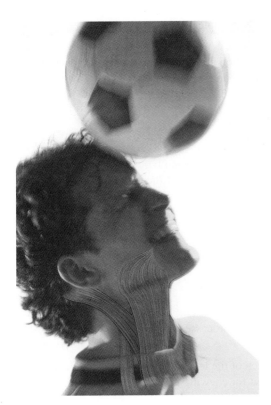

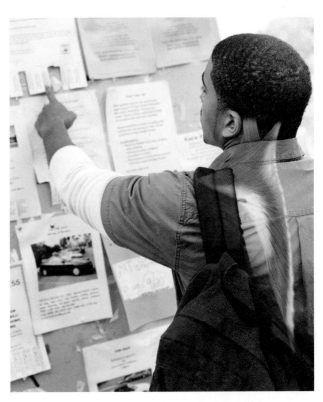

Hitting a header. Soccer is a sport that requires the head and neck to perform powerful forward movements. The deep muscles such as rectus capitis anterior, longus capitis, and longus colli angle the forehead and stabilize the spine. Superficial muscles on the front of the neck such as anterior scalene, sternocleidomastoid, and platysma drive the movement.

Looking up. Coordinated efforts of the deep, intermediate, and superficial muscles on the back of the neck enable us to look up. Deep muscles, such as the suboccipitals, angle the head while the intermediate semispinalis and splenii muscles bend the neck back and stabilize the vertebrae. Superficial muscles such as the levator scapula and trapezius connect the head and shoulders.

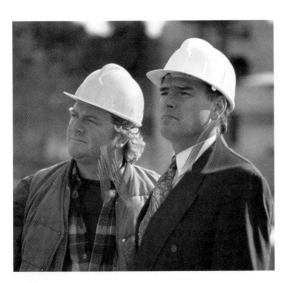

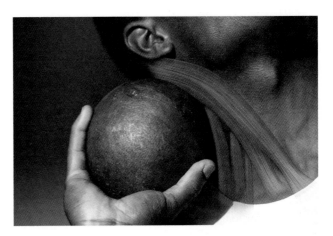

Tuning in. Cocking the head to one side activates several muscles on the front and back of the neck. The small, deep rectus capitis lateralis and obliquus capitis superior tip the head while the semispinalis, splenii, longus colli, scalenes, sternocleidomastoid, and trapezius muscles create larger movements at the head and neck.

Rotating the head. Turning your head to look over your shoulder is a critical movement when driving or taking a breath when swimming. The deep suboccipitals help pivot the head while semispinalis and splenii muscles govern gross neck rotation. The scalenes, levator scapula, sternocleidomastoid, and trapezius anchor the head and neck to the ribcage and shoulder girdle during these movements, levering the head from these stable structures.

SUMMARY

- The cranium is made up of 8 bones (one frontal bone, two parietal bones, one occipital bone, two temporal bones, one sphenoid bone, and one ethmoid bone) held together by several sutures.
- The skull also contains 12 facial bones (two lacrimal bones, two nasal bones, two maxilla bones, two zygomatic bones, two palatine bones, a vomer, and a mandible) that protect openings for the respiratory and digestive tracts.
- The cervical spine consists of 7 vertebrae that allow gliding movements in the head and neck and protect the spinal cord.
- The first two cervical vertebrae are uniquely shaped and allow rotational movements in the head and neck.
- The head and neck contain several special structures including the parotid and thyroid glands, salivary glands, trachea, cervical lymph nodes, and several large arteries, veins, and nerves.
- Multiple layers of small and large muscles work together to create the myriad of fine and powerful movements of the head and neck.
- Several muscles attach to the hyoid bone below the jaw and contribute to chewing and swallowing.
- Several small suboccipital muscles maintain exact alignment between the skull and the vertebral column.
- The mandible articulates with the skull at the temporomandibular joint. Movements of this joint are essential to speaking, eating, and expressing emotion.
- Together, the muscles of the head, neck, and face allow us to bend and twist the head as we look at and listen to the world around us.

FOR REVIEW

Answers to review questions can be found in Appendix A.

Multiple Choice

1. The medial border of the posterior triangle is formed by the:
   A. sternocleidomastoid muscle
   B. clavicle
   C. trapezius muscle
   D. mandible

2. A ligament that bridges the occiput and spinous process of C7 and forms a strong posterior muscle attachment is the:
   A. anterior longitudinal ligament
   B. transverse ligament
   C. ligamentum nuchae
   D. ligamenta flava

3. The joints between the bones of the cranium are:
   A. freely movable
   B. immovable
   C. slightly movable
   D. synovial

4. The intersection between the two parietal bones and the occipital bone is called the:
   A. external occipital protuberance
   B. sagittal suture
   C. coronal suture
   D. lambda

5. A ligament that holds the pivoting dens against the interior anterior surface of the atlas is the:
   A. tectoral membrane
   B. transverse ligament
   C. apical ligament
   D. ligamentum nuchae

6. The u-shaped uncovertebral joints are formed by the articulation of two:
   A. vertebral bodies
   B. spinous processes
   C. transverse processes
   D. facets

7. The branch of the trigeminal nerve that regulates movement for chewing and swallowing is the:
   A. maxillary division
   B. mandibular division
   C. ophthalmic division
   D. none of the above

8. The transverse foramina of the cervical vertebrae contain the:
   A. carotid arteries
   B. jugular veins
   C. vertebral arteries and veins
   D. spinal cord

9. The only pivot joint in the spine is located between the:
   A. 6th and 7th cervical vertebrae
   B. 1st and 2nd cervical vertebrae
   C. atlas and axis
   D. both B and C are correct

10. The vertebral foramina of the cervical vertebrae contain the:
    A. carotid arteries
    B. jugular veins
    C. vertebral arteries
    D. spinal cord

Matching

Different muscle attachments are listed below. Match the correct muscle with its attachment.

11. _____ Anterior surfaces of C2–C6.

12. _____ Lateral surface of the greater wing and infratemporal crest of the sphenoid.

13. _____ Between the superior and inferior nuchal lines of the occiput and spinous processes of C2–T4.

14. _____ Ligamentum nuchae and the spinous processes of C7–T3.

15. _____ Posterior tubercles of the transverse processes of C2–3.

16. _____ Tubercle on the posterior arch of C2.

17. _____ First and second ribs.

18. _____ Underside of the mandible and styloid process of the temporal bone.

19. _____ Superior surface of the transverse process of C2.

20. _____ Coronoid process and anterior border of the ramus of the mandible.

A. Semispinalis
B. Splenius cervicis
C. Temporalis
D. Longus colli
E. Splenius capitis
F. Rectus capitis lateralis
G. Suprahyoids
H. Lateral pterygoid
I. Rectus capitis posterior minor
J. Scalenes

Different muscle actions are listed below. Match the correct muscle with its action. Answers may be used more than once.

21. _____ Flexes the head and neck

22. _____ Extends the head and neck

23. _____ Laterally flexes the head and neck

24. _____ Rotates the head and neck to the same side

25. _____ Rotates the head and neck to the opposite side

26. _____ Elevates the mandible

27. _____ Depresses the mandible

28. _____ Retracts the mandible

29. _____ Protracts the mandible

30. _____ Laterally moves the mandible

A. Sternocleidomastoid
B. Lateral Pterygoid
C. Splenius capitis
D. Longus capitis
E. Temporalis
F. Medial pterygoid
G. Rectus capitis lateralis
H. Digastric
I. Scalenes
J. Obliquus capitis superior

Short Answer

31. Briefly describe how the atlas and axis are different from the other cervical vertebrae. What movements are made possible by the articulation between these two joints?

32. Briefly describe what structures travel through the cervical vertebrae and why proper alignment between the skull and cervical vertebrae is so important.

33. Make a list of muscles that rotate the head and neck to the same side and another of muscles that rotate the head and neck to the opposite side. What do the muscles of each list have in common?

Try This!

Activity: Find a partner and have him or her perform one of the skills identified in the *Putting It in Motion* segment. Identify the specific actions of the neck that make up this skill. Write them down. Use the synergist list to identify which muscles work together to create this movement. Make sure you put the actions in the correct sequence. See if you can discover which muscles are stabilizing or steering the joints into position and which are responsible for powering the movement.

Suggestions: Switch partners and perform a different skill from *Putting It in Motion*. Repeat the steps above. Confirm your findings with the *Putting It in Motion* segment on the student CD included with your textbook. To further your understanding, practice this activity with skills not identified in *Putting It in Motion*.

SUGGESTED READINGS

Chek P. Corrective postural training and the massage therapist. *Massage Therapy Journal*. 1995;34(3):83.

Falla D, Jull G, Russell T, et al. Effect of neck exercise on sitting posture in patients with chronic neck pain. *Physical Therapy*. 2007;87:408–417.

Mansell J, Tierney RT, Sitler MR, et al. Resistance training and head-neck segment dynamic stabilization in male and female collegiate soccer players. *J Athl Train*. 2005;40(4):310–319.

Muscolino J. The effects of postural distortion. *J Massage Ther*. 2006;45(2):167.

Passero PL, Wyman BS, Bell JW, et al. Temporomandibular joint dysfunction syndrome: a clinical report. *Physical Therapy*. 1985;65:1203–1207.

Trunk

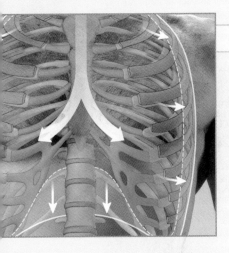

Learning Objectives

After working through the material in this chapter, you should be able to:

- Identify the main structures of the trunk, including bones, joints, special structures, and deep and superficial muscles.

- Identify normal curvatures of the spine, including the cervical, thoracic, and lumbar regions.

- Label and palpate the major surface landmarks of the trunk.

- Draw, label, palpate, and fire the superficial and deep muscles of the trunk.

- Locate the attachments and nerve supply of the muscles of the trunk.

- Identify and demonstrate all actions of the muscles of the trunk.

- Demonstrate resisted range of motion of the trunk.

- Describe the unique functional anatomy and relationships between each muscle of the trunk.

- Identify both the synergists and antagonists involved in each movement of the trunk (flexion, extension, etc.).

- Identify the muscles of breathing and their functions in inhalation and exhalation.

- Identify muscles used in performing four coordinated movements of the trunk: pushing, lifting, bending, and twisting.

▶ OVERVIEW OF THE REGION

The trunk is the body region that includes the thorax (the chest) and the abdomen. It is formed by the ribcage, spine, and the most superior portion of the pelvic girdle. These skeletal structures provide protection for the thoracic organs, primarily the heart, lungs, spleen, and spinal cord, as well as attachments for a complex network of muscles. Layers of strong abdominal muscles protect the abdominal organs.

The trunk is often referred to as the "core" of the body. Many movements are initiated in this region. Forces produced in the lower body must also transfer through the trunk before extending into the arms. We see this type of transfer with movements such as throwing and pushing.

When all of its structures are healthy, balanced, and functionally sound, the trunk is a dynamic, powerful tool that allows us to bend, twist, stand straight, and produce powerful, full-body movements. However, improper development, alignment, and use patterns can easily disrupt this functional equilibrium. Understanding the function of each muscle and its relationship to other structures helps us prevent pathology and enhance performance of work tasks, exercise, sports, and activities of daily living, both for ourselves and for our clients.

▶ SURFACE ANATOMY OF THE TRUNK

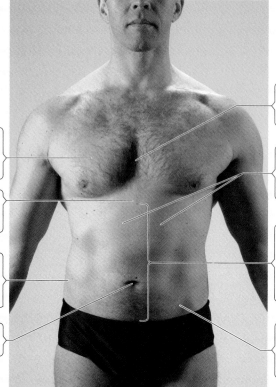

Pectoralis major dominates the superior, anterior trunk. Its primary actions are on the shoulder.

The **xiphoid process** is a tiny diamond-shaped bone at the inferior end of the sternum.

Many muscles attach to the thick superior edge of the ilium, called the **iliac crest**. It marks the most inferior, lateral portion of the trunk.

The **umbilicus** is also called the navel.

The **intersternal notch** is a depression between the right and left pectoralis major.

Rectus abdominis is a paired, superficial muscle that extends from the anterior ribcage to the pubic region.

The **linea alba** segments the fibers of the rectus abdominis vertically. It runs from the xiphoid process to the pubic bone and marks the midline of the anterior trunk.

The obliquely angled **inguinal ligament** is the inferior border of the aponeurosis of the external oblique muscle.

7-1A. Anterior view.

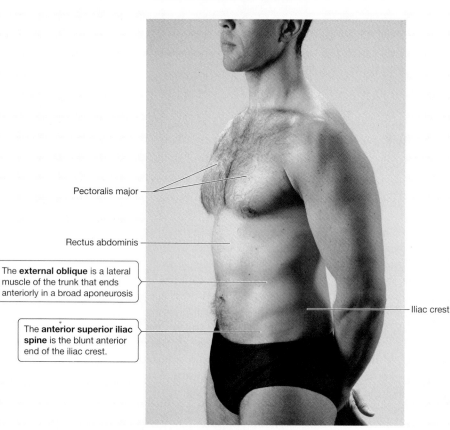

Pectoralis major

Rectus abdominis

The **external oblique** is a lateral muscle of the trunk that ends anteriorly in a broad aponeurosis

The **anterior superior iliac spine** is the blunt anterior end of the iliac crest.

Iliac crest

7-1B. Anterolateral view.

▶ SURFACE ANATOMY OF THE TRUNK

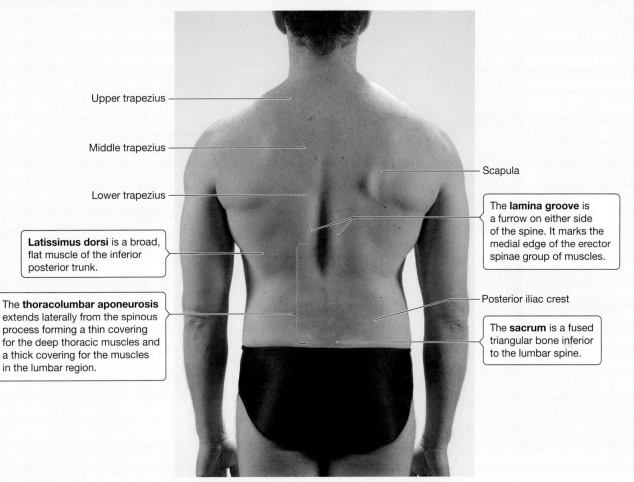

Upper trapezius

Middle trapezius

Lower trapezius

Scapula

The **lamina groove** is a furrow on either side of the spine. It marks the medial edge of the erector spinae group of muscles.

Latissimus dorsi is a broad, flat muscle of the inferior posterior trunk.

The **thoracolumbar aponeurosis** extends laterally from the spinous process forming a thin covering for the deep thoracic muscles and a thick covering for the muscles in the lumbar region.

Posterior iliac crest

The **sacrum** is a fused triangular bone inferior to the lumbar spine.

7-1C. Posterior view.

▶ SKELETAL STRUCTURES OF THE TRUNK

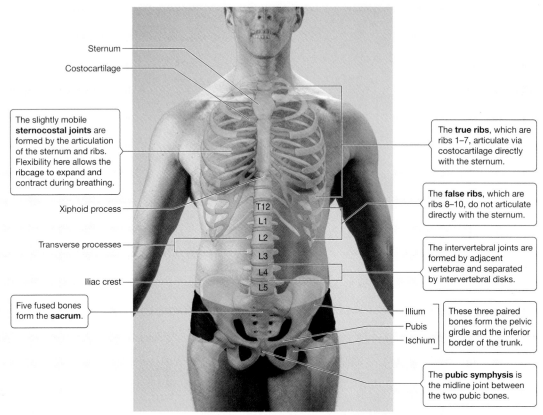

Sternum

Costocartilage

The slightly mobile **sternocostal joints** are formed by the articulation of the sternum and ribs. Flexibility here allows the ribcage to expand and contract during breathing.

Xiphoid process

Transverse processes

Iliac crest

Five fused bones form the **sacrum**.

The **true ribs**, which are ribs 1–7, articulate via costocartilage directly with the sternum.

The **false ribs**, which are ribs 8–10, do not articulate directly with the sternum.

The intervertebral joints are formed by adjacent vertebrae and separated by intervertebral disks.

T12
L1
L2
L3
L4
L5

Illium
Pubis
Ischium

These three paired bones form the pelvic girdle and the inferior border of the trunk.

The **pubic symphysis** is the midline joint between the two pubic bones.

7-2A. Bones of the trunk: anterior view.

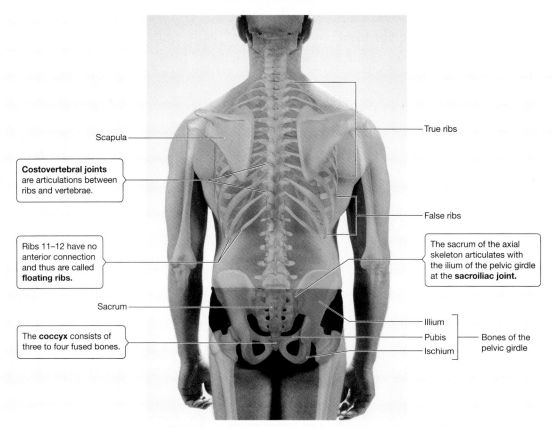

Scapula

Costovertebral joints are articulations between ribs and vertebrae.

Ribs 11–12 have no anterior connection and thus are called **floating ribs.**

Sacrum

The **coccyx** consists of three to four fused bones.

True ribs

False ribs

The sacrum of the axial skeleton articulates with the ilium of the pelvic girdle at the **sacroiliac joint.**

Illium
Pubis
Ischium

Bones of the pelvic girdle

7-2B. Bones of the trunk: posterior view.

▶ SKELETAL STRUCTURES OF THE TRUNK

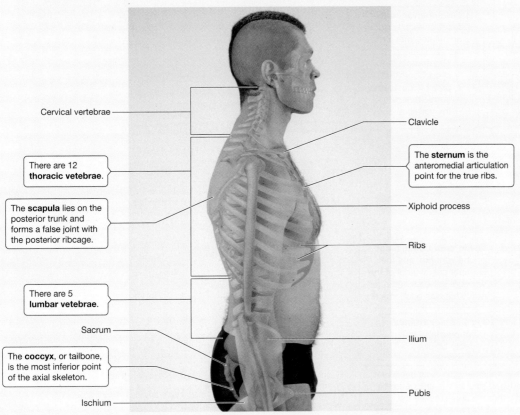

Cervical vertebrae

Clavicle

The **sternum** is the anteromedial articulation point for the true ribs.

There are 12 **thoracic vetebrae**.

Xiphoid process

The **scapula** lies on the posterior trunk and forms a false joint with the posterior ribcage.

Ribs

There are 5 **lumbar vetebrae**.

Sacrum

Ilium

The **coccyx**, or tailbone, is the most inferior point of the axial skeleton.

Ischium

Pubis

7-2C. Bones of the trunk: lateral view.

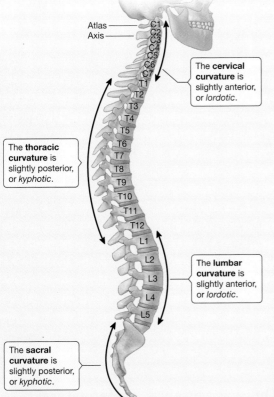

Atlas

Axis

C1
C2
C3
C4
C5
C6
C7
T1
T2
T3
T4
T5
T6
T7
T8
T9
T10
T11
T12
L1
L2
L3
L4
L5

The **cervical curvature** is slightly anterior, or *lordotic*.

The **thoracic curvature** is slightly posterior, or *kyphotic*.

The **lumbar curvature** is slightly anterior, or *lordotic*.

The **sacral curvature** is slightly posterior, or *kyphotic*.

7-2D. Curvatures of the spinal column: lateral view. From this view, the normal curvatures of the spinal column are visible. These characteristic curvatures help maintain erect posture and absorb shock throughout the length of the spinal column. This protects and cushions the axial structures during weight-bearing activities like lifting or walking. Notice that the vertebrae increase in size from superior to inferior to accept more weight.

▶ SKELETAL STRUCTURES OF THE TRUNK

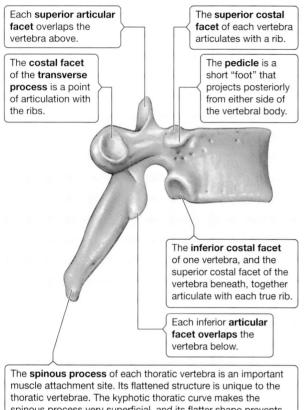

Each **superior articular facet** overlaps the vertebra above.

The **costal facet** of the **transverse process** is a point of articulation with the ribs.

The **superior costal facet** of each vertebra articulates with a rib.

The **pedicle** is a short "foot" that projects posteriorly from either side of the vertebral body.

The **inferior costal facet** of one vertebra, and the superior costal facet of the vertebra beneath, together articulate with each true rib.

Each inferior **articular facet overlaps** the vertebra below.

The **spinous process** of each thoratic vertebra is an important muscle attachment site. Its flattened structure is unique to the thoratic vertebrae. The kyphotic thoratic curve makes the spinous process very superficial, and its flatter shape prevents damage and discomfort when we lie supine.

7-2E. Thoracic vertebra: lateral view.

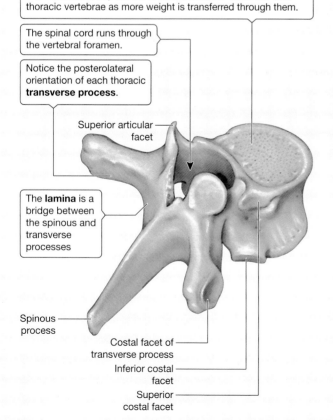

The **vertebral body** increases in size from the 1st to the 12th thoracic vertebrae as more weight is transferred through them.

The spinal cord runs through the vertebral foramen.

Notice the posterolateral orientation of each thoracic **transverse process**.

Superior articular facet

The **lamina** is a bridge between the spinous and transverse processes

Spinous process

Costal facet of transverse process

Inferior costal facet

Superior costal facet

7-2F. Thoracic vertebra: posterolateral oblique view.

◗ SKELETAL STRUCTURES OF THE TRUNK

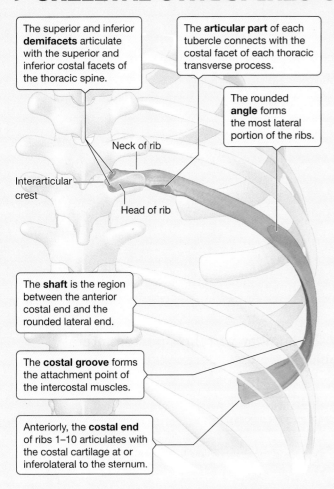

The superior and inferior **demifacets** articulate with the superior and inferior costal facets of the thoracic spine.

The **articular part** of each tubercle connects with the costal facet of each thoracic transverse process.

The rounded **angle** forms the most lateral portion of the ribs.

Neck of rib

Interarticular crest

Head of rib

The **shaft** is the region between the anterior costal end and the rounded lateral end.

The **costal groove** forms the attachment point of the intercostal muscles.

Anteriorly, the **costal end** of ribs 1–10 articulates with the costal cartilage at or inferolateral to the sternum.

7-2G. Features of a typical rib. Each rib differs in size, but all share some common features.

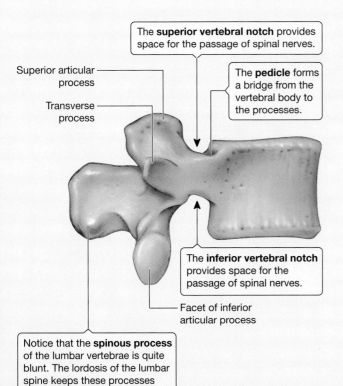

The **superior vertebral notch** provides space for the passage of spinal nerves.

The **pedicle** forms a bridge from the vertebral body to the processes.

Superior articular process

Transverse process

The **inferior vertebral notch** provides space for the passage of spinal nerves.

Facet of inferior articular process

Notice that the **spinous process** of the lumbar vertebrae is quite blunt. The lordosis of the lumbar spine keeps these processes deep, affording them protection.

7-2H. Lumbar vertebra: lateral view.

▶ SKELETAL STRUCTURES OF THE TRUNK

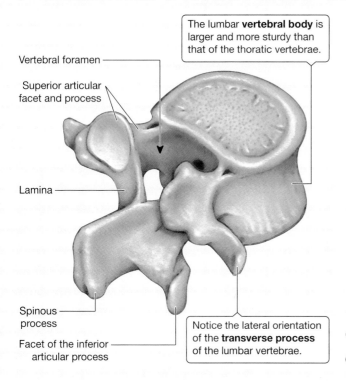

The lumbar **vertebral body** is larger and more sturdy than that of the thoratic vertebrae.

Vertebral foramen

Superior articular facet and process

Lamina

Spinous process

Facet of the inferior articular process

Notice the lateral orientation of the **transverse process** of the lumbar vertebrae.

7-2I. Lumbar vertebra: posterolateral oblique view.

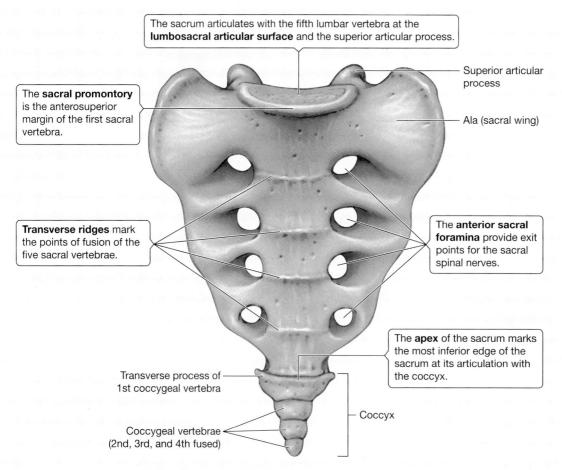

The sacrum articulates with the fifth lumbar vertebra at the **lumbosacral articular surface** and the superior articular process.

The **sacral promontory** is the anterosuperior margin of the first sacral vertebra.

Superior articular process

Ala (sacral wing)

Transverse ridges mark the points of fusion of the five sacral vertebrae.

The **anterior sacral foramina** provide exit points for the sacral spinal nerves.

The **apex** of the sacrum marks the most inferior edge of the sacrum at its articulation with the coccyx.

Transverse process of 1st coccygeal vertebra

Coccyx

Coccygeal vertebrae (2nd, 3rd, and 4th fused)

7-2J. Sacrum: anterior view.
The anterior, or pelvic, surface of the sacrum is concave in shape.

▶ SKELETAL STRUCTURES OF THE TRUNK

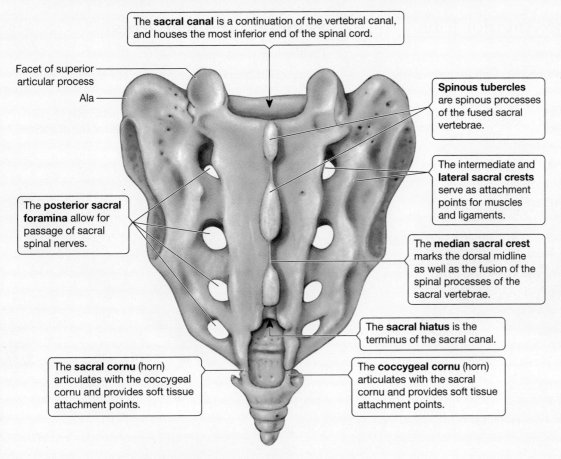

The **sacral canal** is a continuation of the vertebral canal, and houses the most inferior end of the spinal cord.

Facet of superior articular process

Ala

Spinous tubercles are spinous processes of the fused sacral vertebrae.

The intermediate and **lateral sacral crests** serve as attachment points for muscles and ligaments.

The **posterior sacral foramina** allow for passage of sacral spinal nerves.

The **median sacral crest** marks the dorsal midline as well as the fusion of the spinal processes of the sacral vertebrae.

The **sacral hiatus** is the terminus of the sacral canal.

The **sacral cornu** (horn) articulates with the coccygeal cornu and provides soft tissue attachment points.

The **coccygeal cornu** (horn) articulates with the sacral cornu and provides soft tissue attachment points.

7-2K. Sacrum: posterior view. The posterior, or dorsal, surface of the sacrum is convex in shape.

▶ BONY LANDMARKS OF SKELETAL STRUCTURES

Palpating the Anterior Ribs

Positioning: client supine.

1. Locate your client's sternum with the pads of your fingers.
2. Slide your fingertips laterally onto the surfaces of the anterior ribs.

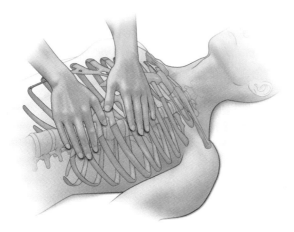

7-3A. **Anterior Ribs**

Palpating the Xiphoid Process of the Sternum

Positioning: client supine.

1. Locate the inferior edge of your client's anterior ribcage with your fingertips.
2. Follow the inferior edge medially onto the diamond-shaped xiphoid process.

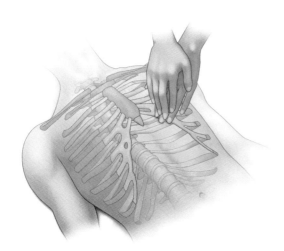

7-3B. **Xiphoid Process of the Sternum**

Palpating the Iliac Crest

Positioning: client supine.

1. Locate the lateral surfaces of your client's trunk with the palms of your hands.
2. Slide your hands inferiorly until the ulnar side of your hand contacts the broad, rounded ridge of the iliac crest.

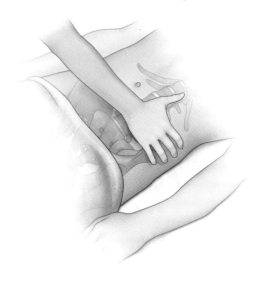

7-3C. **Iliac Crest**

Palpating the Pubis

Positioning: client supine.

1. Place your palm on your client's abdomen between the navel and pelvis.
2. Slide your hand inferiorly until the ulnar side of your hand contacts the horizontal ridge of the pubis.

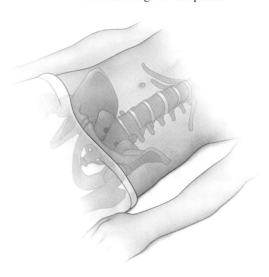

7-3D. **Pubis**

Palpating the Posterior Ribs

Positioning: client prone.

1. Locate the midline of the thoracic region with the pads of your fingers.
2. Slide your fingers laterally onto the surfaces of the posterior ribs.

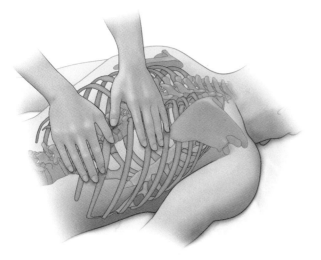

7-3E. Posterior Ribs

Palpating the Spinous Processes

Positioning: client prone.

1. Locate the midline the posterior trunk with the pads of your fingers.
2. Palpate deeply onto the vertically elongated spinous processes of the thoracic spine or blunt spinous processes of the lumbar spine.

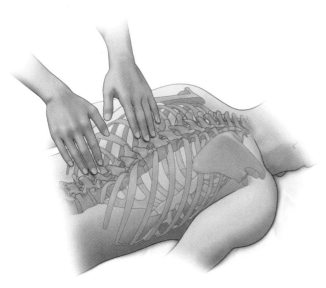

7-3F. Spinous Processes

Palpating the Lamina Groove

Positioning: client prone.

1. Locate the spinous processes with your fingertips.
2. Slide your fingertips slightly lateral and deep into the depression between the spinous and transverse processes of the vertebrae.

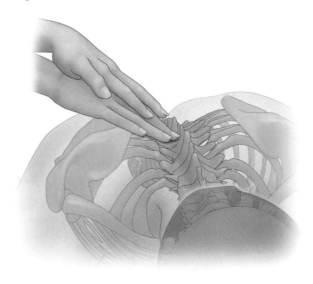

7-3G. Lamina Groove

Palpating the Twelfth Rib

Positioning: client prone.

1. Locate the space between the posterior ilium and ribcage with the pads of your fingers.
2. Slide your fingers superiorly and palpate the shortened twelfth rib near the spine.

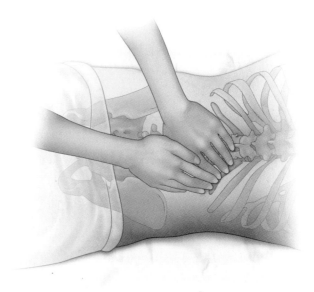

7-3H. Twelfth Rib

Palpating the Transverse Processes

Positioning: client prone.

1. Locate the spinous processes with your fingertips.
2. Slide fingers laterally and deeply past the lamina groove onto the laterally protruding transverse processes.

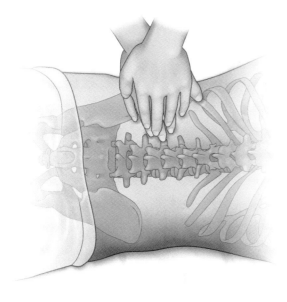

7-3I. **Transverse Processes**

Palpating the Posterior Superior Iliac Spine

Positioning: client prone.

1. Locate the iliac crest with your fingertips.
2. Follow the iliac crest posteriorly onto the posterior superior iliac spine; the most prominent projection just lateral to the sacrum.

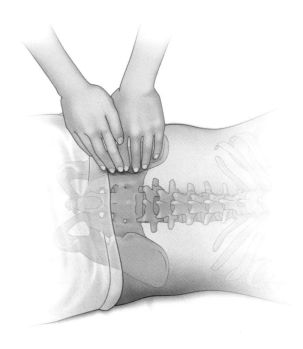

7-3J. **Posterior Superior Iliac Spine**

Palpating the Sacral Spinous Tubercles

Positioning: client prone.

1. Locate the lumbar spinous processes with the pads of your fingers.
2. Palpate inferiorly between the right and left ilium onto the dorsal surface of the sacrum, noting the bumpy spinous tubercles as you palpate inferiorly.

Palpating the Sacral Crests

Positioning: client prone.

1. Locate the dorsal surface of the sacrum with your fingertips.
2. Slide your fingertips laterally onto the vertical ridges the form the intermediate and lateral sacral crests.

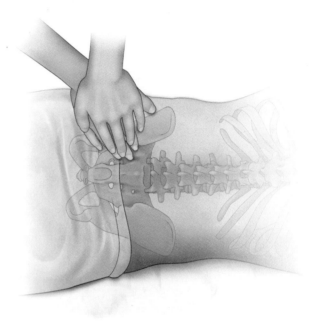

7-3L. **Sacral Crests**

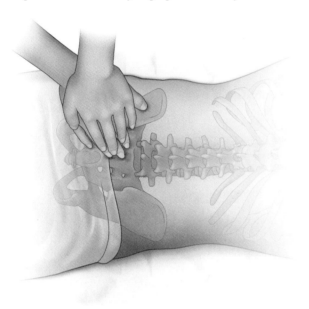

7-3K. **Sacral Spinous Tubercles**

◗ MUSCLE ATTACHMENT SITES

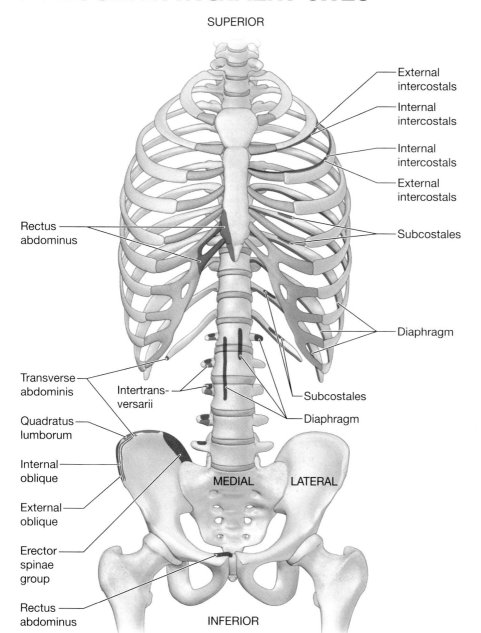

SUPERIOR

External intercostals

Internal intercostals

Internal intercostals

External intercostals

Rectus abdominus

Subcostales

Diaphragm

Transverse abdominis

Intertrans-versarii

Quadratus lumborum

Subcostales

Diaphragm

Internal oblique

MEDIAL   LATERAL

External oblique

Erector spinae group

Rectus abdominus

INFERIOR

7-4A. **Muscle attachments of the trunk:** anterior view.

▶ MUSCLE ATTACHMENT SITES

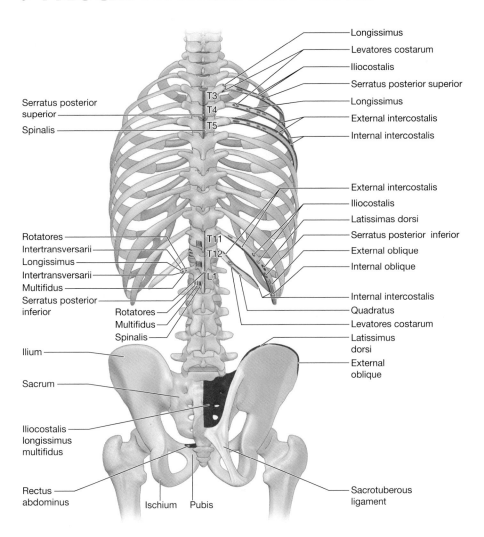

Longissimus
Levatores costarum
Iliocostalis
Serratus posterior superior
Longissimus
External intercostalis
Internal intercostalis

Serratus posterior superior
Spinalis

T3
T4
T5

External intercostalis
Iliocostalis
Latissimas dorsi
Serratus posterior inferior
External oblique
Internal oblique

Rotatores
Intertransversarii
Longissimus
Intertransversarii
Multifidus
Serratus posterior inferior

T11
T12
L1

Internal intercostalis
Quadratus
Levatores costarum
Latissimus dorsi
External oblique

Rotatores
Multifidus
Spinalis

Ilium
Sacrum

Iliocostalis
longissimus
multifidus

Rectus abdominus

Ischium   Pubis

Sacrotuberous ligament

7-4B. Muscle attachments of the trunk: posterior view.

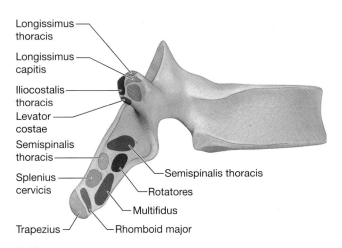

Longissimus thoracis
Longissimus capitis
Iliocostalis thoracis
Levator costae
Semispinalis thoracis
Splenius cervicis
Trapezius

Semispinalis thoracis
Rotatores
Multifidus
Rhomboid major

7-4C. Muscle attachments: a thoracic vertebra. Lateral and posterior close-up views of a typical thoracic vertebra reveal the complex relationships between spinal muscles. Several deep, intermediate, and superficial muscles attach to the spinous and transverse processes. Together, they maintain alignment while allowing fine and powerful movements in the trunk.

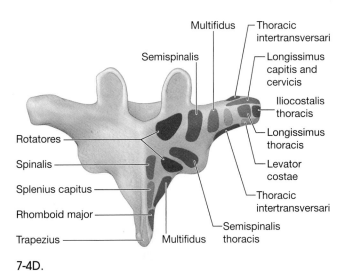

Multifidus   Thoracic intertransversari
Semispinalis
Longissimus capitis and cervicis
Iliocostalis thoracis
Longissimus thoracis
Levator costae
Thoracic intertransversari

Rotatores
Spinalis
Splenius capitus
Rhomboid major
Trapezius   Multifidus

Semispinalis thoracis

7-4D.

❱ LIGAMENTS OF THE TRUNK

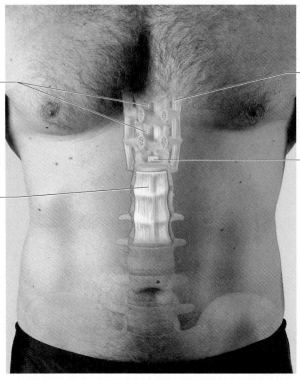

The **ligamentum flavum** is a continuous ligament network connecting the anterior surfaces of the pedicles. This network limits flexion and helps the spinal column return to an upright position.

The **anterior longitudinal ligament** runs vertically along the spine from cervical to sacral regions.

The **intertransverse ligaments** connect adjacent transverse processes and limit lateral flexion of the spine.

The **posterior longitudinal ligament** is a narrow vertical band attaching to the intervertebral disks. Also see B and C.

7-5A. Ligaments of the trunk: Anterior view. Several large ligaments connect the anterior surfaces of the vertebrae.

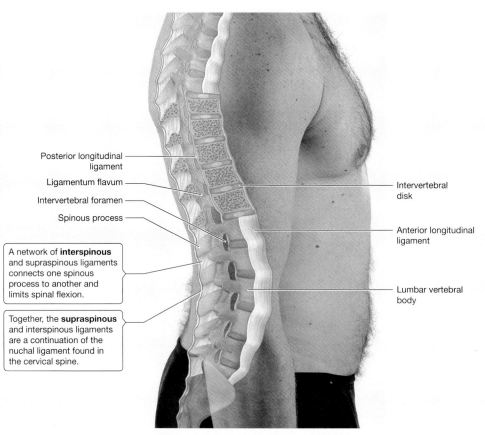

Posterior longitudinal ligament

Ligamentum flavum

Intervertebral foramen

Spinous process

A network of **interspinous** and supraspinous ligaments connects one spinous process to another and limits spinal flexion.

Together, the **supraspinous** and interspinous ligaments are a continuation of the nuchal ligament found in the cervical spine.

Intervertebral disk

Anterior longitudinal ligament

Lumbar vertebral body

7-5B. Ligaments of the trunk: lateral view.

◗ LIGAMENTS OF THE TRUNK

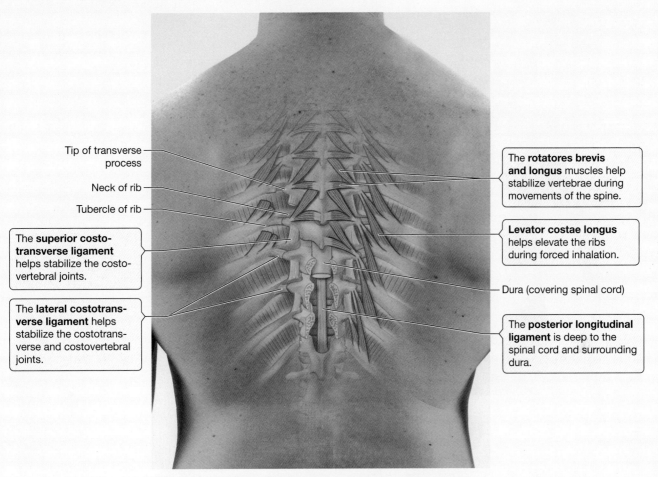

Tip of transverse process

Neck of rib

Tubercle of rib

The **superior costo-transverse ligament** helps stabilize the costo-vertebral joints.

The **lateral costotrans-verse ligament** helps stabilize the costotrans-verse and costovertebral joints.

The **rotatores brevis and longus** muscles help stabilize vertebrae during movements of the spine.

Levator costae longus helps elevate the ribs during forced inhalation.

Dura (covering spinal cord)

The **posterior longitudinal ligament** is deep to the spinal cord and surrounding dura.

7-5C. Ligaments of the trunk: posterior view. Ligaments unique to the thoracic spine help stabilize the costovertebral joints.

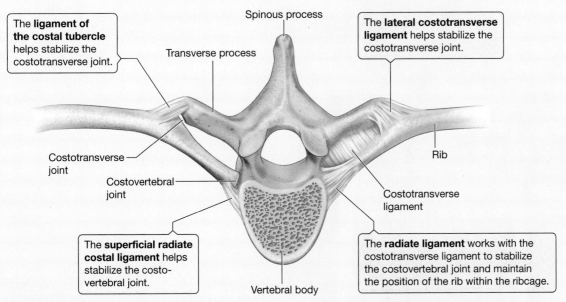

The **ligament of the costal tubercle** helps stabilize the costotransverse joint.

Spinous process

Transverse process

The **lateral costotransverse ligament** helps stabilize the costotransverse joint.

Costotransverse joint

Costovertebral joint

Rib

Costotransverse ligament

The **superficial radiate costal ligament** helps stabilize the costo-vertebral joint.

Vertebral body

The **radiate ligament** works with the costotransverse ligament to stabilize the costovertebral joint and maintain the position of the rib within the ribcage.

7-5D. Ligaments of the trunk: superior view. From this view, the ligaments that stabilize the costovertebral and costotransverse joints are more visible.

▶ SUPERFICIAL MUSCLES OF THE TRUNK

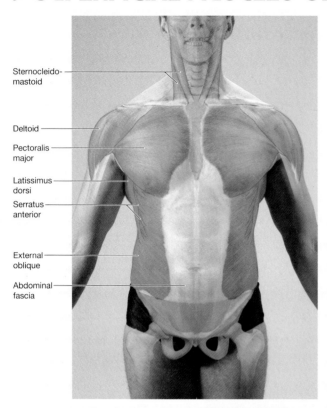

Sternocleido-
mastoid

Deltoid

Pectoralis
major

Latissimus
dorsi

Serratus
anterior

External
oblique

Abdominal
fascia

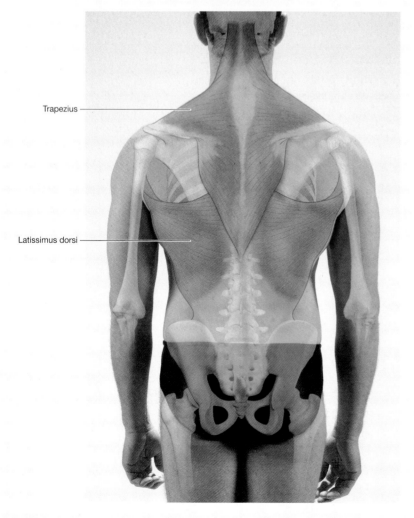

Trapezius

Latissimus dorsi

7-6. Superficial muscles of the trunk.
A. Anterior view. Large, prime movers of the
shoulder girdle and trunk dominate the superficial
trunk. **B. Posterior view.** Spinal muscles are
covered by large shoulder muscles and the fascial
junction at the thoracolumbar aponeurosis.

INTERMEDIATE MUSCLES OF THE TRUNK

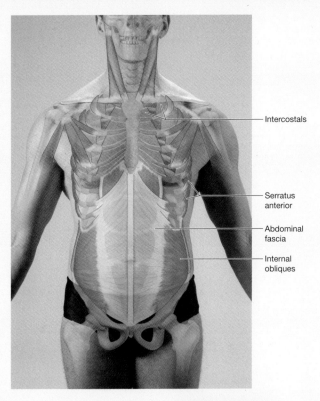

Intercostals

Serratus anterior

Abdominal fascia

Internal obliques

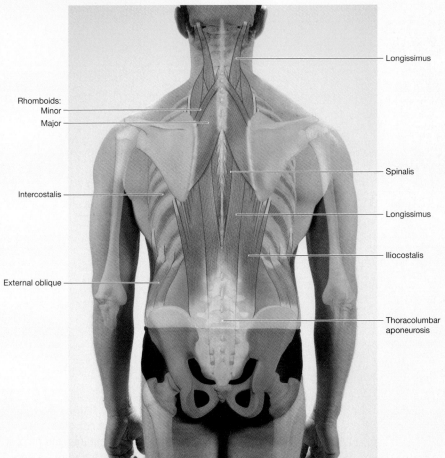

Longissimus

Rhomboids:
  Minor
  Major

Spinalis

Intercostalis

Longissimus

Iliocostalis

External oblique

Thoracolumbar aponeurosis

7-7. Intermediate muscles of the trunk. A. Anterior view. Scapular stabilizers and another layer of protective and prime mover abdominal muscles make up the intermediate layer of the anterior trunk. **B. Posterior view.** More global spinal stabilizers and scapular stabilizers make up the intermediate layer of the posterior trunk.

▌ DEEP MUSCLES OF THE TRUNK

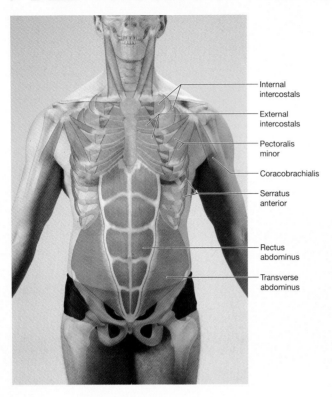

Internal intercostals

External intercostals

Pectoralis minor

Coracobrachialis

Serratus anterior

Rectus abdominus

Transverse abdominus

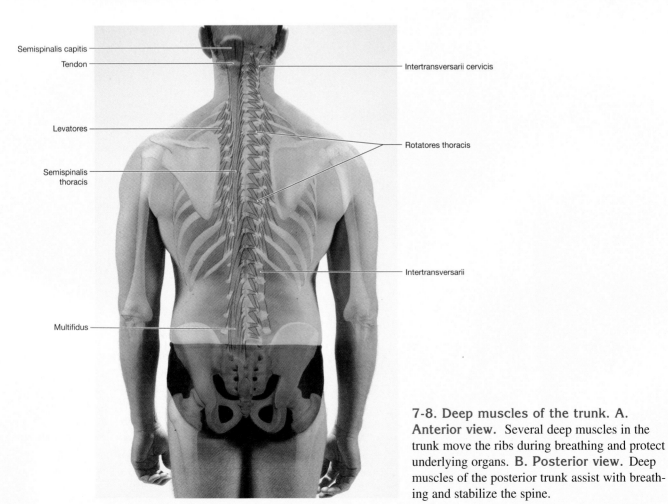

Semispinalis capitis

Tendon

Levatores

Semispinalis thoracis

Multifidus

Intertransversarii cervicis

Rotatores thoracis

Intertransversarii

7-8. Deep muscles of the trunk. A. Anterior view. Several deep muscles in the trunk move the ribs during breathing and protect underlying organs. **B. Posterior view.** Deep muscles of the posterior trunk assist with breathing and stabilize the spine.

▌ MUSCLES OF BREATHING

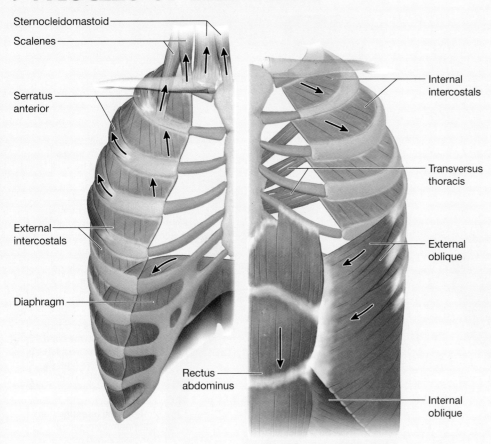

Sternocleidomastoid

Scalenes

Serratus anterior

External intercostals

Diaphragm

Internal intercostals

Transversus thoracis

External oblique

Rectus abdominus

Internal oblique

7-9. Muscles of breathing. Several deep and intermediate muscles work together to produce inhalation and forced exhalation.

▶ SPECIAL STRUCTURES OF THE TRUNK

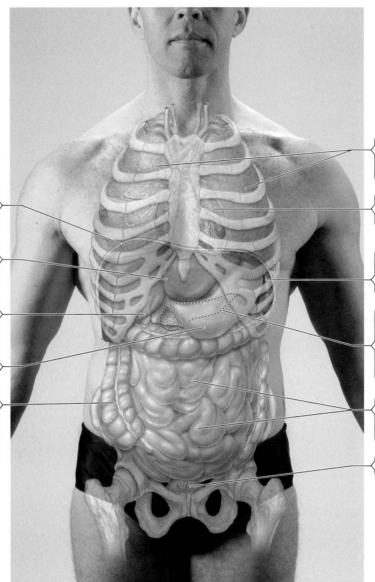

Right and left **lungs** are sheltered by the upper ribs.

The **heart** is protected by the sternum and ribs.

Right dome of the **diaphragm**, the main muscle of breathing.

The **liver** has more than 500 functions, primarily in digestion and metabolism.

The **gallbladder** stores bile, which helps to break down fats.

The **stomach** mixes and begins to digest food.

The large intestine, or **colon**, transports food wastes for elimination from the body.

The **spleen** is a large lymphoid organ posterior to the stomach.

The **pancreas** produces digestive enzymes and hormones that regulate blood glucose. Only its outline is visible here.

The **small intestines** are the primary organ of digestion and absorption.

The **bladder** stores urine.

7-10A. Abdominal and thoracic viscera: anterior view.
The bones and muscles of the trunk protect underlying structures vital to life. Organs of the respiratory, cardiovascular, digestive, and other systems are housed in this region.

❿ SPECIAL STRUCTURES OF THE TRUNK

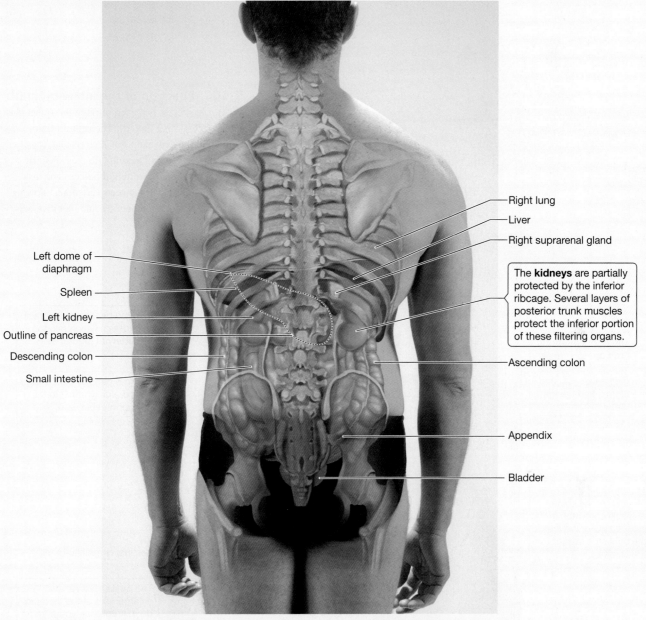

Right lung

Liver

Right suprarenal gland

The **kidneys** are partially protected by the inferior ribcage. Several layers of posterior trunk muscles protect the inferior portion of these filtering organs.

Ascending colon

Appendix

Bladder

Left dome of diaphragm

Spleen

Left kidney

Outline of pancreas

Descending colon

Small intestine

7-10B. Abdominal and thoracic viscera: posterior view. The kidneys are protected partially by the lower ribcage and partially by large muscles of the trunk.

▶ SPECIAL STRUCTURES OF THE TRUNK

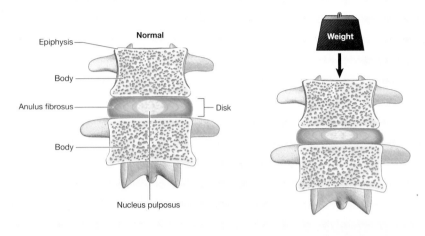

Normal

Epiphysis

Body

Anulus fibrosus

Disk

Body

Nucleus pulposus

Weight

7-10C. Function of the intervertebral disk. As weight is placed through the spine, the intervertebral disk flattens. The central, fluid-containing nucleus pulposus distorts and, together with the surrounding annulus fibrosis, absorbs force, protecting the vertebral bodies. The disk also maintains a gap between vertebrae, allowing passageways for spinal nerves and blood vessels.

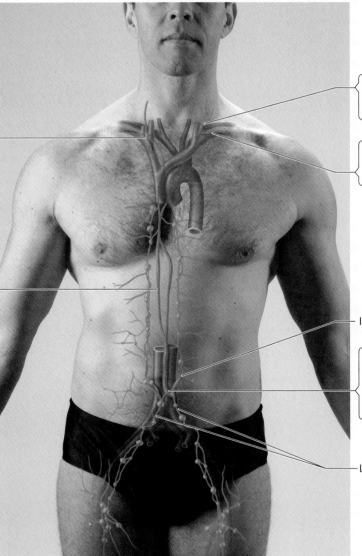

The **right lymphatic duct** collects lymph fom the right side of the head, neck, and thorax, and the right upper extremity.

The **thoracic duct** runs paraellel to the spine and collects lymph from the left side of the and the right side inferior to the diaphragm.

In some people, the thoracic duct drains lymph into the **left internal jugular vein**.

In some people, the thoracic duct drains lymph into the **left subclavian vein**.

Intestinal lymphatic trunk

The **chyle cistern** is an enlargement of the thoracic duct. It collects lymph from the intestinal and lumbar lymphatic trunks.

Lumbar lymphatic trunks

7-10D. Lymphatic vessels and lymph nodes of the trunk.
Several large lymph vessels and clusters of nodes reside deep in the trunk. Both the upper and lower limbs drain lymph into this region to be returned to the circulatory system. Deep breathing can stimulate lymphatic flow in the lower vessels, which are close to the diaphragm.

SPECIAL STRUCTURES OF THE TRUNK

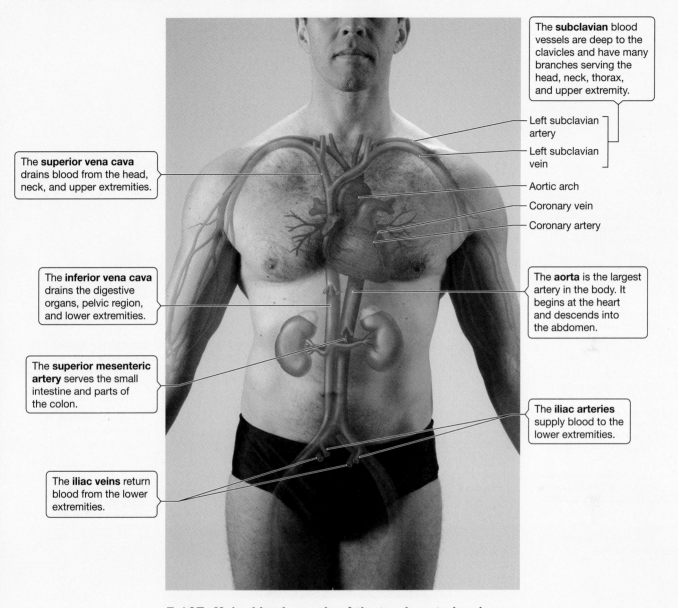

The **subclavian** blood vessels are deep to the clavicles and have many branches serving the head, neck, thorax, and upper extremity.

Left subclavian artery

Left subclavian vein

Aortic arch

Coronary vein

Coronary artery

The **superior vena cava** drains blood from the head, neck, and upper extremities.

The **inferior vena cava** drains the digestive organs, pelvic region, and lower extremities.

The **aorta** is the largest artery in the body. It begins at the heart and descends into the abdomen.

The **superior mesenteric artery** serves the small intestine and parts of the colon.

The **iliac arteries** supply blood to the lower extremities.

The **iliac veins** return blood from the lower extremities.

7-10E. Major blood vessels of the trunk: anterior view.
The aorta and vena cava must pass through the diaphragm muscle (not shown), which separates the thoracic and abdominal cavities.

▶ SPECIAL STRUCTURES OF THE TRUNK

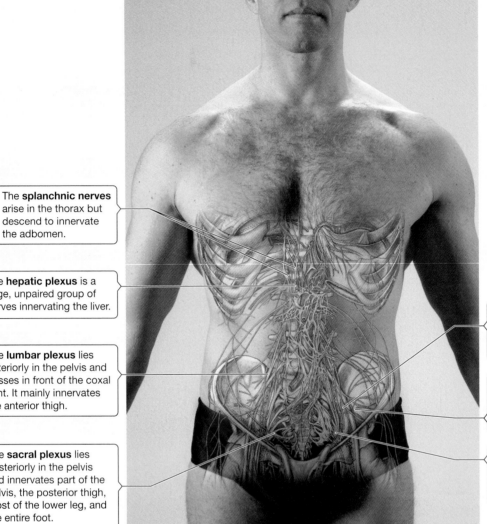

The **splanchnic nerves** arise in the thorax but descend to innervate the adbomen.

The **hepatic plexus** is a large, unpaired group of nerves innervating the liver.

The **lumbar plexus** lies anteriorly in the pelvis and passes in front of the coxal joint. It mainly innervates the anterior thigh.

The **sacral plexus** lies posteriorly in the pelvis and innervates part of the pelvis, the posterior thigh, most of the lower leg, and the entire foot.

The **superior gluteal nerve** innervates the gluteus medius and minimus.

The **inferior gluteal nerve** innervates the gluteus maximus muscle.

The **sciatic nerve** originates near the ischium and descends into the lower extremity.

7-10F. Nerves of the trunk: anterior view. Thoracic, lumbar, and sacral spinal nerves exit the spinal cord and form plexuses, or networks with adjacent blood and lymph vessels. Caution must be used when palpating deep muscles of the abdomen so as not to compress these structures.

▶ SPECIAL STRUCTURES OF THE TRUNK

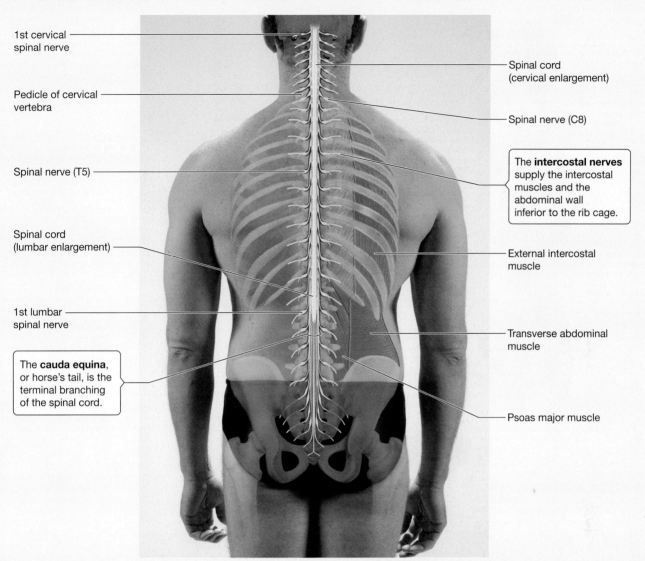

1st cervical
spinal nerve

Pedicle of cervical
vertebra

Spinal nerve (T5)

Spinal cord
(lumbar enlargement)

1st lumbar
spinal nerve

The **cauda equina**,
or horse's tail, is the
terminal branching
of the spinal cord.

Spinal cord
(cervical enlargement)

Spinal nerve (C8)

The **intercostal nerves**
supply the intercostal
muscles and the
abdominal wall
inferior to the rib cage.

External intercostal
muscle

Transverse abdominal
muscle

Psoas major muscle

7-10G. Nerves of the trunk: posterior view. This view reveals
the spinal cord branches at each intervertebral joint forming the 31 pairs of
spinal nerves. These spinal nerves have intimate connections with the vertebrae and surrounding muscles such as the intercostals, transverse abdominus, and psoas major.

▶ POSTURE OF THE TRUNK

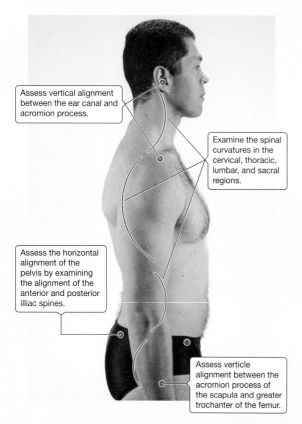

Assess vertical alignment between the ear canal and acromion process.

Examine the spinal curvatures in the cervical, thoracic, lumbar, and sacral regions.

Assess the horizontal alignment of the pelvis by examining the alignment of the anterior and posterior illiac spines.

Assess verticle alignment between the acromion process of the scapula and greater trochanter of the femur.

7-11A. Assessing posture of the trunk: lateral view. Use the lateral view to assess posture in the sagittal plane.

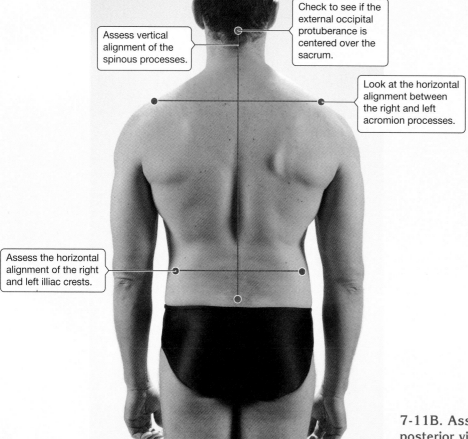

Check to see if the external occipital protuberance is centered over the sacrum.

Assess vertical alignment of the spinous processes.

Look at the horizontal alignment between the right and left acromion processes.

Assess the horizontal alignment of the right and left illiac crests.

7-11B. Assessing posture of the trunk: posterior view. Use the posterior view to assess posture in the frontal and transverse planes.

◗ POSTURE OF THE TRUNK

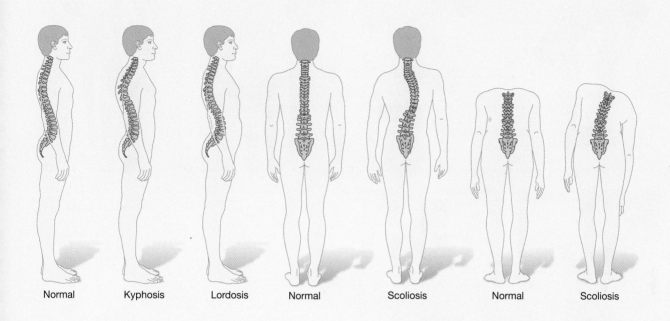

Normal   Kyphosis   Lordosis   Normal   Scoliosis   Normal   Scoliosis

7-12. Common postural deviations. Structural anomalies, muscular imbalances, and poor movement patterns can lead to abnormal or suboptimal posture. Here are several to watch out for when assessing posture. *Kyphosis* is the clinical term for a pathologic exaggeration of the normal thoracic kyphotic curve. It is commonly seen in clients with significant loss of bone density (osteoporosis). *Lordosis* is an exaggeration of the normal lumbar curve. It is common in people who are overweight, and during the later months of pregnancy. *Scoliosis* is a pathologic lateral curvature of the spine. It is typically an inherited condition that becomes most noticeable during the adolescent growth spurt.

▶ MOVEMENTS AVAILABLE: TRUNK

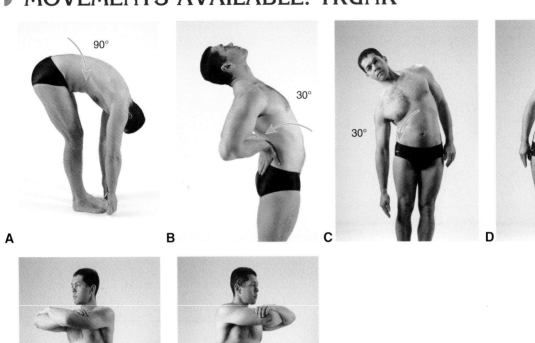

A   B   C   D

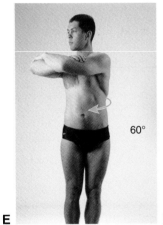 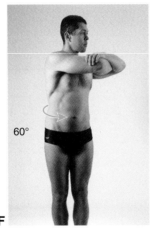

E   F

7-13 **A.** Trunk flexion. **B.** Trunk extension. **C.** Trunk lateral flexion: right. **D.** Trunk lateral flexion: left. **E.** Trunk rotation: right. **F.** Trunk rotation: left.

◗ MOVEMENTS AVAILABLE: BREATHING

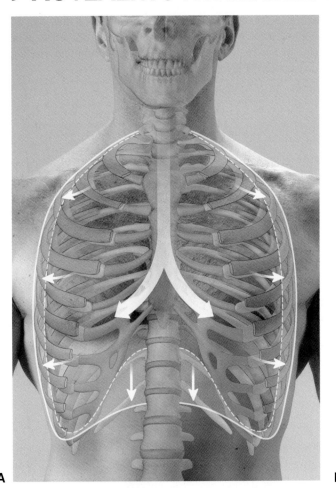

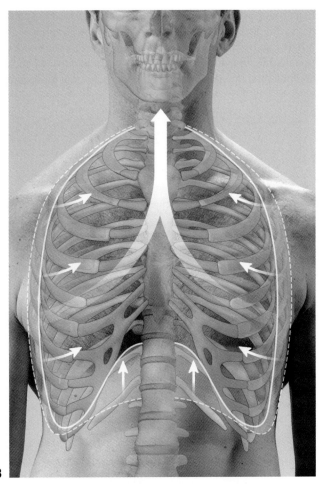

A

B

7-14 A. Inhalation. Expansion of the ribcage decreases air pressure within the thoracic cavity, causing air to rush into the lungs.
B. Exhalation. Compression of the ribcage increases air pressure within the thoracic cavity, causing air to rush out of the lungs.

▶ RESISTED RANGE OF MOTION

Performing resisted range of motion (ROM) for the trunk helps establish the health and function of the dynamic stabilizers and prime movers in this region. Evaluating functional strength and endurance helps you to identify balance and potential imbalance between the muscles that move and stabilize the spine and axial skeleton. Notice that you do not assess passive range of motion as this is not practical or safe in this region. Procedures for performing and grading resisted ROM are outlined in Chapter 3.

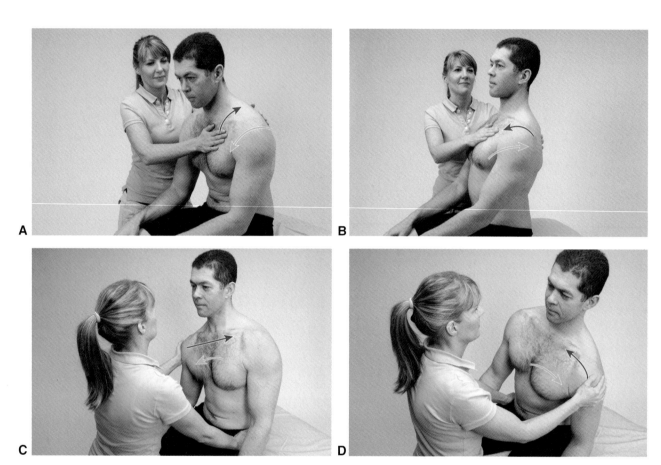

7-15 A. Resisted trunk flexion. The green arrow indicates the direction of movement of the client and the red arrow indicates the direction of resistance from the practitioner. Stand at your seated client's side facing the anterior torso. Place one arm across your client's upper chest and the other across the client's upper back. Instruct the client to meet your resistance by curling the trunk as you gently but firmly straighten the trunk. Assess the strength and endurance of the muscles that flex the trunk. **B. Resisted trunk extension.** Stand at your seated client's side, facing the anterior torso. Place one arm across your client's upper chest and the other across the upper back. Instruct your client to meet your resistance by arching the back as you gently but firmly curl their trunk forward. Assess the strength and endurance of the muscles that extend the trunk. **C. Resisted trunk lateral flexion: right.** Stand in front of your seated client, facing the anterior torso. Place one hand on your client's right lateral shoulder and the other on the side of the left hip. Instruct your client to meet your resistance by tipping the right shoulder toward the right hip as you gently but firmly tip the left shoulder toward the left hip. Assess the strength and endurance of the muscles that laterally flex the trunk to the right. **D. Resisted trunk lateral flexion: left.** Stand in front of your seated client, facing the anterior torso. Place one hand on your client's left lateral shoulder and the other on the side of the right hip. Instruct your client to meet your resistance by tipping the left shoulder toward the left hip as you gently but firmly tip the right shoulder toward the right hip. Assess the strength and endurance of the muscles that laterally flex the trunk to the left. *(continues)*

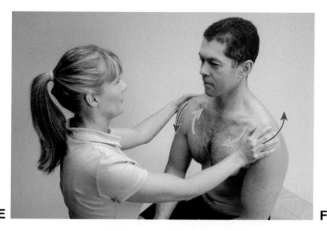

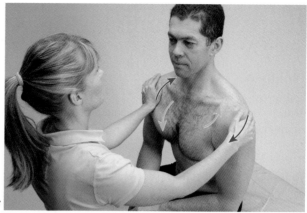

E   **F**

7-15 *(continued)* **E. Resisted trunk rotation: right.** Stand in front of your seated client, facing them. Place one hand on the front of your client's left shoulder and the other on the back of the right. Instruct your client to meet your resistance by turning the upper body to the right as you gently but firmly turn the upper body to the left. Assess the strength and endurance of the muscles that rotate the trunk to the right. **F. Resisted trunk rotation: left.** Stand in front of your seated client, facing them. Place one hand on the front of your client's right shoulder and the other on the back of the left. Instruct your client to meet your resistance by turning the upper body to the left as you gently but firmly turn the upper body to the right. Assess the strength and endurance of the muscles that rotate the trunk to the left.

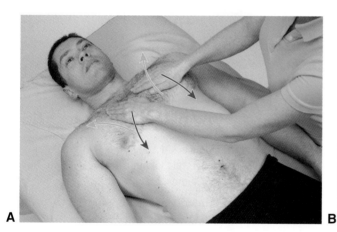

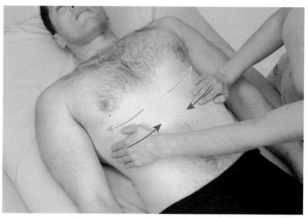

A   **B**

7-16 A. Resisted inhalation: upper ribcage. Stand to the side of your supine client, facing them. Place both your hands on the anterior chest. Instruct your client to meet your resistance by breathing deeply into the chest as you gently but firmly press your hands posteriorly and inferiorly. Assess the strength and endurance of the muscles of inhalation.
B. Resisted inhalation: lower ribcage. Stand to the side of your supine client, facing them. Place one hand on each side of the lower ribcage. Instruct your client to meet your resistance by breathing deeply into the abdomen and sides as you gently but firmly compress the ribcage medially. Assess the strength and endurance of the muscles of inhalation.

Rectus Abdominis • rek′*tus* ab dom′i nis • Latin "**rectus**" *straight* "**abdominus**" *of the abdomen*

Attachments

O: Pubis, crest, and symphysis
I: Ribs 5–7, costal cartilage, and xiphoid process of sternum

Actions

- Flexes the vertebral column (bilateral action)
- Laterally flexes the vertebral column (unilateral action)

Innervation

- T5–T12
- Ventral rami

Functional Anatomy

Rectus abdominis is the most anterior abdominal muscle. It connects the sternum and ribcage to the pubis, and its right and left sides are separated by the vertical linea alba. The fibers of rectus abdominis are also segmented horizontally; each side is divided into five paired sections by a horizontal line of connective tissue. The resulting segments are commonly referred to as a "six pack," since other muscles typically obscure the most superior and inferior segments. Segmentation of rectus abdominis allows for graded movement in the trunk. Sequential contraction of segment pairs creates a rounding effect during trunk flexion.

Besides graded flexion, the rectus abdominis muscles can act unilaterally to assist in lateral flexion. This capacity becomes important during walking. The right rectus abdominis fires with its corresponding right erector spinae muscles to stabilize the trunk as weight is accepted onto the right leg. As weight is shifted onto the left leg, the left rectus abdominis and erector spinae muscles are activated to stabilize the trunk. This unilateral stabilization can be viewed on the student CD included with this text.

Rectus abdominis is also important in maintaining upright posture. It counterbalances the posterior erector spinae muscles, keeping the anterior pelvis fixed superiorly. Weakness in rectus abdominis allows the anterior portion of the pelvis to tip inferiorly (imagine the pelvis as a bowl of water spilling out the front), creating an *anterior pelvic tilt*. This excessively increases the spine's natural lumbar lordosis and can be a cause of low back pain.

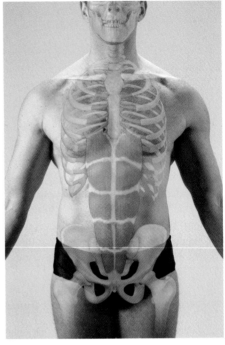

7-17

Palpating Rectus Abdominis

Positioning: client supine.

1. Standing at the client's side, face the abdomen and locate the inferior edge of the anterior ribcage with the palms of both your hands.
2. Slide your hands inferiorly, into the space between the xiphoid process and the anterior pelvis.
3. Locate the segmented fibers of rectus abdominis on either side of the linea alba.
4. Client gently raises both shoulders off of the table to ensure proper location.

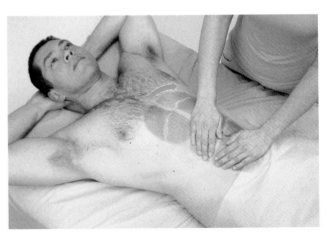

7-18

External Oblique • eks ter'nal o blek • Latin "**extern**" *outward* "**obliquus**" *slanting*

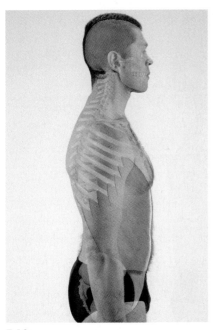

7-19

Palpating External Oblique

Positioning: client supine.

1. Standing at the client's side, face the abdomen and locate the inferior edge of the anterolateral ribcage with the palm of your hand.

2. Slide hand inferiorly into the space between the iliac crest and inferior edge of ribcage.

3. Locate the sloping fibers of external oblique as it angles anteriorly and inferiorly from the lateral ribcage toward the linea alba.

4. Client gently lifts the shoulder of the same side to ensure proper location.

Attachments

O: Ribs 5–12, external surfaces
I: Ilium, anterior crest, inguinal ligament, and linea alba

Actions

- Flexes the vertebral column (bilateral action)
- Laterally flexes the vertebral column (unilateral action)
- Rotates the vertebral column toward opposite side (unilateral action)
- Compresses and supports abdominal organs

Innervation

- T7–T12

Functional Anatomy

The external oblique lies superficial to the internal oblique and lateral to rectus abdominis. It is a thick, strong, prime mover. Its fibers run at an oblique angle from the lateral ribs anteriorly and inferiorly to the ilium, inguinal ligament, and linea alba. The origin of external oblique interdigitates with the costal attachments of serratus anterior (see Chapter 4).

External oblique functions with internal oblique and transverse abdominis to compress and protect the abdominal contents during forced exhalation. When the right and left sides of the external and internal obliques work together, the trunk flexes at the waist. During rotation, the right external oblique teams up with the left internal oblique to turn the trunk to the left. The left external oblique works with the right internal oblique to turn the trunk to the right. During flexion and rotation, these muscles rely on the deep transversospinalis muscles to maintain vertebral alignment. The external and internal obliques are active when we swing an axe, throw overhand, or push with one hand.

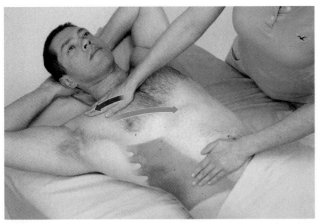

7-20

Internal Oblique

in *ter'nal o blek* • Latin "**intern**" *inward* "**obliquus**" *slanting*

Attachments

O: Thoracolumbar aponeurosis, iliac crest, and lateral inguinal ligament
I: Ribs 10–12, internal surfaces, medial pectineal line of pubis, and linea alba

Actions

- Flexes the vertebral column (bilateral action)
- Laterally flexes the vertebral column (unilateral action)
- Rotates the vertebral column toward same side (unilateral action)
- Compresses and supports abdominal organs

Innervation

- T7–T12, L1
- Iliohypogastric, ilioinguinal, and ventral rami nerves

Functional Anatomy

The internal oblique lies superficial to transverse abdominis, deep to the external oblique, and lateral to rectus abdominis. It is a thick, strong, prime mover muscle. Its fibers run at an oblique angle from the linea alba inferiorly to the ilium and posteriorly to the thoracolumbar aponeurosis.

Internal oblique, external oblique, and transverse abdominis work together to compress and protect the abdominal contents. They are active during forced exhalation. When the right and left sides of the internal and external obliques work together, the trunk flexes, bending the body at the waist. For rotation, the right internal oblique teams up with the left external oblique to turn the trunk to the right. The left internal oblique works with the right external oblique to turn the trunk to the left. These strong trunk rotators rely on the deep transversospinalis muscles to maintain vertebral alignment during movement. The internal and external obliques are responsible for strong rotation and flexion such as in swinging an axe, throwing overhand, and pushing with one hand.

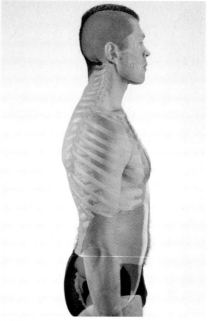

7-21

Palpating Internal Oblique

Positioning: client supine.

1. Standing at the client's side, face the abdomen and locate the inferior edge of the anterolateral ribcage with the palm of your hand.
2. Slide your hand inferiorly, into the space between the iliac crest and inferior edge of ribcage.
3. Locate the sloping fibers of internal oblique as it angles inferiorly and posteriorly from the linea alba toward the lateral iliac crest.
4. Client gently turns the trunk to the same side to ensure proper location.

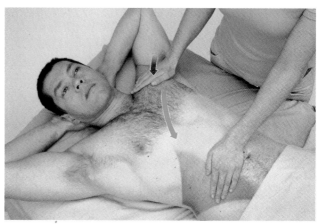

7-22

Transverse Abdominis
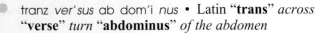
tranz *ver'sus* ab dom'i *nus* • Latin **"trans"** *across* **"verse"** *turn* **"abdominus"** *of the abdomen*

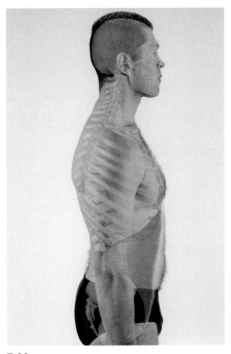

7-23

Palpating Transverse Abdominis

Positioning: client supine.

1. Standing at the client's side, face the abdomen and locate the most lateral edge of the iliac crest with the palms of both your hands, one on each side.

2. Slide your hands superiorly into the space between the iliac crest and inferior edge of ribcage.

3. Locate the horizontal fibers of transverse abdominis with your palms as it wraps around the waist.

4. Client gently exhales while "hissing like a snake" to ensure proper location.

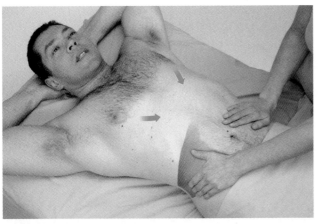

7-24

Attachments

O: Ribs 7–12, costal cartilages, thoracolumbar fascia, internal iliac crest, and lateral inguinal ligament
I: Linea alba and crest and pectineal line of pubis

Actions

• Compresses and supports abdominal organs
• Assists with exhalation

Innervation

• T7–T12, L1
• Lower intercostal, iliohypogastric, and ilioinguinal nerves

Functional Anatomy

Transverse abdominis is the deepest of the abdominal muscles. Its fibers run horizontally and wrap around the waist from the vertebral column to the linea alba. Transverse abdominis is unique in that it has no true action. Instead, it is defined by its function of increasing intra-abdominal pressure. Transverse abdominis joins the internal and external oblique muscles at the abdominal fascia, a sturdy sheath of connective tissue terminating anteriorly at the linea alba and lying superficial to rectus abdominis.

Contraction of transverse abdominis compresses the organs and contents of the abdominal cavity. The resulting increase in pressure within the abdominal cavity serves three functions. First, it assists with expulsion of air during forced exhalation. Second, it assists with expulsion of abdominal contents such as urine and feces, or stomach contents during vomiting. Third, and most importantly to human movement, it supports and stabilizes the lumbar spine. This last function earns transverse abdominus the nickname of "anatomical weightbelt." A strong, functional transverse abdominus will serve the same purpose as the thick belts worn to prevent injury when lifting heavy objects.

Diaphragm ● *di'a* fram • Greek "**dia**" *through* "**phragma**" *partition*

Attachments

O: Ribs 7–12, inner surfaces and costal cartilages, xiphoid
process of sternum, and bodies of L1–L2
I: Central tendon

Actions

• Expands thoracic cavity during inhalation

Innervation

• C3–C5
• Phrenic nerve

Functional Anatomy

The diaphragm is a dome-shaped muscle that forms a seal
around the inferior ribcage and separates the thoracic and
abdominal cavities. It has several openings for blood vessels, nerves, and structures of the digestive system. The
muscle fibers of the diaphragm converge in the center to
form the central tendon. This tendon forms the most superior, medial area of the dome.

The diaphragm is the primary muscle of breathing. As
it contracts, the central tendon is pulled inferiorly toward the
abdominal cavity. This flattens the dome, increasing the volume of the thoracic cavity and decreasing its internal air
pressure. Decreased air pressure within the cavity prompts
environmental air to flow inward to equalize air pressure
(inhalation). This mechanism fills the lungs with air. As the
diaphragm relaxes, resuming its domed shape, the space
within the thoracic cavity decreases. Increased pressure
within the thoracic cavity prompts air to flow out of the
lungs to equalize air pressure (exhalation). Contraction and
relaxation of the diaphragm drives breathing when the body
is relaxed. Other muscles such as the intercostals, subcostales, and serratus posterior muscles are activated to increase the depth of breathing.

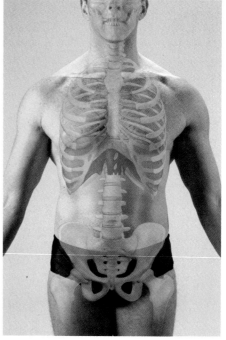

7-25

Palpating the Diaphragm

Positioning: client supine.

1. Standing at the client's side, face the abdomen and locate the inferior edge of the anterolateral ribcage with
your fingertips or pad of your thumb.

2. Instruct your client to take several deep breaths while
you are palpating this muscle.

3. Locate the fibers of the diaphragm by gently sliding
posteriorly and deeply and following the inner surface
of the ribcage.

4. Client inhales to ensure proper location.

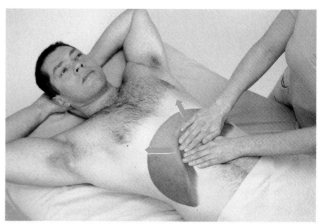

7-26

External Intercostals

eks *ter'nal* in *ter cos'tal* • Latin "**extern**" *outward* "**inter**" *between* "**costal**" *rib*

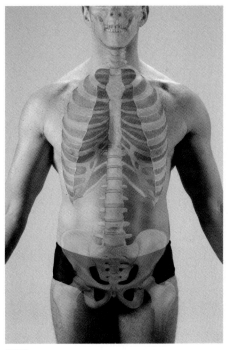

7-27

Palpating External Intercostals

Positioning: client supine.

1. Standing at the client's side, face the abdomen and locate the anterior surface of a rib with the pad of one of your fingers.

2. Slide your finger into the space between this rib and the one immediately superior or inferior.

3. Locate the angled fibers of the external intercostal between the edges of the two ribs.

4. Client forcefully inhales through pursed lips to ensure proper location.

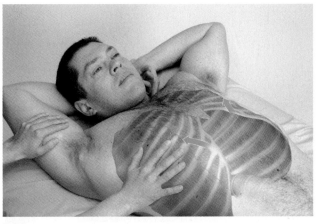

7-28

Attachments

O: Rib, lower border
I: Rib below, upper border

Actions

• Elevate ribs during inhalation

Innervation

• Intercostal nerves

Functional Anatomy

The external intercostals lie between the ribs, superficial to the internal intercostals. Their fibers run at an oblique angle from lateral to medial, like those of the external oblique muscles. The external and internal intercostal muscles help maintain the shape and integrity of the ribcage.

The functional role of the intercostals is controversial. It is clear that they are involved in breathing. Mechanically, the muscles fibers tend to pull the inferior attachment toward the superior attachment, elevating the ribs. This action would assist with inhalation as the ribcage elevates, increasing the space within the thoracic cavity. Activation of the internal and external intercostals seems more significant during activities that require forceful inhalation or exhalation, such as sucking on a straw or blowing out a candle.

Internal Intercostals

in *ter'nal* in *ter* kos'*tal* • Latin "intern" *inward* "**inter**" *between* "**costal**" *rib*

Attachments

O: Rib, inner surface and costal cartilage
I: Rib below, upper borders

Actions

• Depress the ribs during exhalation

Innervation

• Intercostal nerves

Functional Anatomy

The internal intercostals lie between the ribs, deep to the external intercostals. Their fibers run at an oblique angle from medial to lateral, like those of the internal oblique muscles. The internal and external intercostals help maintain the shape and integrity of the ribcage.

As with the external intercostals, there is some controversy about the function of the internal intercostals. It is clear that they are involved in respiration, but it is not clear whether they assist with inhalation, exhalation, or both. Mechanically, the muscle fibers are able to pull their superior attachments toward their inferior attachments to depress the ribs. This action would assist with exhalation as the ribcage depresses, decreasing the space within the thoracic cavity. This ability seems to be more prevalent in the posterior fibers. Anteriorly, the intercostals pull the inferior attachment up toward the superior one. This action assists with inhalation as the ribcage elevates, increasing the space within the thoracic cavity. Activation of the intercostals seems to be more significant during forced breathing activities such as sucking on a straw or blowing out a candle.

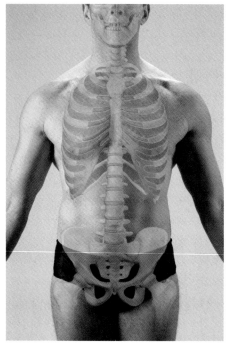

7-29

Palpating Internal Intercostals

Positioning: client supine.

1. Standing at the client's side, face their abdomen and locate the anterior surface of a rib with the pad of one of your fingers.

2. Slide your finger into the space between this rib and the one immediately superior or inferior.

3. Locate the angled fibers of internal oblique between the edges of the two ribs.

4. Client exhales and "hisses like a snake" to ensure proper location.

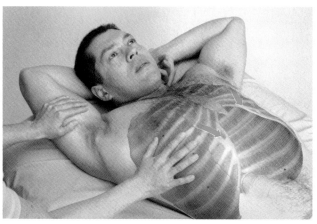

7-30

Iliocostalis
il'e o kos ta'lis • Latin "**ilio**" *of the ilium* "**costalis**" *of the ribs*

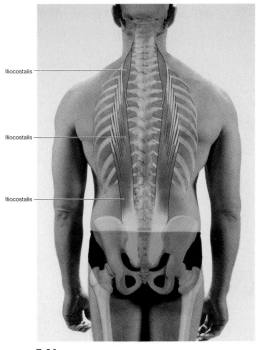

7-31

Palpating Iliocostalis

Positioning: client prone.

1. Standing at the client's side, face the spine and locate the thoracic spinous processes with the fingertips of both your hands.

2. Slide your fingertips laterally, past the lamina groove onto the erector spinae muscles.

3. Strum laterally across the erector spinae muscles with the fingertips of both your hands toward the ribs to find iliocostalis.

4. Client gently lifts the head and extends the trunk to ensure proper location.

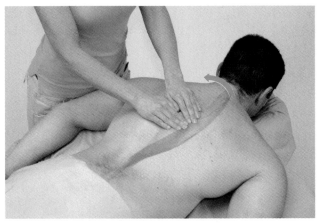

7-32

Attachments

O: sacrum, posterior aspect, medial lip of ilium, and posterior surface of ribs 1–12

I: L1–L3, transverse processes, posterior surface of ribs 1-6, and transverse processes of C4–C7

Actions

• Extends the vertebral column (bilateral action)
• Laterally flexes the vertebral column (unilateral action)

Innervation

• Spinal nerves

Functional Anatomy

The iliocostalis is part of the erector spinae (erect = *upright* and spinae = *spine*) group of muscles. The longissimus and spinalis are also part of this group. These muscles connect the sacrum, ilium, vertebral column, and cranium. They provide broader stabilization and movement than the deeper transversospinalis group. Together, the erector spinae and transversospinalis groups maintain upright posture of the spine against gravity.

Iliocostalis is the most lateral of the three pairs of erector spinae muscles. Its segments extend superiorly and laterally, like the branches of a tree, from the posterior sacrum and ilium to the posterior ribs and transverse processes in the lumbar and cervical spine. These branches give it leverage to extend and strongly laterally flex the vertebral column. Iliocostalis also may contribute to pulling the ribs down during forced exhalation.

Longissimus
lon jis imus • Latin "**longissimus**" *long*

Attachments

O: Thoracolumbar aponeurosis, transverse processes of L5–T1, and articular processes of C4–C7

I: T1–T12, transverse processes, posterior surface of ribs 3–12, transverse processes of C2–C6, and mastoid process of the temporal bone

Actions

- Extends the vertebral column (bilateral action)
- Laterally flexes the vertebral column (unilateral action)
- Rotates the head and neck toward same side (unilateral action of cervical portion)

Innervation

- Spinal nerves

Functional Anatomy

The longissimus is part of the erector spinae group of muscles. The iliocostalis and spinalis are also part of this group, which connects, stabilizes, and allows for broad movements of the sacrum, ilium, vertebral column, and skull. The erector spinae also work with the transversospinalis group to maintain upright posture in the spine against gravity.

Each longissimus lies medial to iliocostalis and lateral to spinalis. This muscle spans the entire axial skeleton and connects the sacrum and cranium: it extends from the sacrum and ilium to the transverse processes of the vertebrae and the mastoid process of the temporal bone. The fibers of longissimus are more vertical than iliocostalis; thus, it is a strong extender and weak lateral flexor of the spine. It also stabilizes and rotates the head and neck by pulling the mastoid process posteriorly and inferiorly toward the spine.

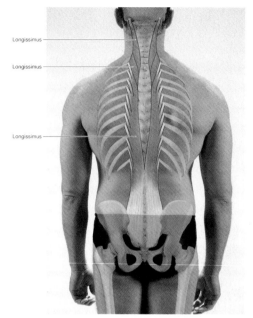

7-33

Palpating Longissimus

Positioning: client prone.

1. Standing at the client's side, face the spine and locate the thoracic spinous processes with fingertips of both your hands.

2. Slide your fingertips laterally, past the lamina groove onto the erector spinae muscles.

3. Strum back and forth across the erector spinae muscles with fingertips of both your hands to differentiate the vertical fibers of longissimus in the center from the lateral, oblique fibers of iliocostalis.

4. Client gently lifts the head and extends the trunk to ensure proper location.

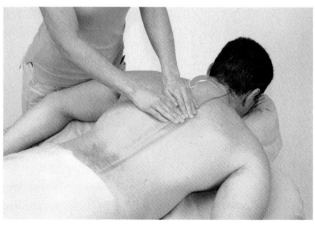

Spinalis ● *spi na'lis* • Latin "**spinalis**" *of the spine*

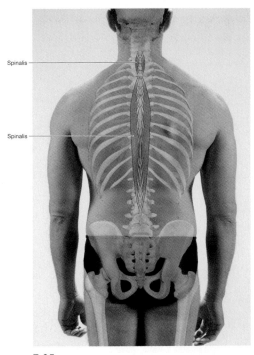

Spinalis

Spinalis

7-35

Palpating Spinalis

Positioning: client prone.

1. Standing at the client's side, face the spine and locate the thoracic spinous processes with the fingertips of both your hands.

2. Slide your fingertips laterally, past the lamina groove onto the erector spinae muscles.

3. Strum back and forth across the erector spinae muscles with the fingertips of both your hands locating the most medial edge formed by spinalis.

4. Client gently lifts the head and extends the trunk to ensure proper location.

Attachments

O: L2–T11, spinous processes, ligamentum nuchae, and spinous processes of T2–C7

I: T1–T8, spinous processes, spinous processes of C2–C4, and between the superior and inferior nuchal lines of the occiput

Actions

- Extends the vertebral column (bilateral action)
- Rotates head and neck toward opposite side (unilateral action)

Innervation

- Spinal nerves

Functional Anatomy

The spinalis is part of the erector spinae group of muscles, which also includes iliocostalis and longissimus. These muscles connect the sacrum, ilium, vertebral column, and cranium, and provide broad stabilization and movement. The erector spinae and transversospinalis group together maintain upright posture in the spine against gravity.

Spinalis is the most medial of the three pairs of erector spinae muscles. It extends from the spinous processes of the lower thoracic and upper lumbar vertebrae to the spinous processes of the upper thoracic and lower cervical vertebrae. Its vertical fibers make it stronger in extension than rotation. In the cervical spine, spinalis joins the semispinalis muscle of the transversospinal group before attaching to the occiput.

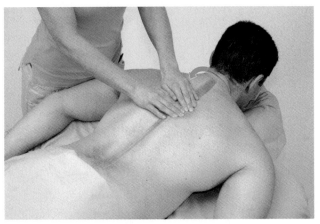

7-36

Quadratus Lumborum

kwah *dra'tus lum bo'rum* • Latin "**quadratus**" *square* "**lumborum**" *of the loins*

Attachments

O: Iliac crest, posterior and iliolumbar ligament
I: L1–L4, transverse processes and inferior border of 12th rib

Actions

- Extends the vertebral column (bilateral action)
- Laterally flexes the vertebral column (unilateral action)
- Depresses/fixes the last rib during inhalation.

Innervation

- T12–L3
- Lumbar plexus

Functional Anatomy

The quadratus lumborum is a deep, multifunctional muscle of the spine. It connects the ilium to the lateral lumbar spine and twelfth rib. The fibers of each quadratus lumborum run slightly diagonal from the rib and spine inferiorly and laterally toward the posterior ilia. Quadratus lumborum lies deep to the erector spinae muscles and posterior to the psoas major, helping form the posterior abdominal wall.

Functionally, the quadratus lumborum muscles position the spine relative to the pelvis when the lower body is fixed. They maintain upright posture, creating fine lateral movements as well as extension when coordinating with the erector spinae muscles. When we stand, the paired quadratus lumborum muscles work with the gluteus medius muscles to position the body over the lower extremities.

During walking, the quadratus lumborum and gluteus medius help stabilize the pelvis as the weight of the body shifts onto one foot, then the other. These muscles prevent the pelvis from shifting laterally and maintain movement in the sagittal plane. Also, quadratus lumborum raises the iliac crest toward the ribcage as weight shifts to the other foot. This action allows the leg to swing forward without the foot hitting the ground.

Quadratus lumborum also assists with breathing. During inhalation, it tethers the 12th rib inferiorly, allowing the ribcage to fully expand. Dysfunction in quadratus lumborum can occur from labored breathing, weakness in gluteus medius, and imbalances in postural muscles such as the erector spinae, abdominals, and psoas.

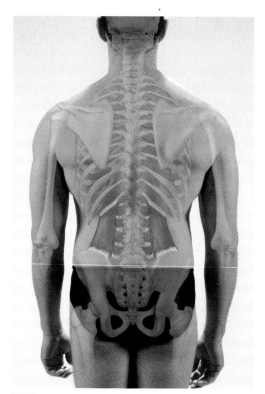

7-37

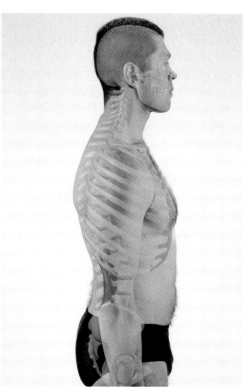

7-38

Quadratus Lumborum *(continued)*

Palpating Quadratus Lumborum

Positioning: client prone.

1. Standing at the client's side, face the spine and locate the lumbar spinous processes with fingertips of both your hands.

2. Slide your fingertips laterally, past the lamina groove and the erector spinae muscles.

3. Palpate deeply between the twelfth rib and ilium to find the angled fibers of quadratus lumborum.

4. Client gently elevates the hip superiorly to ensure proper location.

Positioning: client sidelying with top arm forward or overhead.

1. Standing at the client's side, face the spine and locate the iliac crest of their up-facing hip with your fingertips or elbow.

2. Slide your fingers or elbow superiorly toward the ribcage and laterally to the erector spinae.

3. Palpate deeply between the twelfth rib and ilium to find the angled fibers of quadratus lumborum.

4. Client gently elevates the hip superiorly to ensure proper location.

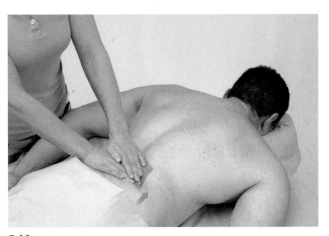

7-39

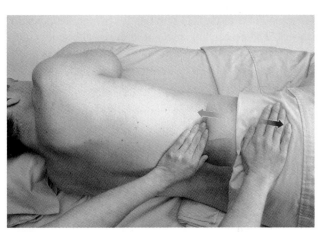

7-40

Serratus Posterior Superior

ser rat′us pos ter′e or su per′e or • Latin "**serra**" *saw* "**posterior**" *toward the back* "**superior**" *above*

Attachments

O: C7–T3, spinous processes and ligamentum nuchae
I: Ribs 2–5, posterior surfaces

Actions

• Elevates ribs during inhalation

Innervation

• Intercostal nerves 2–5

Functional Anatomy

Serratus posterior superior is deep to the rhomboids and trapezius muscles (see Chapter 4). It connects the spine at C7 through T3 to the 2nd through 5th ribs on the posterior ribcage. The descending angle of its fibers allows this muscle to elevate the upper ribs during forced inhalation.

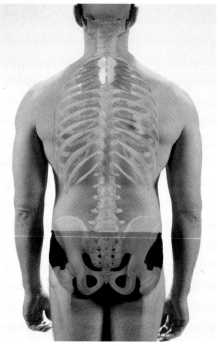

7-41

Palpating Serratus Posterior Superior

Positioning: client prone.

1. Standing at the client's side, face the spine and locate the spinous process of C7–T3 with your fingertips.

2. Slide your fingertips laterally and slightly inferiorly toward the ribs.

3. Locate the inferiorly angled fibers of serratus posterior along the posterior surfaces of ribs 2–12.

4. Client inhales forcefully through pursed lips to ensure proper location.

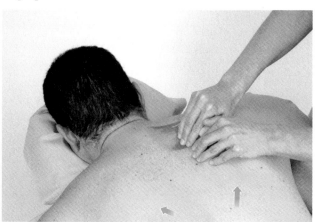

7-42

Serratus Posterior Inferior

ser at'us pos ter'e or su per'e or • Latin "**serra**" *saw* "**posterior**" *toward the back* "**inferior**" *below*

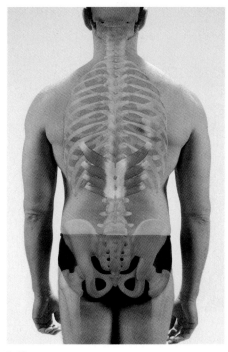

7-43

Attachments

O: T11–L3, spinous processes
I: Ribs 9–12, posterior surfaces

Actions

• Depresses ribs during exhalation

Innervation

• Intercostal nerves

Functional Anatomy

Serratus posterior inferior lies deep to latissimus dorsi (see Chapter 4) and superficial to the erector spinae muscles. It connects the spine at T11 through L3 to the 9th through 12th ribs on the posterior ribcage. The ascending angle of its fibers allows this muscle to depress these ribs. There is some controversy as to this muscle's role in breathing. Most agree that the depression of the lower ribs by serratus posterior inferior assists with forced exhalation.

Palpating Serratus Posterior Inferior

Positioning: client prone.

1. Standing at the client's side, face the spine and locate the spinous process of T11–L3 with your fingertips.

2. Slide your fingertips laterally and slightly superiorly toward the ribs.

3. Locate the superiorly angled fibers of serratus posterior inferior along the posterior surface of the lower ribs.

4. Client exhales and "hisses like a snake" to ensure proper location.

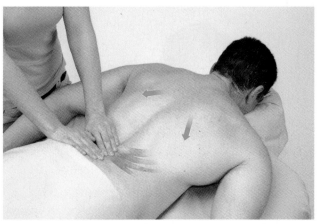

7-44

Semispinalis ● sem′e spi na′lis • Latin "**semi**" *half* "**spinalis**" *of the spine*

Attachments

O: T10–C7, transverse processes and C6–C4 articular processes

I: T4–C2, spinous processes and occiput between superior and inferior nuchal lines

Actions

- Extends the vertebral column (bilateral action)
- Rotates the head and vertebral column toward opposite side (unilateral action)

Innervation

- Spinal nerves

Functional Anatomy

The semispinalis muscles are part of the transversospinalis (transverse = *across* and spinalis = *the spine*) group of muscles. They work with the rotatores and multifidi to stabilize and steer the individual vertebrae as the spinal column moves. But unlike rotatores and multifidi, semispinalis is not present in the lumbar region.

Semispinalis is the most superficial of the transversospinalis muscles. Its fibers connect the transverse process of one vertebra to the spinous process of the vertebra five or six above. Its fiber direction is the most vertical of the transversospinalis muscles; this characteristic gives it the best leverage for extension. All of the transversospinalis muscles rotate the vertebral column to the opposite side by pulling the spinous processes inferiorly toward the transverse processes.

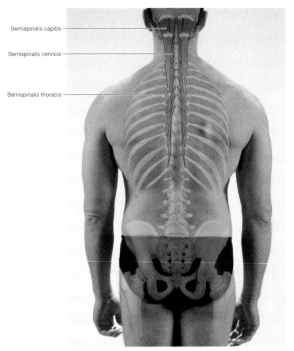

Semispinalis capitis
Semispinalis cervicis
Semispinalis thoracis

7-45

Palpating Semispinalis

Positioning: client prone.

1. Sitting at the client's head, place both your hands palm up under client's head, and find external occipital protuberance with your fingertips.

2. Slide your fingertips inferiorly and laterally into the suboccipital region and lamina groove.

3. Follow the vertical muscle fibers inferiorly within the lamina groove as the client tucks their chin to slack superficial structures.

4. Client gently resists tipping the head back to ensure proper location.

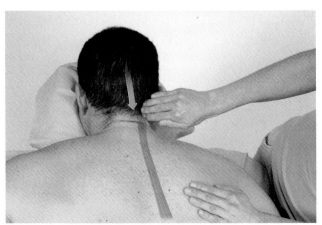

7-46

Multifidi ● *mu'l tif'i di* • Latin "**mult**" *many* "**findus**" *divided*

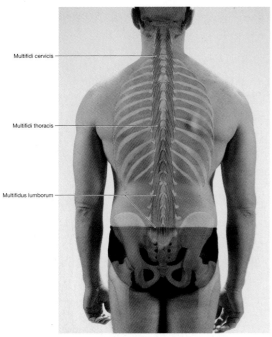

Multifidi cervicis

Multifidi thoracis

Multifidus lumborum

7-47

Palpating Multifidi

Positioning: client prone.

1. Standing at the client's side, face the spine and locate the lumbar spinous processes with fingertips of both your hands.

2. Slide your fingertips laterally and deeply toward the transverse processes or sacrum and into the lamina groove.

3. Locate the multifidi with your fingertips between the spinous processes and transverse processes or sacrum directly below.

4. Client gently lifts the head and one shoulder off the table to ensure proper location.

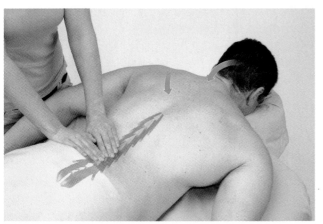

7-48

Attachments

O: L5–C4, transverse processes, posterior sacrum, and posterior iliac spine
I: L5–C2, spinous process 2–4 vertebrae above

Actions

• Extends the vertebral column (bilateral action)
• Rotates vertebra toward opposite side (unilateral action)

Innervation

• Spinal nerves

Functional Anatomy

The multifidi are part of the transversospinalis group of muscles. Together with the rotatores and semispinalis muscles, they form a network connecting the transverse and spinous processes of different vertebrae. They also stabilize and steer the vertebrae as the spinal column moves.

The multifidi lie deep to the semispinalis and superficial to the rotatores. They are present in all segments of the spine. Their fibers connect the transverse process of one vertebra to the spinous process of the vertebrae three or four above. The multifidi lie slightly more vertically than the rotatores, allowing them better leverage to extend the vertebral column. All of the transversospinalis muscles rotate the vertebral column to the opposite side. This is accomplished by pulling the spinous processes toward the transverse processes immediately inferior.

Rotatores ● *ro ta to'rez* • Latin "**rotatores**" *rotators*

Attachments

O: L5–C1, transverse processes
I: Vertebra above, spinous process

Actions

- Extends the vertebral column (bilateral action)
- Rotates vertebra toward opposite side (unilateral action)

Innervation

- Spinal nerves

Functional Anatomy

The rotatores are part of the transversospinalis group of muscles. The multifidi and semispinalis muscles are also part of this group. The deep, small muscles of the transversospinalis group form a network connecting the transverse and spinous processes of different vertebrae. They work together to stabilize and steer the individual vertebrae as the spinal column moves.

The rotatores are the deepest muscles of the transversospinalis group. They're present in all segments of the spine, but most developed in the thoracic spine. Each muscle has two parts: the first connects the transverse process of one vertebra to the spinous process of the vertebra immediately superior, and the second connects the transverse process to the spinous process of the vertebra that is two vertebrae superior. Rotatore's nearly horizontal fiber direction gives it good leverage for rotation, but less for extension. The multifidi and semispinalis muscles are more vertically oriented. All of the transversospinalis muscles rotate the vertebral column to the opposite side. This is accomplished by pulling the spinous processes toward the transverse processes immediately inferior.

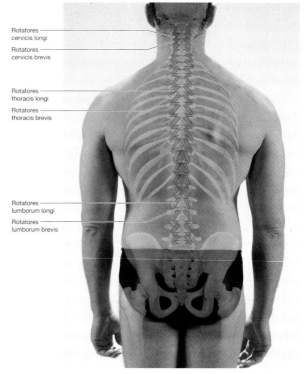

Rotatores cervicis longi
Rotatores cervicis brevis
Rotatores thoracis longi
Rotatores thoracis brevis
Rotatores lumborum longi
Rotatores lumborum brevis

7-49

Palpating Rotatores

Positioning: client prone.

1. Standing at the client's side facing the spine, locate the spinous processes with your fingertips. Use both hands.

2. Slide your fingertips laterally and deeply toward the transverse processes and into the lamina groove.

3. Locate rotatores with your fingertips between the spinous processes and transverse processes directly inferior.

4. Client resists slight trunk rotation to ensure proper location.

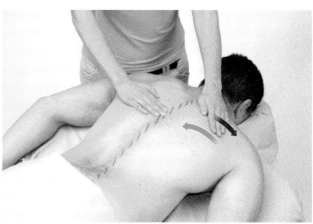

7-50

Interspinalis   in′ter spi na′lez • Latin "**inter**" *between* "**spinalis**" *of the spine*

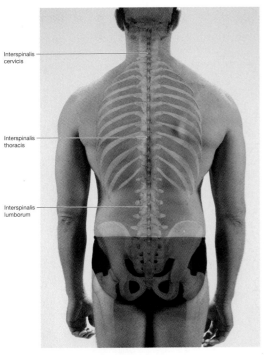

Interspinalis
cervicis

Interspinalis
thoracis

Interspinalis
lumborum

7-51

Palpating Interspinalis

Positioning: client prone over pillow.

1. Standing at the client's side, face the spine and locate the spinous processes with your fingertips.

2. Slide your fingertips between one spinous process and the one below; your client remains relaxed.

3. Locate the vertical fibers of interspinalis centrally between the two spinous processes (one on the right and one on the left of midline).

4. Client gently extends the trunk to ensure proper location.

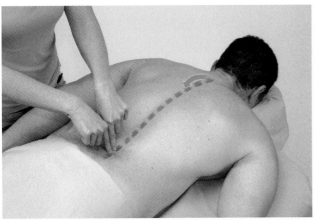

7-52

Attachments

O: L5–T12, spinous processes and T3–C2, spinous processes
I: Vertebra above, spinous process

Actions

• Extends the vertebral column (bilateral action)

Innervation

• Spinal nerves

Functional Anatomy

The interspinalis are small, deep muscles that connect the spinous process of one vertebra to the spinous process of the vertebra immediately superior. They work in pairs, one on each side of the interspinous ligament. Their main function is to monitor and maintain front-to-back posture when the body is upright against gravity. Their muscle fibers are on the posterior, medial vertebral column and run vertically. This position allows them to contract isometrically and maintain the spine upright in the sagittal plane.

The interspinalis muscles are not present throughout the thoracic spine. There is less mobility in this region of the spine due to the stabilizing action of the ribcage and thus less need for stabilizing muscles like the interspinalis.

Intertransversarii

in'ter tranz *ver sa're* i • Latin "**inter**" *between* "**trans**" *across* " **vers**" *turn* "**ari**" *much*

Attachments

O: L5–C1, transverse processes
I: Vertebrae above, transverse processes

Actions

• Laterally flexes the vertebral column (unilateral action)

Innervation

• Spinal nerves

Functional Anatomy

The intertransversari are small, deep muscles that connect the transverse process of one vertebra to the tranverse process of the vertebra immediately superior. So as you might guess, their muscle fibers are laterally oriented on the vertebral column, and run vertically. This position allows them to contract isometrically and maintain the spine upright in the frontal plane. Indeed, their main function is to maintain side-to-side posture against gravity when the body is upright.

The intertransversari of the thoracic spine are indistinguishable from the intercostal muscles between the ribs. There is less call for lateral stabilization by the intertransversari as the ribcage limits movement in this region.

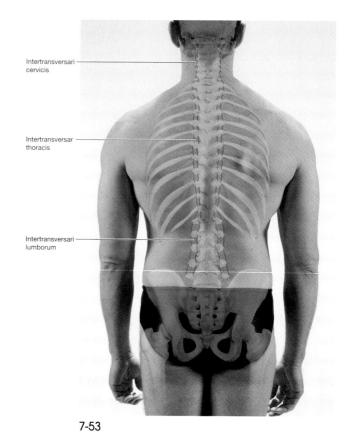

Intertransversari cervicis

Intertransversar thoracis

Intertransversari lumborum

7-53

Palpating Intertransversarii

The intertransversarii muscles are very small and too deep to palpate.

▶ TABLE 7-1. OTHER MUSCLES INVOLVED IN BREATHING

Muscle	Origin	Insertion	Function
Levator costarum	C7–T11 Transverse Processes	Ribs 1–12, angle of rib below	Elevates rib during forced inhalation
Subcostales	Ribs 10–12, near angle	Ribs 8–10, near angle	Depresses ribs 8–10 during forced exhalation
Transversus Thoracis	Xiphoid process and sternum	Ribs 2–6, costal cartilage	Depresses ribs 2–6 during forced exhalation

▶ SYNERGISTS/ANTAGONISTS: TRUNK

Trunk Motion	Muscles Involved	Trunk Motion	Muscles Involved
Flexion 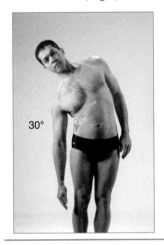 (image shows 90°)	Rectus Abdominis External oblique Internal oblique	Extension 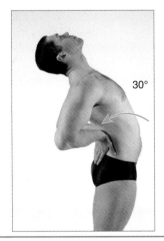 (image shows 30°)	Iliocostalis Longissimus Spinalis Quadratus lumborum Semispinalis Rotatores Multifidi Interpinalis
Lateral Flexion (Right) 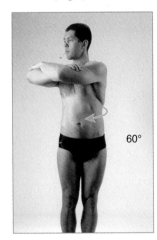 (image shows 30°)	Right rectus abdominus Right external oblique Right internal oblique Right iliocostalis Right longissimus Right quadratus Lumborum Right intertransversarii	Lateral Flexion (Left) 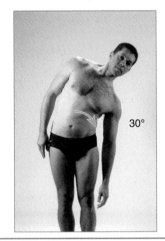 (image shows 30°)	Left rectus abdominus Left external oblique Left internal oblique Left iliocostalis Left longissimus Left quadratus lumborum Left intertransversarii
Rotation (Right) 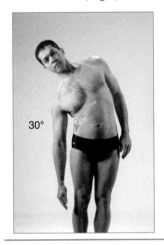 (image shows 60°)	Right external oblique Left internal oblique Left semispinalis Left multifidi Left rotatores	Rotation (Left) 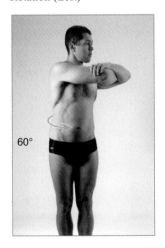 (image shows 60°)	Left external oblique Right internal oblique Right semispinalis Right multifidi Right rotatores

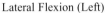

▶ SYNERGISTS/ANTAGONISTS: BREATHING

Thoracic Motion	Muscles Involved	Thoracic Motion	Muscles Involved
Inhalation	Diaphragm	Exhalation	Internal intercostals
	External intercostals		Serratus posterior inferior
	Serratus posterior superior		Transverse abdominus
	Levator costarum		Internal oblique
	Quadratus lumborum		External oblique
	Scalenes (see Ch 6)		Rectus abdominus
	Pectoralis minor (see Ch 4)		Subcostales
	Serratus anterior (see Ch 4)		Transverse thoracis

▶ PUTTING IT IN MOTION

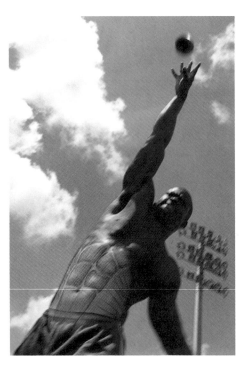

Pushing. The abdominal muscles are capable of powerful forward movements of the trunk. The arms and trunk flexors work together when pushing anteriorly and overhead such as with this throwing motion.

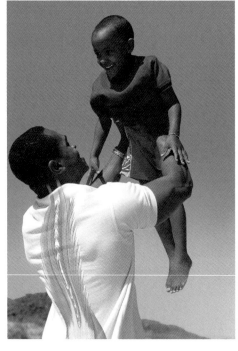

Lifting. Maintaining erect posture and re-establishing this posture after bending is a primary function of the trunk extensors. The erector spinae group is a main contributor to this function, particularly when carrying or moving loads in the front of the body.

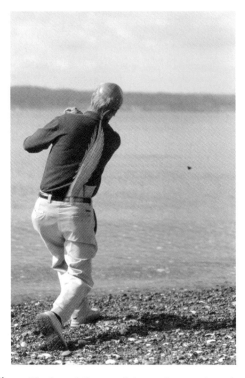

Bending. The lateral flexors of the trunk are active when bending toward one side of the body. Deep stabilizers, such as the quadratus lumborum and erector spinae muscles, maintain posture while the abdominals power the movement of bending to the side.

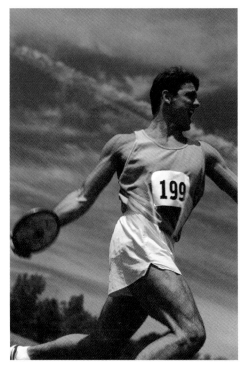

Twisting. Rotational movements such as throwing require coordination of the deep spinal stabilizers and superficial prime movers of rotation. The rotatores and multifidi muscles maintain spinal alignment while the obliques turn the body and generate force in the trunk.

SUMMARY

- The bones of the trunk include the thoracic and lumbar vertebrae, sacrum, and coccyx, the 12 ribs, the sternum, and the paired ilium, ischium, and pubis.
- The ribcage contains anterior costosternal joints and posterior costovertebral joints while the spinal column consists of overlapping intervertebral joints.
- The spinal column has four curved divisions: the lordotic cervical spine, kyphotic thoracic spine, lordotic lumbar spine, and kyphotic sacral region.
- Each spinal division has unique bony and soft tissue features that regulate mobility and function.
- Deep muscles such as the rotatores and multifidi stabilize spinal segments while large superficial muscles like the obliques and erector spinae powerfully move the trunk.
- Complex networks of nerves branch from the spinal cord and form plexuses in the trunk. Trunk bones and muscles are nourished and drained by circulatory and lymphatic vessels.
- Movements available in the trunk include flexion, extension, lateral flexion, and rotation.
- The motions responsible for inhalation and exhalation occur in the trunk and are controlled mainly by the diaphragm, intercostals, and abdominals.
- Coordinated movement of the trunk muscles creates smooth, efficient motions such as pushing, lifting, bending, and twisting.

FOR REVIEW

Multiple Choice

1. Lordotic curvatures are normally found in the:
   A. cervical and thoracic spine
   B. cervical and lumbar spine
   C. thoracic and lumbar spine
   D. cervical and sacral regions

2. Kyphotic curvatures are normally found in the:
   A. cervical and thoracic spine
   B. cervical and lumbar spine
   C. thoracic and sacral regions
   D. lumbar and sacral regions

3. The floating ribs are named for lack of attachment to the:
   A. sternum
   B. costocartilage
   C. vertebral body
   D. transverse processes

4. Organs that are protected by the ribcage include the:
   A. heart, liver, and small intestine
   B. small intestine, spleen, and liver
   C. colon, stomach, and spleen
   D. heart, spleen, and lungs

5. An enlargement at the end of the thoracic duct that collects lymph from lumbar lymphatic trunks is called the:
   A. right lymphatic duct
   B. chyle cistern
   C. abdominal aorta
   D. intestinal lymphatic trunk

6. Large vessels that return blood from the arms, legs, and head to the heart are the:
   A. aorta and chyle cistern
   B. renal vein and artery
   C. inferior vena cava and superior vena cava
   D. aorta and inferior vena cava

7. The gelatinous center of the intervertebral disk absorbs force and is called the:
   A. vertebral body
   B. transverse process
   C. anulus fibrosus
   D. nucleus pulposus

8. The spinal cord branches to form _____ distinct pairs of spinal nerves.
   A. 31
   B. 21
   C. 51
   D. 10

9. The muscle primarily responsible for relaxed breathing is the:
   A. rectus abdominis
   B. transverse abdominis
   C. derratus posterior superior
   D. diaphragm

10. A muscle that has no true action or movement, but functions to compress and support the abdominal organs, is the:
    A. rectus abdominis
    B. transverse abdominis
    C. serratus posterior superior
    D. diaphragm

Matching

Different muscle attachments are listed below. Match the correct muscle with its attachment.

11. _____ T1–T8, spinous processes, spinous processes of C2–C4, and between the superior and inferior nuchal lines of the occiput

12. _____ Ribs 5–12, external surfaces

13. _____ Ribs 7–12, inner surfaces and costal cartilages, xiphoid process of sternum, and bodies of L1–L2

14. _____ L5–C2, spinous process 2–4 vertebrae above

15. _____ Linea alba and crest and pectineal line of pubis

16. _____ Ribs 2–5, posterior surfaces

17. _____ Thoracolumbar fascia, iliac crest, and lateral inguinal ligament

18. _____ Vertebrae above, transverse processes

19. _____ Vertebra above, spinous process

20. _____ Thoracolumbar aponeurosis, transverse processes of L5–T1, and articular processes of C4–C7

A. Serratus posterior superior
B. Intertransversarii
C. Spinalis
D. Multifidi
E. Longissimus
F. Transverse abdominis
G. Rotatores
H. Diaphragm
I. Internal oblique
J. External oblique

Different muscle actions are listed below. Match the correct muscle with its action. Answers may be used more than once.

21. _____ Right internal oblique

22. _____ Left intertransversarii

23. _____ Rectus abdominis

24. _____ Diaphragm

25. _____ Right external oblique

26. _____ Transverse abdominis

27. _____ Serratus posterior inferior

28. _____ Left rotatores

29. _____ Right quadratus lumborum

30. _____ Longissimus

A. Trunk flexion
B. Trunk extension
C. Trunk right lateral flexion
D. Trunk left lateral flexion
E. Trunk right rotation
F. Trunk left rotation
G. Inhalation
H. Exhalation

Short Answer

31. Compare and contrast the structures of the thoracic and lumbar vertebrae. What do they have in common and what is different about them? Briefly explain the purpose or cause of their differences.

32. Draw or explain the structures of the ribcage. Include all bones, articulations, and muscles. Describe how this structure is able to expand and contract to create breathing.

33. Make a list of all the muscles of the trunk that attach to the spine. Briefly describe the function of each.

Try This!

Activity 1: Find a partner. Study the person's standing posture from the side. Write down what you observe about their postural alignment. Repeat this process, this time looking from the back. If you notice any deviations, use your knowledge of muscle functions and relationships to determine which muscles might be out of balance. See if you can figure out which muscles are tight. Switch partners and repeat the process. Compare your findings.

Activity 2: Find a partner and have him or her perform one of the skills identified in the *Putting It in Motion* segment. Identify the specific actions of the trunk that make up this skill. Write them down. Use the synergist list to identify which muscles work together to create this movement. Make sure you put the actions in the correct sequence. See if you can discover which muscles are stabilizing or steering the joints into position and which are responsible for powering the movement.

Suggestions: Switch partners and perform a different skill from *Putting It in Motion*. Repeat the steps above. Confirm your findings with the *Putting It in Motion* segment on the student CD included with your textbook. To further your understanding, practice this activity with skills not identified in *Putting It in Motion*.

Activity 3: Make your own diaphragm model! First, cut the bottom end off of a plastic bottle (a 2-liter bottle works well). Next, cut a piece of exercise band large enough to cover the newly opened end of the bottle. Tape the band to the bottle securely so that it seals that end. Be sure there are no gaps. Finally, place a small balloon inside the top end of the bottle so it sits inside and seals the top of the bottle. Now you can pull down on the center of the bottom seal. What happens to the balloon? What happens when you push up on the bottom seal? How is this like the action of the diaphragm and the lungs?

SUGGESTED READINGS

Chek P. Corrective postural training and the massage therapist. *J Massage Ther.* 1995;34(3):83.

Drysdale CL, Earl JE, Hertel J. Surface electromyographic activity of the abdominal muscles during pelvic-tilt and abdominal hollowing exercises. *J Athl Train.* 2004;39(1):32–36.

Konrad P, Schmitz K, Denner S. Neuromuscular evaluation of trunk-training exercises. *J Athl Train.* 2001;36(2):109–118.

Scannell JP, McGill SM. Lumbar posture-should it and can it be modified? A study of passive tissue stiffness and lumbar position during activities of daily living. *Phys Ther.* 2003;83:907–917.

Udermann BE, Mayer JM, Graves JE, et al. Quantitative assessment of lumbar paraspinal muscle endurance. *J Athl Train.* 2003;38(3):259–262.

Pelvis, Thigh, and Knee

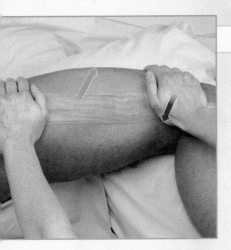

Learning Objectives

After working through the material in this chapter, you should be able to:

- Identify the main structures of the pelvis, thigh, and knee, including bones, joints, special structures, and deep and superficial muscles.

- Label and palpate the major surface landmarks of the pelvis, thigh, and knee.

- Identify normal posture and postural deviations of the pelvis, thigh, and knee.

- Identify and demonstrate all actions of the muscles of the pelvis, thigh, and knee.

- Demonstrate passive and resisted range of motion of the pelvis, thigh, and knee.

- Draw, label, palpate, and fire the superficial and deep muscles of the pelvis, thigh, and knee.

- Locate the attachments and nerve supply of the muscles of the pelvis, thigh, and knee.

- Describe the unique functional anatomy and relationships between each muscle of the pelvis, thigh, and knee.

- Identify both the synergists and antagonists involved in each movement of the hip and knee (flexion, extension, etc.).

- Identify muscles used in performing four coordinated movements of the hip and knee: running, lifting, throwing, and kicking.

▶ OVERVIEW OF THE REGION

The pelvic girdle is similar to the shoulder girdle, but has a few structural and functional differences. Both the shoulder and pelvic girdles provide anchors for the extremities. The shoulder girdle is highly mobile, increasing movement possibilities in the upper extremity. The pelvic girdle is more stable, bearing the weight of the trunk and upper body. It also receives and transmits forces generated in the lower extremity.

The hip joint parallels the shoulder joint in the upper extremity. Each allows multiplanar movements, but the hip must bear the body's weight and therefore requires more stability. This stability is achieved through deeper joint articulations, strong ligament networks, and multilayered muscle groups.

The knee is a modified hinge and includes articulations between the femur, tibia, and patella. Its unique anatomy balances stability for weight bearing with rotational mobility for direction changes such as pivoting around a planted foot. Several unique structures help support and cushion the knee.

▶ SURFACE ANATOMY OF THE PELVIS, THIGH, AND KNEE

The **iliac crest** is the superior edge of the wing of the coxal bone.

The **femoral triangle** is formed by the inguinal ligament, sartorius, and adductor longus.

Tensor fascia latae is a small hip flexor visible on the anterior thigh.

Rectus femoris is a prime mover for hip flexion and knee extension.

Vastus lateralis is part of the quadriceps and forms the bulk of the lateral thigh.

Vastus medialis is part of the quadriceps and has a teardrop shape just superior and medial to the knee.

The **patella** is commonly called the kneecap.

The **patellar tendon** joins the quadriceps muscles, crosses the patella and attaches to the tibia tuberosity.

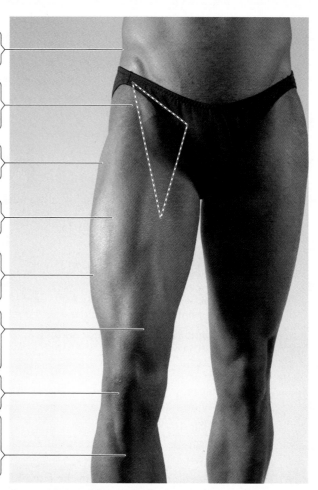

8-1A. Anterior view.

▶SURFACE ANATOMY OF THE PELVIS, THIGH, AND KNEE

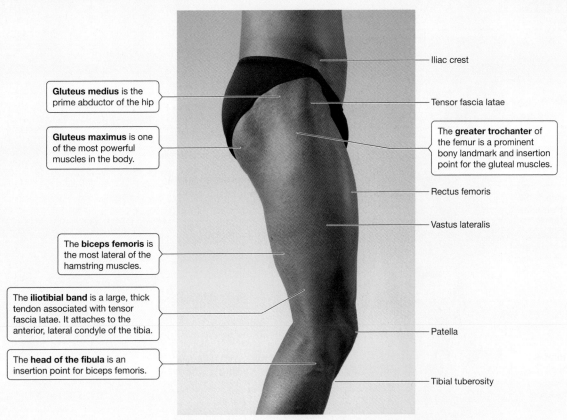

Gluteus medius is the prime abductor of the hip

Gluteus maximus is one of the most powerful muscles in the body.

The **biceps femoris** is the most lateral of the hamstring muscles.

The **iliotibial band** is a large, thick tendon associated with tensor fascia latae. It attaches to the anterior, lateral condyle of the tibia.

The **head of the fibula** is an insertion point for biceps femoris.

Iliac crest

Tensor fascia latae

The **greater trochanter** of the femur is a prominent bony landmark and insertion point for the gluteal muscles.

Rectus femoris

Vastus lateralis

Patella

Tibial tuberosity

8-1B. Lateral view.

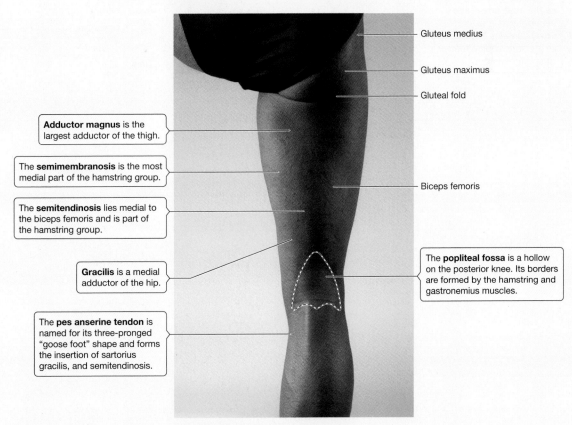

Adductor magnus is the largest adductor of the thigh.

The **semimembranosis** is the most medial part of the hamstring group.

The **semitendinosis** lies medial to the biceps femoris and is part of the hamstring group.

Gracilis is a medial adductor of the hip.

The **pes anserine tendon** is named for its three-pronged "goose foot" shape and forms the insertion of sartorius gracilis, and semitendinosis.

Gluteus medius

Gluteus maximus

Gluteal fold

Biceps femoris

The **popliteal fossa** is a hollow on the posterior knee. Its borders are formed by the hamstring and gastronemius muscles.

8-1C. Posterior view.

▶ SKELETAL STRUCTURES OF THE PELVIS, THIGH, AND KNEE

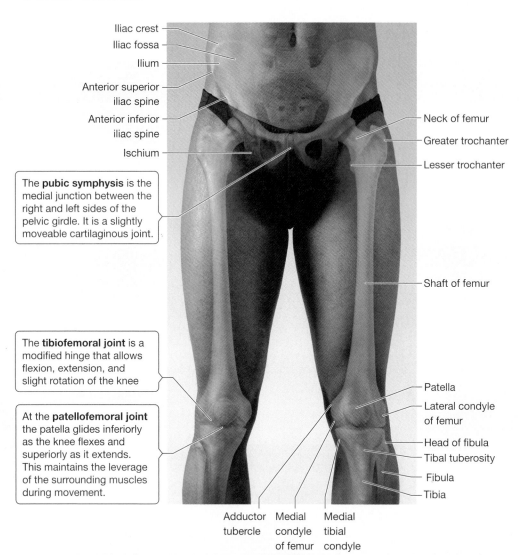

Iliac crest

Iliac fossa

Ilium

Anterior superior iliac spine

Anterior inferior iliac spine

Ischium

Neck of femur

Greater trochanter

Lesser trochanter

The **pubic symphysis** is the medial junction between the right and left sides of the pelvic girdle. It is a slightly moveable cartilaginous joint.

Shaft of femur

The **tibiofemoral joint** is a modified hinge that allows flexion, extension, and slight rotation of the knee

At the **patellofemoral joint** the patella glides inferiorly as the knee flexes and superiorly as it extends. This maintains the leverage of the surrounding muscles during movement.

Patella

Lateral condyle of femur

Head of fibula

Tibal tuberosity

Fibula

Tibia

Adductor tubercle

Medial condyle of femur

Medial tibial condyle

8-2A. Anterior view.

▶SKELETAL STRUCTURES OF THE PELVIS, THIGH, AND KNEE

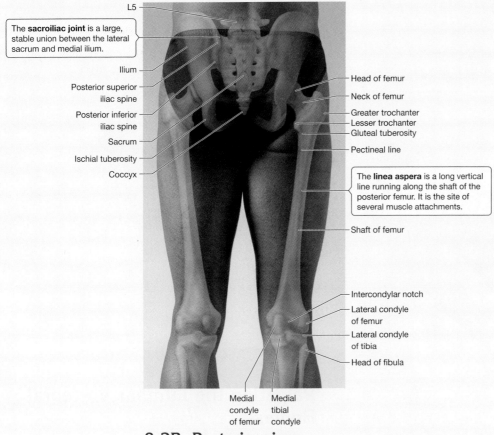

L5

The **sacroiliac joint** is a large, stable union between the lateral sacrum and medial ilium.

Ilium

Posterior superior iliac spine

Posterior inferior iliac spine

Sacrum

Ischial tuberosity

Coccyx

Head of femur

Neck of femur

Greater trochanter

Lesser trochanter

Gluteal tuberosity

Pectineal line

The **linea aspera** is a long vertical line running along the shaft of the posterior femur. It is the site of several muscle attachments.

Shaft of femur

Intercondylar notch

Lateral condyle of femur

Lateral condyle of tibia

Head of fibula

Medial condyle of femur   Medial tibial condyle

8-2B. Posterior view.

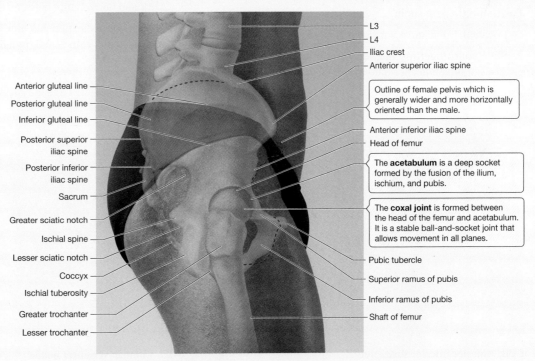

L3

L4

Iliac crest

Anterior superior iliac spine

Outline of female pelvis which is generally wider and more horizontally oriented than the male.

Anterior inferior iliac spine

Head of femur

The **acetabulum** is a deep socket formed by the fusion of the ilium, ischium, and pubis.

The **coxal joint** is formed between the head of the femur and acetabulum. It is a stable ball-and-socket joint that allows movement in all planes.

Pubic tubercle

Superior ramus of pubis

Inferior ramus of pubis

Shaft of femur

Anterior gluteal line

Posterior gluteal line

Inferior gluteal line

Posterior superior iliac spine

Posterior inferior iliac spine

Sacrum

Greater sciatic notch

Ischial spine

Lesser sciatic notch

Coccyx

Ischial tuberosity

Greater trochanter

Lesser trochanter

8-2C. Lateral view.

▶ BONY LANDMARKS OF SKELETAL STRUCTURES

Palpating the Anterior Superior Iliac Spine (ASIS)

Positioning: client supine.

1. Locate the iliac crest with your fingertips.
2. Slide your fingertips anteriorly and inferiorly onto the anteriorly protruding ASIS.

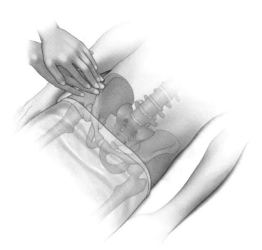

8-3A. Anterior superior iliac spine.

Palpating the Anterior Inferior Iliac Spine (AIIS)

Positioning: client supine.

1. Locate the iliac crest with your fingertips.
2. Slide your fingertips anteriorly and inferiorly past the ASIS and then deeper onto the AIIS.

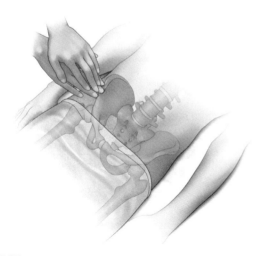

8-3B. Anterior inferior iliac spine.

Palpating the Iliac Fossa

Positioning: client supine.

1. Locate the iliac crest with your fingertips.
2. Slide your fingertips medially, inferiorly, and deeply onto the concave surface of the iliac fossa.

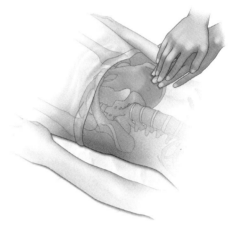

8-3C. Iliac fossa.

Palpating the Lumbar Vertebral Bodies

Positioning: client supine with hip slightly flexed.

1. Locate a spot vertically between the pubic symphesis and ASIS and horizontally between the umbilicus and pubis.
2. Deepen your palpation and aim your fingertips medially until you contact the solid, rounded bodies of the lumbar vertebrae.

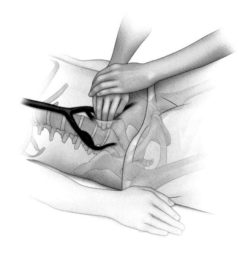

8-3D. Lumbar vertebral bodies.

Palpating the Rami of the Pubis

Positioning: client supine.

1. Locate the iliac crest with your fingertips.
2. Slide your fingertips medially and slightly inferiorly onto the broad, flat surfaces of the pubic rami.

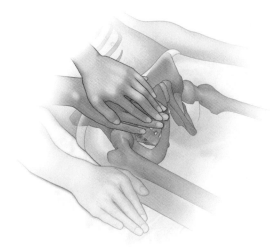

8-3E. **Rami of the pubis.**

Palpating the Adductor Tubercle

Positioning: client supine.

1. Locate the patella on the anterior knee with your thumb.
2. Slide your thumb medially onto the rounded prominence of the adductor tubercle.

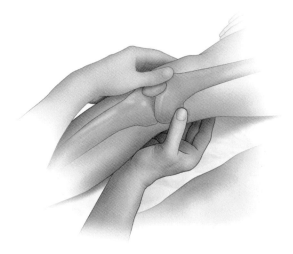

8-3F. **Adductor tubercle.**

Palpating the Medial Femoral Condyle

Positioning: client supine.

1. Locate the patella on the anterior knee with your thumb.
2. Slide your thumb medially and slightly inferiorly onto the broad, rounded medial femoral condyle.

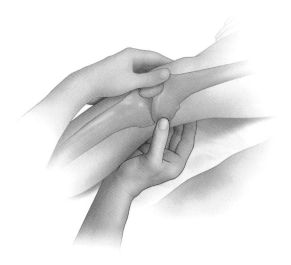

8-3G. **Medial femoral condyle.**

Palpating the Lateral Femoral Condyle

Positioning: client supine.

1. Locate the patella on the anterior knee with your thumb.
2. Slide your thumb laterally and slightly inferiorly onto the broad, rounded medial femoral condyle.

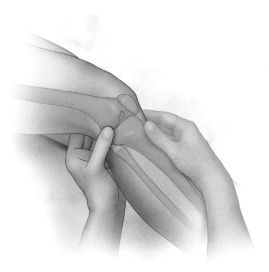

8-3H. **Lateral femoral condyle.**

Palpating the Medial Tibial Condyle

Positioning: client supine.

1. Locate the patella on the anterior knee with your thumb.
2. Slide your thumb medially and inferiorly past the tibiofemoral joint line and onto the curved medial tibial condyle.

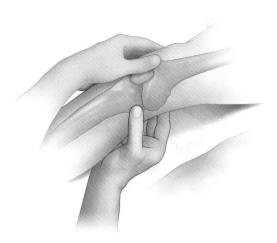

8-3I. **Medial tibial condyle.**

Palpating the Fibular Head

Positioning: client supine.

1. Locate the lateral tibiofemoral joint line with your thumb.
2. Slide your thumb inferiorly and posteriorly onto the laterally protruding, rounded head of the fibula.

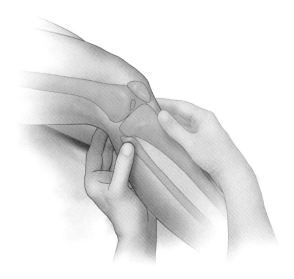

8-3K. **Fibular head.**

Palpating the Lateral Tibial Condyle

Positioning: client supine.

1. Locate the patella on the anterior knee with your thumb.
2. Slide your thumb laterally and inferiorly past the tibiofemoral joint line and onto the curved lateral tibial condyle.

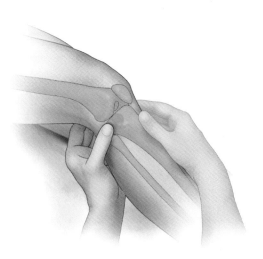

8-3J. **Lateral tibial condyle.**

Palpating the Tibial Tuberosity

Positioning: client supine.

1. Locate the patella on the anterior knee with your thumb.
2. Slide your thumb inferiorly following the patellar tendon and onto the slight bump of the tibial tuberosity.

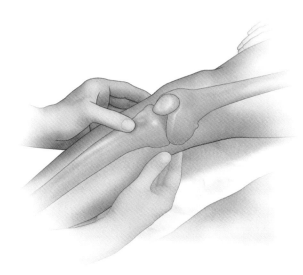

8-3L. **Tibial tuberosity.**

Palpating the Posterior Superior Iliac Spine (PSIS)

Positioning: client prone.

1. Locate the lumbar spinous processes with your fingertips.
2. Slide your fingertips inferiorly onto the round, prominent PSIS.

Palpating the Sacrum

Positioning: client prone.

1. Locate the lumber spinous processes with your fingertips.
2. Slide your fingertips inferiorly between the right and left PSIS and onto the posterior surface of the sacrum.

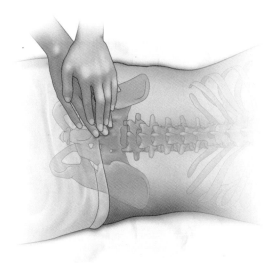

8-3N. **Sacrum.**

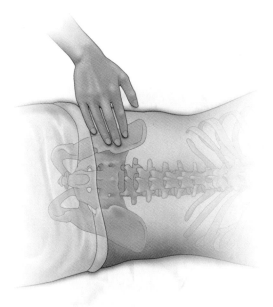

8-3M. **Posterior superior iliac spine.**

Palpating the Greater Trochanter of the Femur

Positioning: client prone.

1. Locate the iliac crest with your fingertips.
2. Slide your fingertips several inches inferiorly onto the large, rounded protrusion of the greater trochanter.

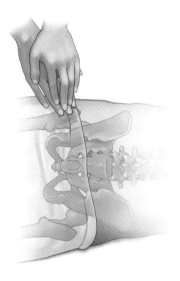

8-3O. Greater trochanter of the femur.

Palpating the Ischial Tuberosity

Positioning: client prone.

1. Locate the superior, posterior thigh with your fingertips.
2. Slide your fingertips anteriorly and superiorly, underneath the gluteal fold and onto the large, rounded ischial tuberosity.

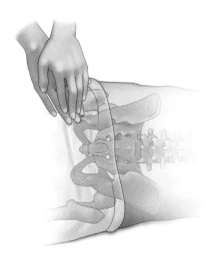

8-3P. Ischial tuberosity.

MUSCLE ATTACHMENT SITES

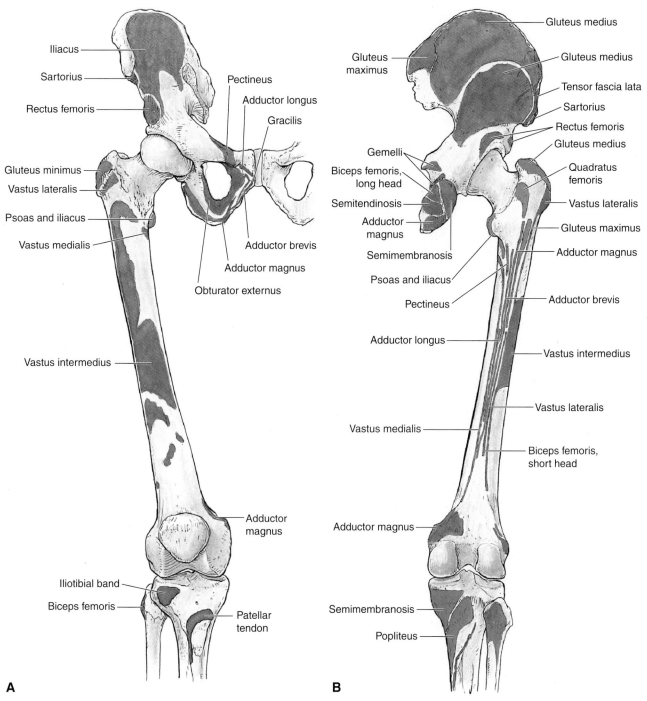

8-4 Muscle attachments of the pelvis, thigh, and knee. A. Anterior view. **B.** Posterior view.

LIGAMENTS OF THE PELVIS, THIGH, AND KNEE

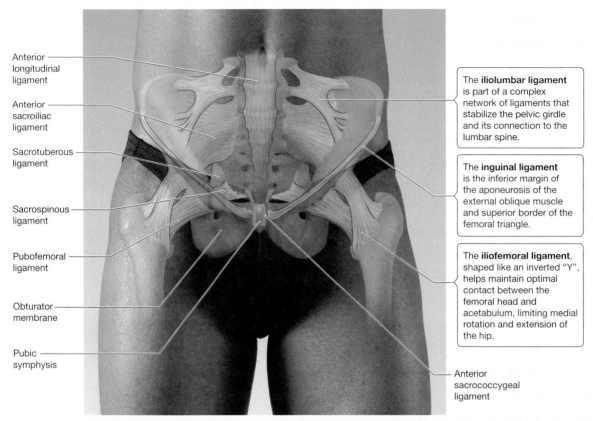

Anterior longitudinal ligament

Anterior sacroiliac ligament

Sacrotuberous ligament

Sacrospinous ligament

Pubofemoral ligament

Obturator membrane

Pubic symphysis

The **iliolumbar ligament** is part of a complex network of ligaments that stabilize the pelvic girdle and its connection to the lumbar spine.

The **inguinal ligament** is the inferior margin of the aponeurosis of the external oblique muscle and superior border of the femoral triangle.

The **iliofemoral ligament**, shaped like an inverted "Y", helps maintain optimal contact between the femoral head and acetabulum, limiting medial rotation and extension of the hip.

Anterior sacrococcygeal ligament

8-5A. Ligaments of the pelvis and hip: anterior view.

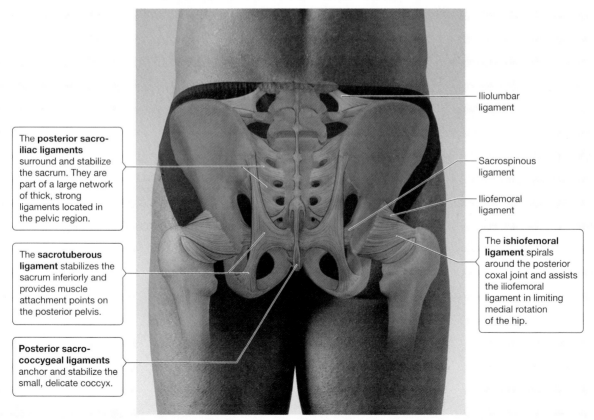

Iliolumbar ligament

Sacrospinous ligament

Iliofemoral ligament

The **posterior sacro-iliac ligaments** surround and stabilize the sacrum. They are part of a large network of thick, strong ligaments located in the pelvic region.

The **sacrotuberous ligament** stabilizes the sacrum inferiorly and provides muscle attachment points on the posterior pelvis.

Posterior sacro-coccygeal ligaments anchor and stabilize the small, delicate coccyx.

The **ishiofemoral ligament** spirals around the posterior coxal joint and assists the iliofemoral ligament in limiting medial rotation of the hip.

8-5B. Ligaments of the pelvis and hip: posterior view.

▶ LIGAMENTS OF THE PELVIS, THIGH, AND KNEE

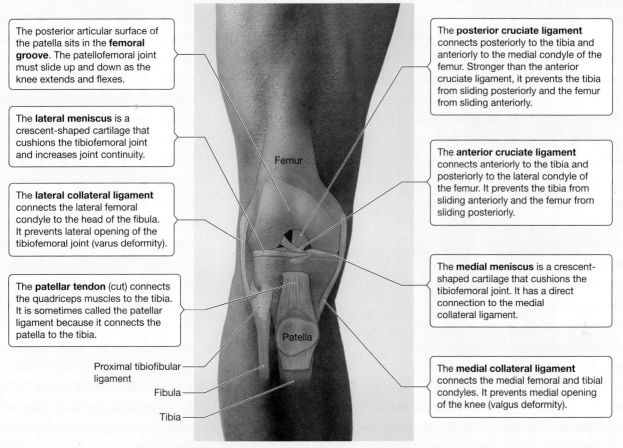

The posterior articular surface of the patella sits in the **femoral groove**. The patellofemoral joint must slide up and down as the knee extends and flexes.

The **lateral meniscus** is a crescent-shaped cartilage that cushions the tibiofemoral joint and increases joint continuity.

The **lateral collateral ligament** connects the lateral femoral condyle to the head of the fibula. It prevents lateral opening of the tibiofemoral joint (varus deformity).

The **patellar tendon** (cut) connects the quadriceps muscles to the tibia. It is sometimes called the patellar ligament because it connects the patella to the tibia.

The **posterior cruciate ligament** connects posteriorly to the tibia and anteriorly to the medial condyle of the femur. Stronger than the anterior cruciate ligament, it prevents the tibia from sliding posteriorly and the femur from sliding anteriorly.

The **anterior cruciate ligament** connects anteriorly to the tibia and posteriorly to the lateral condyle of the femur. It prevents the tibia from sliding anteriorly and the femur from sliding posteriorly.

The **medial meniscus** is a crescent-shaped cartilage that cushions the tibiofemoral joint. It has a direct connection to the medial collateral ligament.

The **medial collateral ligament** connects the medial femoral and tibial condyles. It prevents medial opening of the knee (valgus deformity).

Femur

Patella

Proximal tibiofibular ligament

Fibula

Tibia

8-5C. Ligaments of the knee: anterior view.

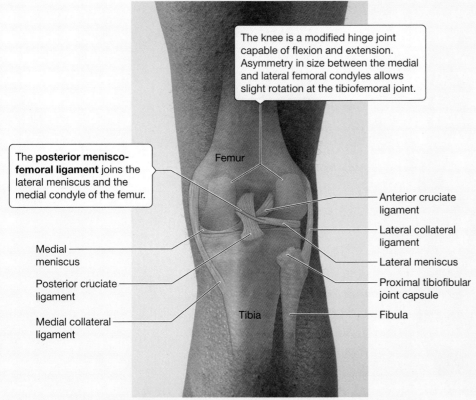

The knee is a modified hinge joint capable of flexion and extension. Asymmetry in size between the medial and lateral femoral condyles allows slight rotation at the tibiofemoral joint.

The **posterior meniscofemoral ligament** joins the lateral meniscus and the medial condyle of the femur.

Femur

Anterior cruciate ligament

Lateral collateral ligament

Lateral meniscus

Proximal tibiofibular joint capsule

Fibula

Medial meniscus

Posterior cruciate ligament

Medial collateral ligament

Tibia

8-5D. Ligaments of the knee: posterior view.

▶ SUPERFICIAL MUSCLES OF THE PELVIS, THIGH, AND KNEE

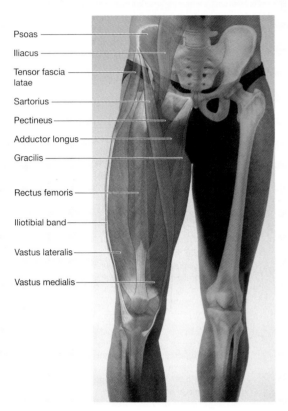

Psoas
Iliacus
Tensor fascia latae
Sartorius
Pectineus
Adductor longus
Gracilis
Rectus femoris
Iliotibial band
Vastus lateralis
Vastus medialis

8-6A. Anterior view.

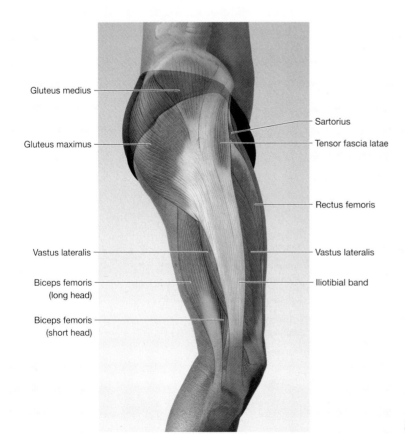

Gluteus medius
Gluteus maximus
Sartorius
Tensor fascia latae
Rectus femoris
Vastus lateralis
Vastus lateralis
Biceps femoris (long head)
Iliotibial band
Biceps femoris (short head)

8-6B. Lateral view.

SUPERFICIAL MUSCLES OF THE PELVIS, THIGH, AND KNEE

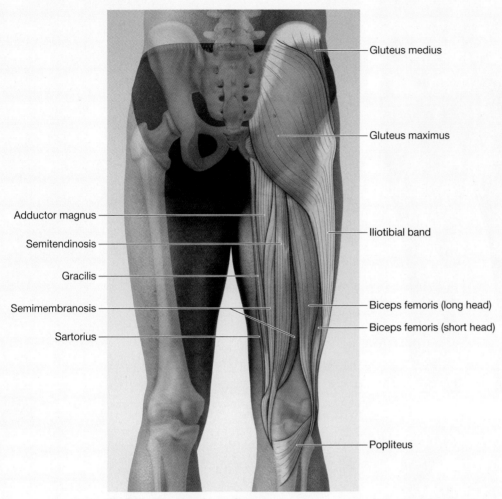

8-6C. Posterior view.

Gluteus medius

Gluteus maximus

Iliotibial band

Biceps femoris (long head)

Biceps femoris (short head)

Popliteus

Adductor magnus

Semitendinosis

Gracilis

Semimembranosis

Sartorius

▌ DEEP MUSCLES OF THE PELVIS, THIGH, AND KNEE

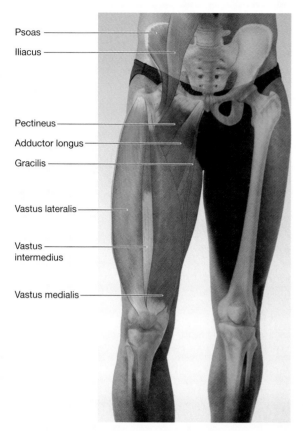

Psoas

Iliacus

Pectineus

Adductor longus

Gracilis

Vastus lateralis

Vastus intermedius

Vastus medialis

8-7A. Anterior view.

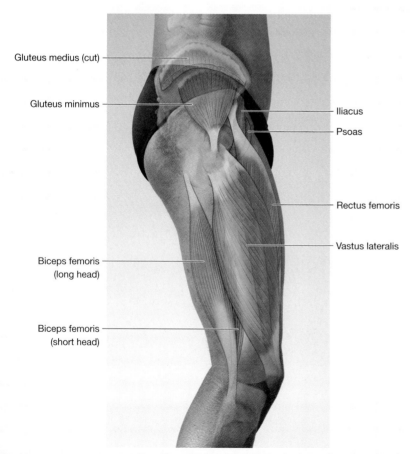

Gluteus medius (cut)

Gluteus minimus

Iliacus

Psoas

Rectus femoris

Vastus lateralis

Biceps femoris (long head)

Biceps femoris (short head)

8-7B. Lateral view.

▶ DEEP MUSCLES OF THE PELVIS, THIGH, AND KNEE

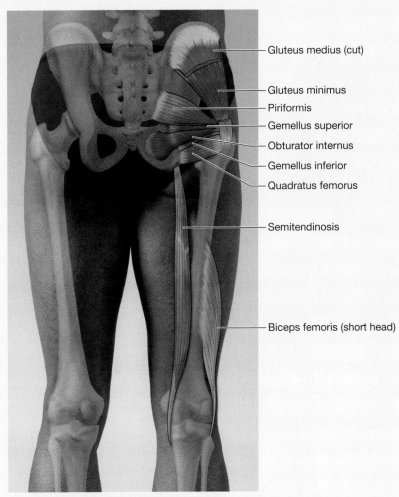

- Gluteus medius (cut)
- Gluteus minimus
- Piriformis
- Gemellus superior
- Obturator internus
- Gemellus inferior
- Quadratus femorus
- Semitendinosis
- Biceps femoris (short head)

8-7C. Posterior view.

▶ SPECIAL STRUCTURES OF THE PELVIS, THIGH, AND KNEE

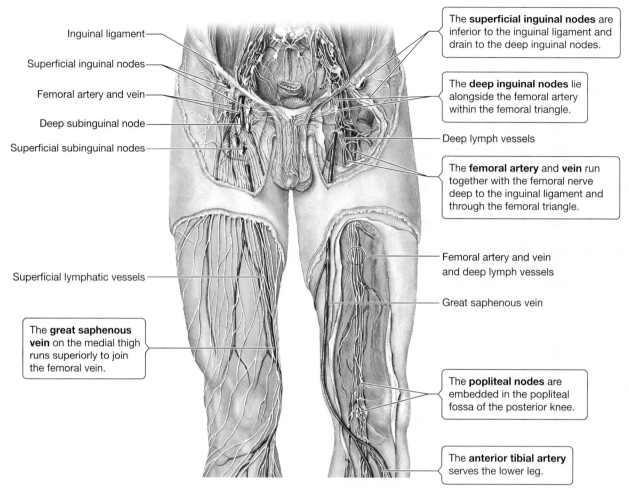

Inguinal ligament

Superficial inguinal nodes

Femoral artery and vein

Deep subinguinal node

Superficial subinguinal nodes

Superficial lymphatic vessels

The **great saphenous vein** on the medial thigh runs superiorly to join the femoral vein.

The **superficial inguinal nodes** are inferior to the inguinal ligament and drain to the deep inguinal nodes.

The **deep inguinal nodes** lie alongside the femoral artery within the femoral triangle.

Deep lymph vessels

The **femoral artery** and **vein** run together with the femoral nerve deep to the inguinal ligament and through the femoral triangle.

Femoral artery and vein and deep lymph vessels

Great saphenous vein

The **popliteal nodes** are embedded in the popliteal fossa of the posterior knee.

The **anterior tibial artery** serves the lower leg.

8-8. Blood vessels and lymphatics of the pelvis, thigh, and knee: anterior view.

► SPECIAL STRUCTURES OF THE PELVIS, THIGH, AND KNEE

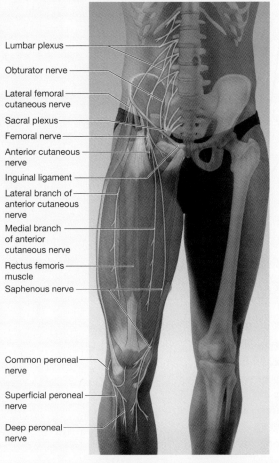

Lumbar plexus

Obturator nerve

Lateral femoral cutaneous nerve

Sacral plexus

Femoral nerve

Anterior cutaneous nerve

Inguinal ligament

Lateral branch of anterior cutaneous nerve

Medial branch of anterior cutaneous nerve

Rectus femoris muscle

Saphenous nerve

Common peroneal nerve

Superficial peroneal nerve

Deep peroneal nerve

8-9A. Nerves of the pelvis, thigh, and knee: anterior view.

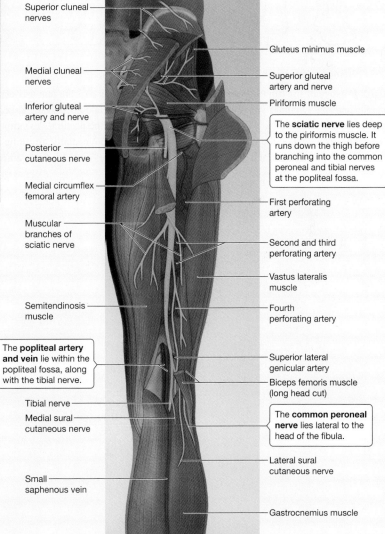

Superior cluneal nerves

Medial cluneal nerves

Inferior gluteal artery and nerve

Posterior cutaneous nerve

Medial circumflex femoral artery

Muscular branches of sciatic nerve

Semitendinosis muscle

The **popliteal artery and vein** lie within the popliteal fossa, along with the tibial nerve.

Tibial nerve

Medial sural cutaneous nerve

Small saphenous vein

Gluteus minimus muscle

Superior gluteal artery and nerve

Piriformis muscle

The **sciatic nerve** lies deep to the piriformis muscle. It runs down the thigh before branching into the common peroneal and tibial nerves at the popliteal fossa.

First perforating artery

Second and third perforating artery

Vastus lateralis muscle

Fourth perforating artery

Superior lateral genicular artery

Biceps femoris muscle (long head cut)

The **common peroneal nerve** lies lateral to the head of the fibula.

Lateral sural cutaneous nerve

Gastrocnemius muscle

8-9B. Nerves of the pelvis, thigh, and knee: posterior view.

▶ POSTURE OF THE HIP AND KNEE

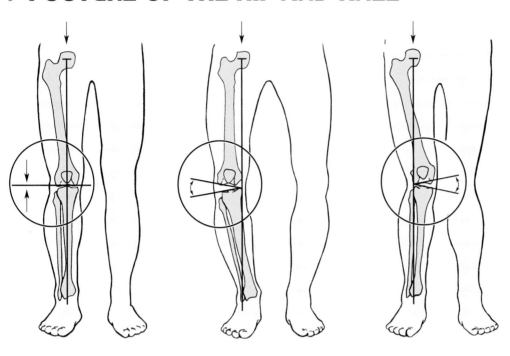

Normal alignment   Genu varum   Genu valgum

8-10. Posture of the hip and knee: anterior view.   The head of the femur is centered over the patella and tibiofemoral joint in normal alignment of the hip and knee. If the knee is lateral to the femoral head, the knee will "open" laterally, resulting in the postural deviation *genu varum*. If the knee is medial to the femoral head, the knee will "open" medially, resulting in the postural deviation *genu valgum*. Each deviation causes specific stresses on tendons, ligaments, and articulating surfaces.

▶ MOVEMENTS AVAILABLE: HIP

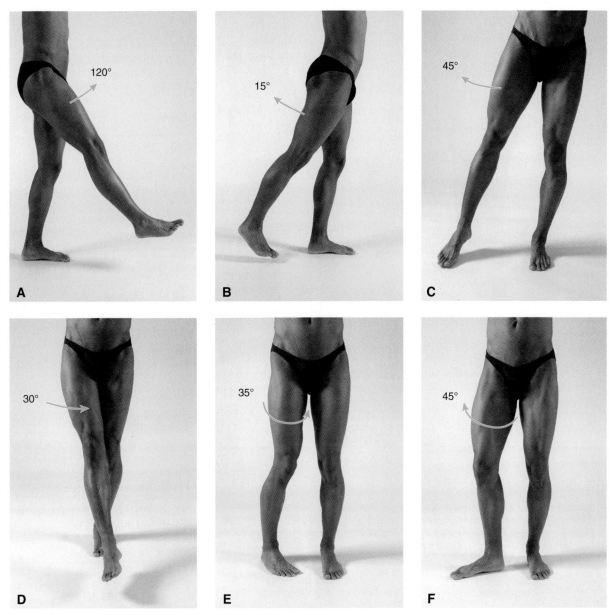

8-11 A. Hip flexion. **B.** Hip extension. **C.** Hip abduction. **D.** Hip adduction. **E.** Hip internal rotation. **F.** Hip external rotation.

▌ MOVEMENTS AVAILABLE: KNEE

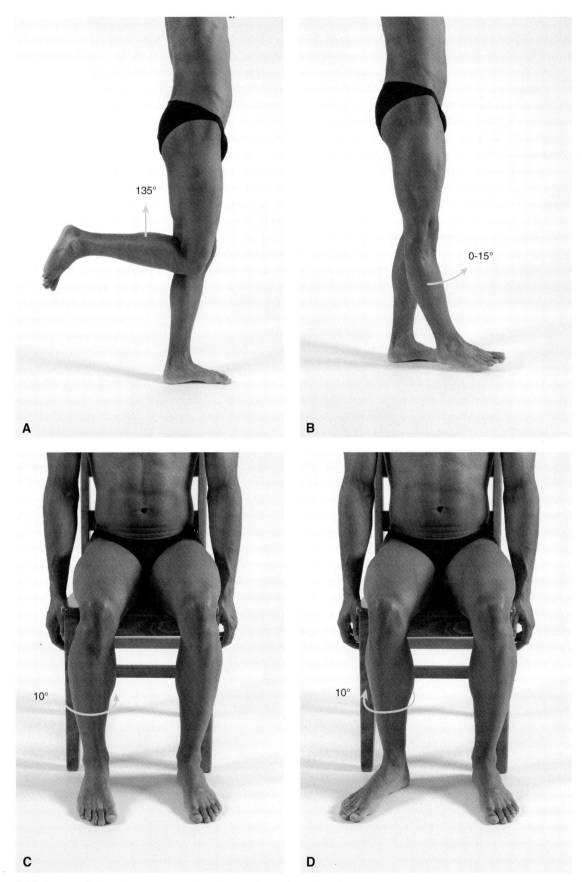

8-12 **A.** Knee flexion. **B.** Knee extension. **C.** Knee internal rotation. **D.** Knee external rotation.

❱ PASSIVE RANGE OF MOTION

Performing passive range of motion (ROM) in the coxal and tibiofemoral joints helps establish the health and function of inert structures such as the joint capsules and ligaments.

The client should be lying on a massage or examination table. Ask the client to relax and allow you to perform the ROM exercises without the client "helping." For each of the movements illustrated below, take the leg through to endfeel while watching for compensation (extraneous movement) in the trunk. Procedures for performing passive ROM are described toward the end of Chapter 3.

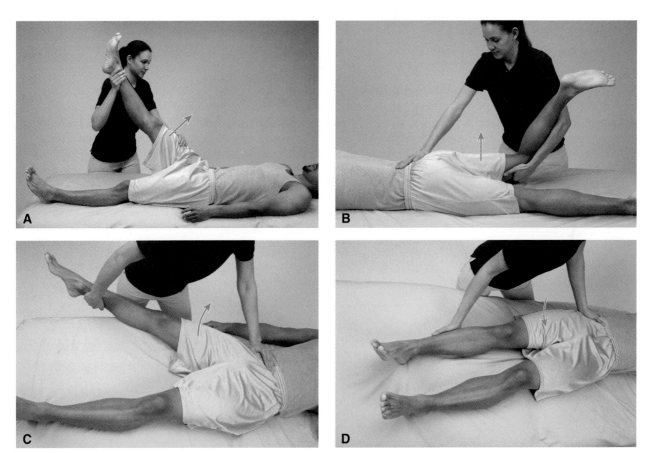

8-13 A. Passive hip flexion. The blue arrow indicates the direction of movement. Stand at the supine client's side. Grasp the lower leg with one hand and stabilize the thigh with the other. Instruct the client to remain relaxed as you move their leg. Maintain a straight knee while you move the client's leg from the table toward their chest. Assess the ROM of the posterior hip ligaments, joint capsule, and muscles that extend the hip. **B. Passive hip extension.** Stand at the prone client's side. Grasp under the thigh with one hand and stabilize the pelvis with the other. Instruct the client to remain relaxed as you move their leg. Lift the client's leg straight up from the table. Assess the ROM of the anterior hip ligaments, joint capsule, and muscles that flex the hip. **C. Passive hip abduction.** Stand at the supine client's side. Grasp the lower leg with one hand and stabilize the opposite side of the pelvis with the other. Instruct the client to remain relaxed as you move their leg. Maintain a straight knee as you move the leg to the side, away from the body, as far as is comfortable. Assess the ROM of the medial hip ligaments, joint capsule, and muscles that adduct the hip. **D. Passive hip adduction.** Stand at the supine client's side. Grasp the lower leg with one hand and stabilize the same side of the pelvis with the other. Instruct the client to remain relaxed as you move their leg. Maintain a straight knee as you move the leg inward, toward the body, as far as is comfortable. Assess the ROM of the lateral hip ligaments, joint capsule, and muscles that abduct the hip. *(continues)*

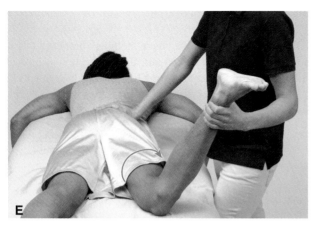

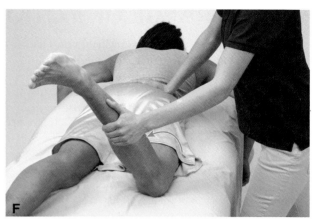

8-13 *(continued)* **E. Passive hip internal rotation.** Stand at the prone client's side. Grasp the lower leg with one hand and stabilize the center of the pelvis with the other. Instruct the client to remain relaxed as you move their leg. Maintain a 90-degree flexed knee as you pivot the leg so the foot moves out, away from the body, as far as is comfortable. Assess the ROM of the hip ligaments, joint capsule, and muscles that externally rotate the hip. **F. Passive hip external rotation.** Stand at the prone client's side. Grasp the lower leg with one hand and stabilize the center of the pelvis with the other. Instruct the client to remain relaxed as you move their leg. Maintain a 90-degree flexed knee as you pivot the leg so the foot moves inward, toward the body, as far as is comfortable. Assess the ROM of the hip ligaments, joint capsule, and muscles that internally rotate the hip.

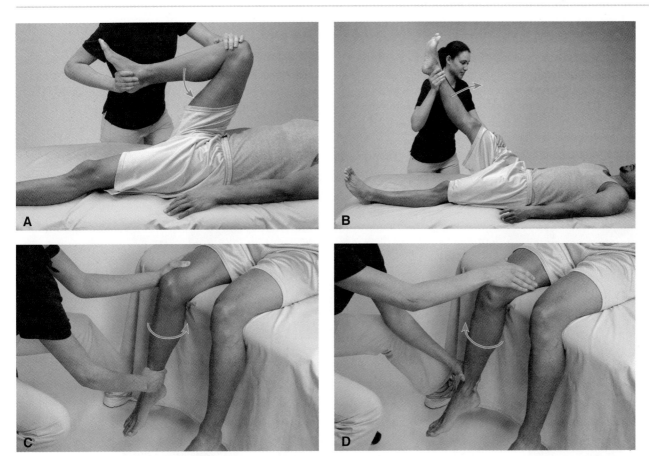

8-14 A. Passive knee flexion. Stand at the supine client's side. Grasp the bottom of the foot with one hand and stabilize the knee with the other. Instruct the client to remain relaxed as you move their leg. Bend the knee while you move the client's leg from the table toward their chest. Assess the ROM of the anterior knee ligaments, joint capsule, and muscles that extend the knee. **B. Passive knee extension.** Stand at the supine client's side. Grasp the ankle with one hand and stabilize the thigh with the other. Instruct the client to remain relaxed as you move their leg. Straighten the knee while you move the client's leg from the table toward their chest. Assess the ROM of the posterior knee ligaments, joint capsule, and muscles that flex the knee. **C. Passive knee internal rotation.** Sit in front of the seated client. Grasp the ankle with one hand and stabilize the knee with the other. Instruct the client to remain relaxed as you move their lower leg. Pivot the leg inward, toward the body, as far as is comfortable. Assess the ROM of the joint capsule and muscles that externally rotate the knee. **D. Passive knee external rotation.** Sit in front of the seated client. Grasp the ankle with one hand and stabilize the knee with the other. Instruct the client to remain relaxed as you move their lower leg. Pivot the leg outward, away from the body, as far as is comfortable. Assess the ROM of the joint capsule and muscles that internally rotate the knee.

❱ RESISTED RANGE OF MOTION

Performing resisted range of motion (ROM) for both the coxal joint and tibiofemoral joint helps establish the health and function of the dynamic stabilizers and prime movers in this region. Evaluating functional strength and endurance helps you to identify balance and potential imbalance between the muscles that steer and power the lower extremity. Procedures for performing and grading resisted ROM are outlined in Chapter 3.

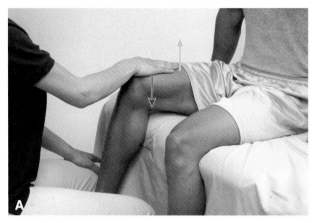

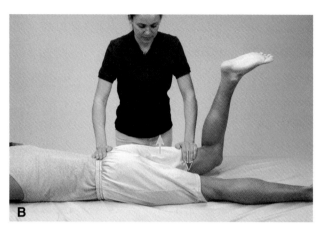

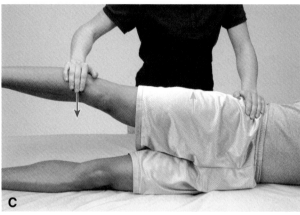

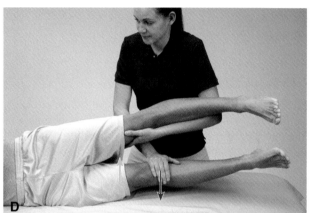

8-15 A. Resisted hip flexion. The green arrow indicates the direction of movement of the client and the red arrow indicates the direction of resistance from the practitioner. Sit facing the seated client. Place the palm of one hand on top of the client's thigh. Instruct the client to meet your resistance by lifting the thigh up as you gently but firmly press the thigh down. Assess the strength and endurance of the muscles that flex the hip. **B. Resisted hip extension.** Stand facing the prone client. Place the palm of your hand on top of the client's thigh as you stabilize the pelvis with the other hand. Instruct the client to meet your resistance by lifting their thigh off the table as you gently but firmly press the thigh down. Assess the strength and endurance of the muscles that extend the hip. **C. Resisted hip abduction.** Stand behind the sidelying client. Place the palm of one hand on the client's lower leg as you stabilize the pelvis with the other hand. Instruct the client to meet your resistance by lifting their thigh away from the other as you gently but firmly press the thigh down. Assess the strength and endurance of the muscles that abduct the hip. **D. Resisted hip adduction.** Stand behind the sidelying client. Place the palm of one hand on the client's bottom upper leg as you support the other leg with the other hand. Instruct the client to meet your resistance by lifting their bottom thigh away from the table as you gently but firmly press the thigh down. Assess the strength and endurance of the muscles that adduct the hip. *(continues)*

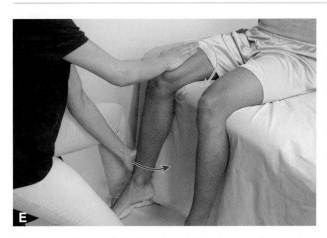
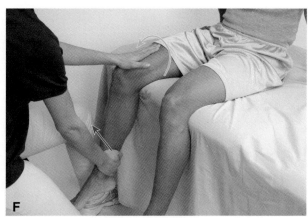

8-15 *(continued)* **E. Resisted hip internal rotation.** Sit facing the seated client. Place the palm of one hand on the outside of the client's lower leg as you stabilize the knee with the other hand. Instruct the client to meet your resistance by pivoting their leg away from the other as you gently but firmly press the leg inward. Assess the strength and endurance of the muscles that internally rotate the hip. **F. Resisted hip external rotation.** Sit facing the seated client. Place the palm of one hand on the inside of the client's lower leg as you stabilize the knee with the other hand. Instruct the client to meet your resistance by pivoting their leg toward the other as you gently but firmly press the leg outward. Assess the strength and endurance of the muscles that externally rotate the hip.

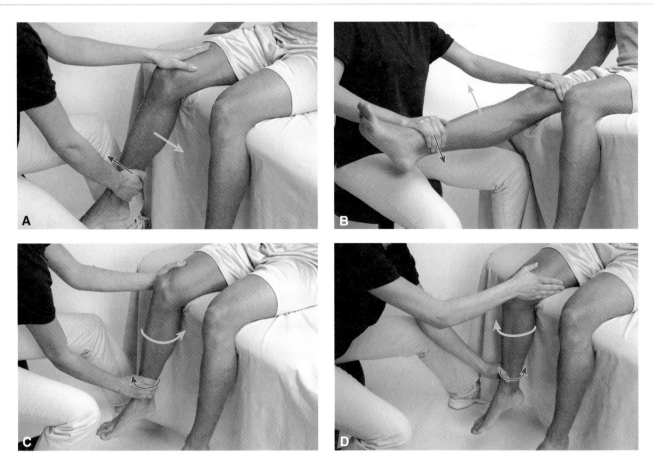

8-16 A. Resisted knee flexion. Sit facing the seated client. Place one hand around the back of the ankle as you stabilize the knee with the other hand. Instruct the client to meet your resistance by pulling their heel back as you gently but firmly pull it forward. Assess the strength and endurance of the muscles that flex the knee. **B. Resisted knee extension.** Sit facing the side of the seated client. Place one hand on top of the straightened leg as you stabilize the thigh with the other hand. Instruct the client to meet your resistance by maintaining a straight knee as you gently but firmly push it down. Assess the strength and endurance of the muscles that extend the knee. **C. Resisted knee internal rotation.** Sit facing the seated client. Place one hand around the inside of the ankle as you stabilize the knee with the other hand. Instruct the client to meet your resistance by pivoting their lower leg in as you gently but firmly pivot it out. Assess the strength and endurance of the muscles that internally rotate the knee. **D. Resisted knee external rotation.** Sit facing the seated client. Place one hand around the outside of the ankle as you stabilize the knee with the other hand. Instruct the client to meet your resistance by pivoting their lower leg out as you gently but firmly pivot it in. Assess the strength and endurance of the muscles that externally rotate the knee.

Psoas   *so as.* • **"psoa"** Greek *of the loins*

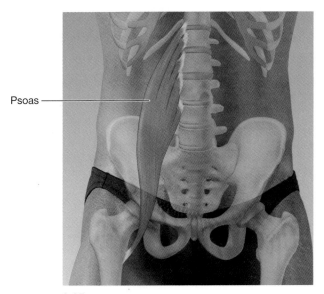

Psoas ———

8-17

Palpating Psoas

Positioning: client supine with hip and knee flexed.

1. Standing at the client's side facing the abdomen, locate the anterior iliac crest with your fingertips. Use both hands.

2. Slide your fingertips superiorly, medially, and deeply toward the lateral vertebral bodies of the lumbar spine. *(Caution: the abdominal aorta is located in this region. To avoid compressing this structure be sure and palpate from lateral to medial.)*

3. Allow your fingers to gently sink onto the oblique fibers of the psoas, strumming them back and forth to identify the tube-shaped muscle.

4. Client gently resists flexion of the hip to ensure proper location.

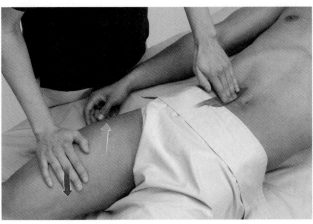

8-18

Attachments

O: T12–L5 vertebrae, transverse processes, lateral bodies and corresponding intevertberal disks.

I: Femur, lesser trochanter

Actions

- Flexes the hip
- Externally rotates the hip

Innervation

- Lumbar plexus
- L1–L4

Functional Anatomy

Psoas major and minor create a connection between the trunk and lower extremity. Originating on the lateral aspect of the lumbar vertebrae, they stabilize the lower spine when the body is upright. The fibers of psoas converge at and must bend around the anterior edge of the pelvic girdle. Finally, they insert on the lesser trochanter of the femur next to the iliacus.

Both the psoas and iliacus flex the hip during activities like walking, running, and jumping. Because of their shared actions and insertion, the psoas major, psoas minor, and iliacus are combines to form the *iliopsoas* group. Because they have separate functions in addition to their shared actions, the psoas and iliacus will be addressed separately here.

The psoas plays a unique role in posture. When the body is standing, the psoas, along with quadratus lumborum and the erector spinae group, tilts the pelvis forward. These muscles must oppose the forces of the abdominals and gluteals, which tilt the pelvis backward. Together, these muscle groups maintain alignment between the trunk and pelvis.

Imbalances between these pelvic postural muscles are common, creating pain and dysfunction in the core of the body. The psoas often becomes tight and shortened in people who sit or drive for prolonged periods. Standing upright with a shortened psoas tilts the pelvis forward excessively, compressing the lumbar spine. This posture is called *anterior pelvic tilt,* which is commonly associated with exaggerated lumbar lordosis (see Chapter 7) and low back pain.

Iliacus • il e a′kus • "ilia" Latin *flank, loin*

Attachments
O: Ilium, iliac fossa and ala of sacrum
I: Femur, lesser trochanter

Actions
- Flexes the hip
- Externally rotates the hip

Innervation
- Femoral nerve
- L1–L4

Functional Anatomy

The iliacus is a prime mover for hip flexion and external rotation. Its origin is spread across the inner surface of the ilium and its fibers join the psoas at the lesser trochanter of the femur. The main function of iliacus is to flex the hip during movements such as walking, running, jumping, and kicking.

The iliacus assists with pulling the pelvis forward when the lower extremity is weight bearing. However, because of its origin on the ilium, it does not have the same effect on the spine as psoas. Maintaining strength, flexibility, and balance in iliacus is critical to proper posture and lower extremity function.

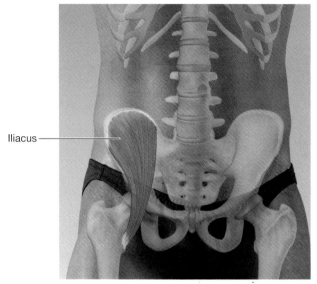

Iliacus

8-19

Palpating Iliacus

Positioning: client supine with hip and knee flexed.

1. Standing at the client's side facing the abdomen, locate the anterior iliac crest with your fingertips. Use both hands.

2. Slide your fingertips inferiorly, medially, and deep along the anterior surface of the ilium. (*Caution: the abdominal organs are located in this region so be sure and palpate from lateral to medial, scooping laterally and posterior to the intestines, avoiding painful compression of these organs.*)

3. Allow your fingers to gently sink onto the fan-shaped fibers of iliacus.

4. Client gently resists flexion of the hip to ensure proper location.

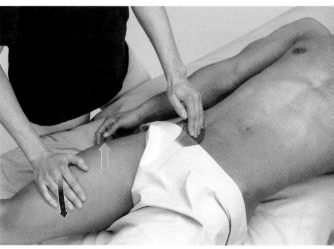

8-20

Rectus Femoris   • rek'tus fem'or is • "**recti**" Latin *straight* "**femoro**" Latin *thigh*

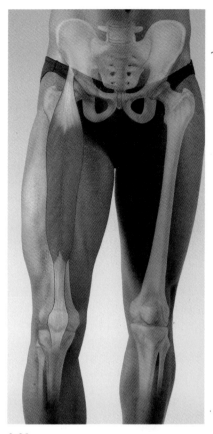

8-21

Palpating Rectus Femoris

Positioning: client supine.

1. Standing at the client's side facing the thigh, locate the anterior superior iliac spine with your fingertips.

2. Slide your fingertips inferiorly between tensor fascia latae and sartorius.

3. Allow your fingers to remain superficial on the thigh to find the feather-like fibers of rectus femoris.

4. Client gently resists flexion of the hip and extension of the knee to ensure proper location.

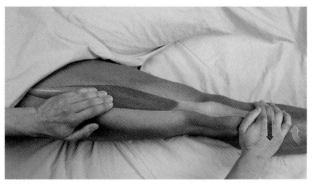

8-22

Attachments

O: Ilium, anterior inferior iliac spine (AIIS) and upper rim of acetabulum
I: Tibia, tibial tuberosity via the patellar tendon

Actions

• Flexes the hip
• Extends the knee

Innervation

• Femoral nerve
• L2–L4

Functional Anatomy

Rectus femoris bisects the front of thigh between the sartorius and tensor fasciae latae. It is the only quadriceps muscle that crosses the hip joint. The fibers of rectus femoris are bipennate and function as a prime mover for hip flexion and knee extension.

During walking and running the rectus femoris pulls the femur forward while kicking out the lower leg. This places the foot in position to contact the ground and accept the weight of the body. This muscle is stronger in knee extension than hip flexion but still assists muscles like psoas, iliacus, sartorius, and tensor fasciae latae in moving the hip. Because of its origin at the anterior inferior iliac spine, the rectus femoris also has some ability to tilt the pelvis anteriorly.

The rectus femoris, vastus lateralis, vastus intermedius, and vastus medialis form the quadriceps group and straighten the knee during standing and lifting with the legs. The vastus muscles are much more powerful than rectus femoris in this action. The strength of the vastus muscles is generated by their large cross-sectional area, increased leverage created by the patella, and single purpose of extending the knee.

Tightness in the rectus femoris is a common problem and can lead to knee pain. This pain is caused by compression of the articular surface of the patella into the femoral groove. Prolonged compression can wear away the articular cartilage, causing chronic knee problems. Adequate flexibility in the rectus femoris can help prevent this type of knee pathology.

Sartorius • sar *to're us* • "**sartori**" Latin *tailor*

Attachments

O: Ilium, anterior superior iliac spine (ASIS)
I: Tibia, medial shaft via the pes anserine tendon

Actions

- Flexes the hip
- Abducts the hip
- Externally rotates the hip
- Flexes the knee
- Internally rotates the knee

Innervation

- Femoral nerve
- L3–L4

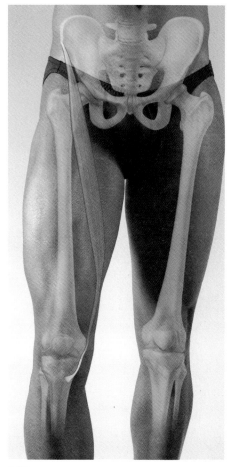

8-23

Sartorius *(continued)*

Functional Anatomy

Sartorius is the longest muscle in the human body and is often referred to as the "tailor's muscle." It is so named for the cross-legged working position utilized in that profession where the ankle of one leg rests on top of the knee of the other leg. *(The tailor's position is seen in Figure 1-12).* Achieving this position utililizes the actions of sartorius. In order to sit cross-legged, one must flex, abduct, and externally rotate the hip while flexing the knee.

Sartorius is long, slender, and very superficial in the thigh. Along with tensor fasciae latae, it forms an upside down "v" on the front of the thigh. Both muscles flex the hip, but rotate in opposite directions. This relationship helps control rotational movements in the hip and knee, such as planting and pivoting the lower extremity.

Sartorius joins the gracilis and semitendinosis at the pes anserine tendon. *Pes anserine* means "goose foot" and is named for its three-pronged shape. The three muscles converge at the inside of the knee and insert on the medial shaft of the tibia. Together they form a tripod of dynamic stabilizers for the medial knee. Sartorius descends from the front, gracilis from the middle, and semitendonosis from the back of the thigh. Ligament injuries to the underlying medial collateral ligament are very common, particularly when these three muscles are weak or imbalanced.

Palpating Sartorius

Positioning: client supine with hip externally rotated and knee flexed.

1. Standing at the client's side facing the thigh, locate the anterior superior iliac spine with your fingertips.

2. Slide your fingertips inferiorly and medially along the lateral edge of the femoral triangle. *(Caution: the femoral triangle lies just medial to the sartorius and contains lymph nodes as well as the femoral nerve, artery, and vein. To avoid these structures, palpate lateral to the inguinal crease.)*

3. Allow your fingers to remain superficial on the thigh to find the strap-like fibers of sartorius.

4. Client gently resists flexion and external rotation of the hip to ensure proper location.

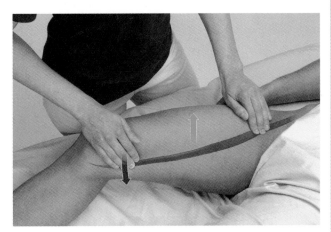

8-24

Tensor Fasciae Latae

ten'sor fash'e e la te • Latin "**tensor**" *tightener*
"**fasci**" *bundle or band* "**lati**" *wide*

Attachments

O: Ilium, anterolateral lip of iliac crest
I: Tibia, lateral condyle via the iliotibial band

Actions

* Flexes the hip
* Abducts the hip
* Internally rotates the hip

Innervation

* Superior gluteal nerve
* L4–S1

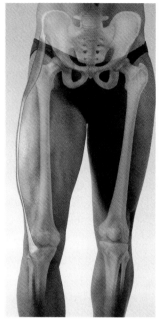

8-25

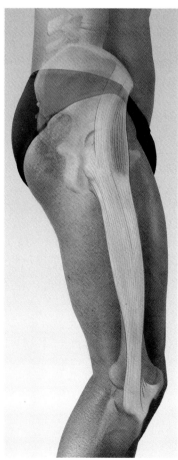

8-26

Tensor Fasciae Latae *(continued)*

Functional Anatomy

Tensor fasciae latae is a small muscle on the lateral edge of the anterior hip. It forms the other half of the "v" with sartorius on the front of the thigh. Both of these muscles flex the hip while rotating in opposite directions. Tensor fasciae latae and sartorius are both active when the lower extremity pivots over a planted foot.

The large, thick tendon associated with the tensor fasciae is a very important structure in the lower extremity. Called the *iliotibial band,* it is a primary stabilizer for the hip and lateral knee. Both tensor fasciae latae (anterior) and gluteus maximus (posterior) descend laterally into the iliotibial band. This thick band transcends the lateral thigh and attaches to the anterior, lateral condyle of the tibia. Its distal fibers assist the lateral collateral ligament in preventing separation between the lateral femoral and tibial condyles.

Tightness in the tensor fasciae latae, gluteus maximus, and associated iliotibial band can create friction proximally on the greater trochanter or distally on the lateral condyle of the femur. This excessive friction often results in injury to the bursa or tendon. Maintaining flexibility in the iliotibial band and strength balance between the adductors and abductors of the hip helps prevent this problem.

Palpating Tensor Fasciae Latae

Positioning: client supine with hip internally rotated.

1. Standing at the client's side facing the thigh, locate the anterior superior iliac spine with your fingertips.

2. Slide your fingertips laterally and inferiorly toward the outside of the thigh.

3. Palpate along the fibers of tensor fasciae latae as it becomes thicker and smoother at the iliotibial band.

4. Client gently resists abduction and flexion of the hip to ensure proper location.

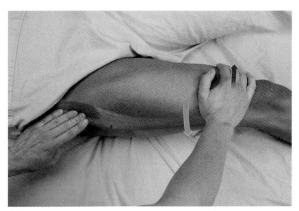

8-27

Palpating the Iliotibial Band

Positioning: client sidelying with hip and knee slightly flexed.

1. Standing at the client's side facing the thigh, locate the lateral femoral condyle with the palm of one hand.

2. Slide your palm proximally toward the greater trochanter.

3. Palpate along the fibers of the iliotibial band along the lateral thigh.

4. Client gently resists abduction of the hip to ensure proper location.

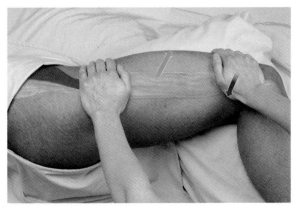

8-28

Vastus Lateralis ● vas'tus lat er a'lis • "**vast**" Latin *huge* "**lateral**" Latin *side*

Attachments

O: Femur, greater trochanter, gluteal tuberosity and proximal, lateral lip of the linea aspera
I: Tibia, tibial tuberosity via the patellar tendon

Actions

• Extends the knee

Innervation

• Femoral nerve
• L2–L4

Functional Anatomy

Vastus lateralis is one of the quadriceps muscles. Its fibers wrap around the outside of the thigh beginning at the lateral linea aspera, a vertical ridge on the posterior femur. The thick, oblique fibers of vastus lateralis are deep to the iliotibial band and join the rest of the quadriceps muscles anteriorly at the patellar tendon. It is not uncommon for the iliotibial band to become adhered to the myofascia of the underlying vastus lateralis.

Vastus lateralis, vastus intermedius, and vastus medialis have the single function of extending the knee. Rectus femoris is also recruited for this action. Standing, lifting, jumping, and powerful kicking require strong, well-balanced quadricep muscles.

Vastus lateralis is often well developed compared to vastus medialis. This imbalance can lead to improper tracking of the patella as the knee flexes and extends. Specifically, the patella can be pulled laterally in the femoral groove causing pain and wear in the articular cartilage. If severe imbalance is present the patella can be pulled out of the groove entirely, causing patellar *dislocation*. This is more common in individuals that have a high *quadriceps* (or *Q*) *angle*. This angle measures bend in the patellar tendon and is determined by the way the femur sits atop the tibia and the location of the tibial tuberosity. Normal Q angle is 5 to 15 degrees and tends to be higher in females compared to males, due to a wider pelvis.

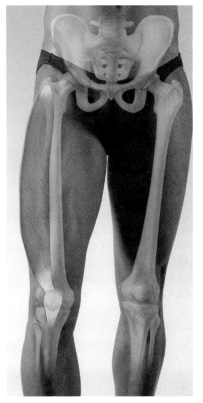

8-29

Palpating Vastus Lateralis

Positioning: client supine with hip externally rotated and knee flexed.

1. Standing at the client's side facing the thigh, locate the greater trochanter with the palm of your hand.

2. Slide your hand distally onto the lateral thigh.

3. Palpate the oblique fibers of vastus lateralis anterior and posterior to the iliotibial band.

4. Client gently resists extension of the knee to ensure proper location.

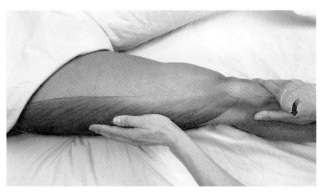

8-30

Vastus Medialis ● *vas′tus me de a′lis* • Latin "**vast**" *huge* "**medi**" *middle*

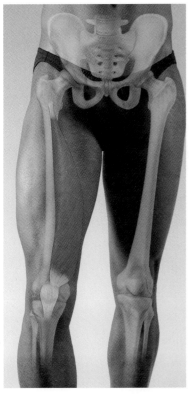

8-31

Palpating Vastus Medialis

Positioning: client supine.

1. Standing at the client's side facing the thigh, locate the proximal patella with your fingertips.

2. Slide your fingertips medially and proximally toward the sartorius.

3. Palpate deep to the sartorius following the oblique fibers of vastus medialis proximally and posteriorly.

4. Client gently resists extension of the knee to ensure proper location.

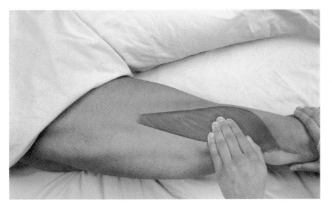

8-32

Attachments

O: Femur, intertrochanteric line and medial lip of linea aspera
I: Tibia, tibial tuberosity via the patellar tendon

Actions

Innervation

- Femoral nerve
- L2–L4

Functional Anatomy

Vastus medialis is one of the quadriceps muscles. Its fibers wrap around the inside of the thigh beginning at the medial linea aspera, a vertical ridge on the posterior femur. The thick, oblique fibers of vastus medialis form a teardrop shape on the anteromedial knee when well developed.

Like vastus lateralis and intermedius, vastus medialis has the single function of extending the knee. Its fibers are more medially oriented and balance the outward pull of vastus lateralis. Balanced strength and flexibility between vastus medialis and vastus lateralis contributes to proper patellar tracking in the femoral groove. Standing, lifting, jumping, and powerful kicking require strong, well-balanced quadriceps muscles. The single purpose of extending the knee, large cross-sectional area, and fulcrum action of the patella contribute to the strength of the vastus muscles.

Vastus Intermedius

vas'tus in'ter me'de us • Latin "**vast**" *huge* "**inter**" *between* "**medi**" *middle*

Attachments

O: Femur, proximal two-thirds of anterior shaft and distal, lateral lip of the linea aspera

I: Tibia, tibial tuberosity via the patellar tendon

Actions

• Extends the knee

Innervation

• Femoral nerve

• L2–L4

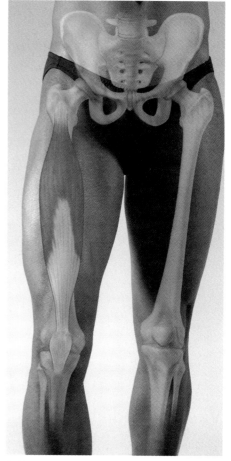

8-33

Vastus Intermedius *(continued)*

Functional Anatomy

Vastus intermedius is one of the quadriceps muscles lying directly deep to the rectus femoris. It is strongly anchored to the front of the femur, allowing it to pull powerfully on that bone. Vastus intermedius is somewhat continuous with the vastus lateralis and medialis, but its fibers are less obliquely oriented. This muscle pulls vertically rather than at oblique angles like its lateral and medial counterparts.

Like the other vastus muscles of the quadriceps, vastus intermedius has the sole function of extending the knee. It is smaller that vastus lateralis and medialis, but still powerful in its action. All of the vastus muscles are essential in powerful movements like running, jumping, and kicking as well as static stabilization of the knee. The strength of the vastus muscles is generated by their large cross-sectional area, increased leverage created by the patella, and single purpose of extending the knee.

Palpating Vastus Intermedius

Positioning: client supine with hip externally rotated and knee flexed.

1. Standing at the client's side facing the thigh, locate the proximal patella with your fingertips.

2. Slide your fingertips proximally from either the lateral or medial side, pushing rectus femoris aside.

3. Palpate deep to the rectus femoris aiming at the femoral shaft.

4. Client gently resists extension of the knee to ensure proper location.

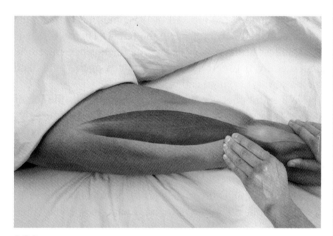

8-34

Pectineus   pek tin'e us • "**pectin**" Latin *comb*

Attachments
O: Pubis, superior ramus
I: Femur, pectineal line

Actions
- Adducts the hip
- Flexes the hip

Innervation
- Femoral and obturator nerves
- L2–L4

Functional Anatomy

The pectineus is part of the adductor group of the thigh. It joins the adductor brevis, longus, and magnus as well as gracilis in adducting the hip. All of these muscles connect the inferior, medial pelvic girdle to the femur. The pectineus is the smallest of these muscles and its fibers slope inferiorly and laterally between the superior ramus of the pubis and the posterior, proximal end of the femur.

When the foot is not planted, pectineus pulls the femur in and forward as it rotates externally. This motion helps position the lower extremity for heel strike when walking and running. Pectineus is also utilized for kicking in activities like soccer or football. When the foot is planted the function of pectineus differs: it helps stabilize the pelvis over the femur and allows changes in the direction of movement. Without it and the other adductors, the pelvis would shift medially over the knee, compromising stability and alignment in the lower extremity.

The role of pectineus and the other adductors also changes with the position of the femur. When the hip is flexed and the femur is forward, the adductors will extend the hip to bring the pelvis over the foot. When the hip is extended and the femur is back, the adductors will flex the hip to swing the leg forward. This alternating function is consistent with the dynamics of walking or running.

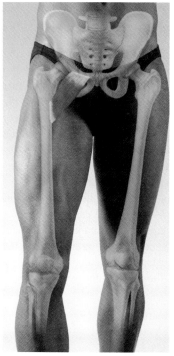

8-35

Palpating Pectineus

Positioning: client supine.

1. Standing at the client's side facing the thigh, locate the superior ramus of the pubus with the lateral edge of your palm.

2. Slide your hand laterally and distally toward the sartorius.

3. Palpate between the iliopsoas and medial adductors following the descending fibers of pectineus.

4. Client gently resists flexion and adduction of the hip to ensure proper location.

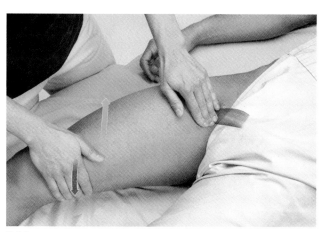

8-36

Adductor Brevis   *a duk'tor brev'is* • Latin *"ad" toward* **"ducere"** *to pull* **"brevis"** *short*

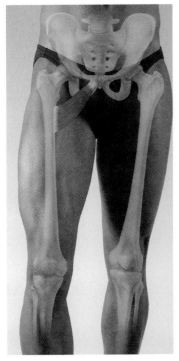

8-37

Palpating Adductor Brevis

Positioning: client supine with hip externally rotated.

1. Standing at client's side facing the thigh, locate the lateral edge of the pubis with the lateral edge of your palm.

2. Slide your hand laterally and distally toward the sartorius.

3. Palpate between the pectineus and medial adductors following the descending fibers of adductor brevis.

4. Client gently resists flexion and adduction of the hip to ensure proper location.

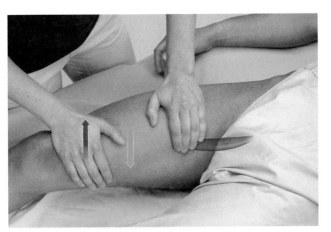

8-38

Attachments

O: Pubis, outer surface of inferior ramus
I: Femur, pectineal line and proximal one-half of medial lip of linea aspera

Actions

• Adducts the hip
• Flexes the hip
• Externally rotates the hip

Innervation

• Obturator nerve
• L2–L4

Functional Anatomy

Adductor brevis joins pectineus, adductor longus, adductor magnus, and gracilis in adducting the hip. It is a direct synergist to pectineus as both muscles adduct, flex, and externally rotate the hip. These muscles share similar origins and fiber directions with adductor brevis having a broader insertion on the femur. Adductor brevis is deep to both the pectineus and adductor longus.

When the foot is not planted, adductor brevis pulls the femur medially and anteriorly as it rotates externally. This motion helps position the lower extremity for heel strike when walking and running. Adductor brevis is also used for kicking in activities such as soccer or football. When the foot is planted, the function of adductor brevis differs: it helps stabilize the pelvis over the femur and allows us to change the direction of our movement. Without it and the other adductors, the pelvis would shift medially over the knee, compromising stability and alignment in the lower extremity.

The role of adductor brevis and the other adductors also changes with the position of the femur. When the hip is flexed and the femur is forward, the adductors will extend the hip to bring the pelvis over the foot. When the hip is extended and the femur is back, the adductors will flex the hip to swing the leg forward.

Adductor Longus   ● *a duk'tor long'gus* • Latin "**ad**" *toward* "**ducere**" *to pull* "**longi**" *long*

Attachments

O: Pubis, between pubic crest and symphysis
I: Femur, middle one-third of medial lip of linea aspera

Actions

• Adducts the hip
• Flexes the hip

Innervation

• Obturator nerve
• L2–L4

Functional Anatomy

Adductor longus is part of the adductor group of the thigh. It joins the pectineus, adductor brevis, adductor magnus, and gracilis in adducting the hip. All of these muscles connect the inferior, medial pelvic girdle to the femur.

When the foot is not planted adductor longus pulls the femur in and forward. This motion helps position the lower extremity for heel strike when walking and running. Adductor longus is also used in kicking in activities like soccer or football. The function of adductor longus differs when the foot is planted. Here it helps stabilize the pelvis over the femur as we change the direction of our movement. Without it and the other adductors, the pelvis would shift medially over the knee, compromising stability and alignment in the lower extremity.

The role of adductor longus and the other adductors also changes with the position of the femur. When the hip is flexed and the femur is forward, the adductors will extend the hip to bring the pelvis over the foot. When the hip is extended and the femur is back, the adductors will flex the hip to swing the leg forward. Adductor longus has particularly good leverage for this.

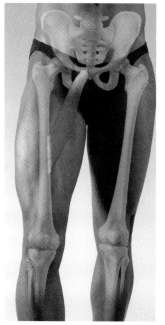

8-39

Palpating Adductor Longus

Positioning: client supine with hip externally rotated.

1. Standing at the client's side facing the thigh, locate the pubis with the lateral edge of your palm.

2. Slide your hand laterally and distally toward sartorius finding the most prominent tendon in the region. *(Caution: the femoral triangle lies just lateral to the adductor longus and contains lymph nodes as well as the femoral nerve, artery, and vein. To avoid compressing these structures, palpate distal to the inguinal crease.)*

3. Palpate and follow the fibers of adductor longus until they run under sartorius.

4. Client gently resists flexion and adduction of the hip to ensure proper location.

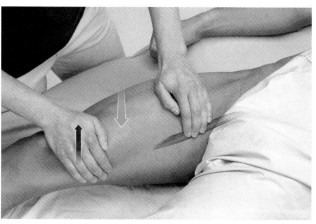

8-40

Gracilis • gras'i lis • "**gracili**" Latin *slender*

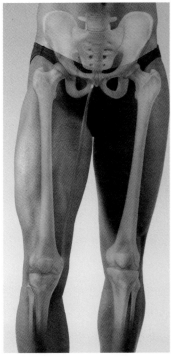

8-41

Palpating Gracilis

Positioning: client supine with hip externally rotated and knee slightly flexed.

1. Standing at the client's side facing the thigh, locate the medial femoral condyle with your palm.

2. Slide your hand proximally toward the pubis finding the most prominent tendon in the region.

3. Palpate and follow the long, slender fibers of gracilis proximally.

4. Client gently resists adduction of the hip and flexion of the knee to ensure proper location.

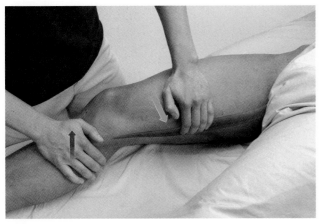

8-42

Attachments

O: Pubis, inferior ramus
I: Tibia, medial shaft via the pes anserine tendon

Actions

- Adducts the hip
- Flexes the knee
- Internally rotates the knee

Innervation

- Obturator nerve
- L2–L4

Functional Anatomy

Gracilis joins pectineus, adductor brevis, adductor longus, and adductor magnus in adducting the hip. It is the most medial adductor and is similar in shape and function to the sartorius. Both muscles cross the hip and the knee, attaching to the tibia at the pes anserine tendon. The origin of gracilis on the pubic ramus allows stronger hip flexion compared to most of the other adductors.

Gracilis forms the center of the tripod of the pes anserine muscles at the knee. Here it is able to flex and internally rotate the knee. All three muscles that converge at the pes anserine help stabilize the lower extremity as the body turns over a planted foot. These structures assist the medial collateral ligament in preventing separation between the medial femoral and tibial condyles. A strong pes anserine group may prevent medial collateral ligament injury, a common knee pathology.

Adductor Magnus

a duk'tor mag'nus • Latin "**ad**" *toward* "**ducere**" *to pull* "**magni**" *great or large*

Attachments

O: Pubis, inferior ramus, ramus of the ischium, and ischial tuberosity

I: Femur, medial lip of linea aspera, medial supracondylar line, and adductor tubercle

Actions

- Adducts the hip
- Flexes the hip (anterior fibers)
- Extends the hip (posterior fibers)

Innervation

- Obturator and sciatic nerves
- L2–S1

Functional Anatomy

Adductor magnus is the largest adductor of the thigh. It joins the pectineus, adductor brevis, adductor longus, and gracilis in adducting the hip. All of these muscles connect the inferior, medial pelvic girdle to the femur. The broad fibers of adductor magnus are nearly continuous following the entire length of the femur, attaching on the medial edge of the linea aspera.

When the foot is not planted adductor magnus strongly pulls the femur inward. This motion helps position the lower extremity for heel strike when walking and running. Adductor magnus is also recruited for kicking in activities like soccer or football. The main function of adductor magnus occurs when the foot is planted. Here it helps stabilize the pelvis over the femur. Adductor magnus can pull the pelvis medially, anteriorly, or posteriorly centering it over the lower extremity. Without it and the other adductors, the pelvis would shift medially over the knee, compromising stability and alignment in the lower extremity.

The role of adductor magnus and the other adductors also changes with the position of the femur. When the hip is flexed and the femur is forward, the adductors will extend the hip to bring the pelvis over the foot. When the hip is extended and the femur is back, the adductors will flex the hip to swing the leg forward. Adductor magnus has particularly good mechanical advantage for both flexion and extension. This is due to its origin on both the pubis and ischium and its long posterior insertion on the femur. The alternating flexing and extending function is consistent with the dynamics of walking or running.

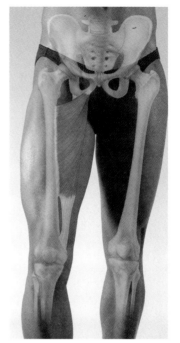

8-43

Palpating Adductor Magnus

Positioning: client prone.

1. Standing at the client's side facing the thigh, locate the ischial tuberosity with your fingertips.

2. Slide your fingers medially and distally toward the medial femoral condyle.

3. Palpate between the gracilis and medial hamstrings following the descending fibers of adductor magnus to the middle of the inner thigh.

4. Client gently resists adduction of the hip to ensure proper location.

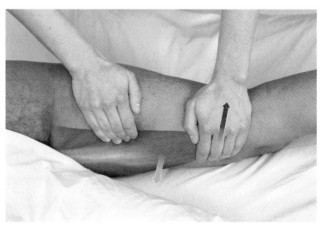

8-44

Gluteus Maximus ● *glu'teus* maks'i mus • **"glute"** Greek *rump* **"maxim"** Latin *largest*

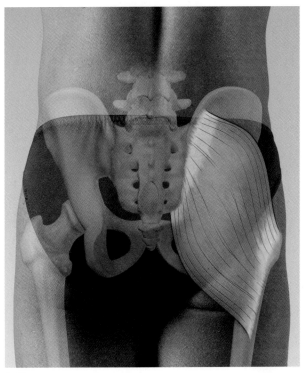

8-45

Palpating Gluteus Maximus

Positioning: client prone.

1. Standing at the client's side facing the hip, locate the lateral edge of the sacrum with your fingertips.

2. Slide your fingertips laterally and distally toward the greater trochanter.

3. Palpate and follow the muscle fibers as they converge and insert into the iliotibial band.

4. Client gently resists extension of the hip to ensure proper location.

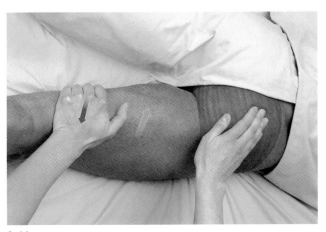

8-46

Attachments

O: Ilium, posterior iliac crest, posterior sacrum, coccyx and lumbar aponeurosis
I: Femur, gluteal tuberosity and lateral tibial condyle via the iliotibial band

Actions

- Extends the hip
- Externally rotates the hip
- Abducts the hip (upper fibers)
- Adductus the hip (lower fibers)

Innervation

- Inferior gluteal nerve
- L5–S2

Functional Anatomy

Gluteus maximus is one of the most powerful muscles in the body. It is superficial to the gluteus medius and its parallel fibers connect the lumbar fascia, ilium, sacrum, and coccyx to the greater trochanter before converging into the iliotibial band. Gluteus maximus is large in size and broad in function.

Dynamically, the gluteus maximus extends the hip during activities such as walking or rising from a sitting position. It also powers movements like running and jumping. When the lower extremity is fixed, the powerful gluteus maximus straightens the body, along with the hamstring muscles, pulling the pelvis back over the knee and foot. This "hip-hinging" function is critical during weight-bearing movements.

Posturally, the gluteus maximus braces the pelvis, hip, and knee. It works with the rectus abdominus (see Chapter 7) to posteriorly tilt the pelvis and counterbalance the quadratus lumborum, psoas, iliacus, and other hip flexors. Weakness in gluteus maximus may lead to anterior pelvic tilt while tightness contributes to posterior tilting of the pelvis. Distally, the glueus maximus stabilizes the lateral hip and knee via the thick iliotibial band. For this reason, ligament injuries are uncommon in these areas.

The upper fibers of gluteus maximus abduct the hip while the lower fibers adduct. These opposing forces enhance the stabilizing forces at the hip, allowing gluteus maximus to focus force production in the sagittal plane, specifically with extension. Gluteus maximus also externally rotates the hip, helping to maintain the position of the femur relative to the tibia during weight-bearing activities.

Gluteus Medius ● *glu'te us me'de us* • "**glute**" Greek *rump* "**medi**" Latin *middle*

Attachments

O: Ilium, external surface between iliac crest and the anterior and posterior gluteal lines
I: Femur, lateral surface of greater trochanter

Actions

- Abducts the hip
- Flexes the hip (anterior fibers)
- Internally rotates the hip (anterior fibers)
- Extends the hip (posterior fibers)
- Externally rotates the hip (posterior fibers)

Innervation

- Superior gluteal nerve
- L4–S1

Functional Anatomy

Gluteus medius lies superficial to gluteus minimus and deep to gluteus maximus. It is the prime abductor of the hip. Gluteus medius parallels the deltoid in the shoulder joint in shape, fiber direction, and function. Like the deltoid, it has multiple actions, including abduction, flexion, extension, internal rotation, and external rotation of the hip. It is a strong and versatile muscle in the lower extremity.

When we stand, the hip is held in by the unified action of the gluteus medius, gluteus mimimus, and quadratus lumborum (see Chapter 7). This action assists in proper alignment of the hip over the rest of the lower extremity. Weakness in these muscles allows the pelvis to shift laterally during standing, walking, or running. When standing on one leg, the client is unable to keep the pelvis centered over the knee and foot. With walking, an inability to maintain sagittal movement results in a "waddling," frontal-oriented gait pattern.

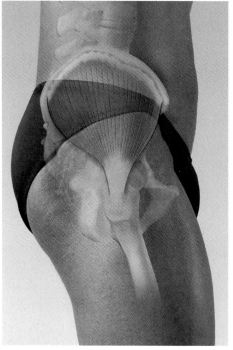

8-47

Palpating Gluteus Medius

Positioning: client prone.

1. Standing at the client's side facing the hip, locate the lateral edge of the iliac crest with your fingertips.

2. Slide your fingertips distally toward the greater trochanter.

3. Palpate and follow the muscle fibers as they converge and insert on the lateral surface of the greater trochanter.

4. Client gently resists abduction of the hip to ensure proper location.

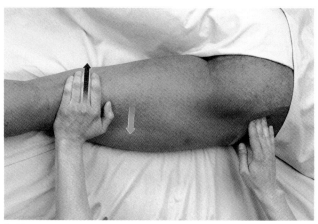

8-48

Gluteus Minimus ● *glu'te us min'i mus* • **"glute"** Greek *rump* **"minim"** Latin *smallest*

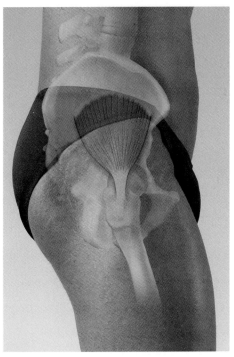

8-49

Palpating Gluteus Minimus

Positioning: client prone.

1. Standing at the client's side facing their hip, locate the anterior, lateral edge of the iliac crest with your fingertips.

2. Slide your fingertips medially and distally toward the greater trochanter.

3. Palpate and follow the muscle fibers as they converge and insert on the anterior border of the greater trochanter.

4. Client gently resists internal rotation of the hip to ensure proper location.

Attachments

O: Ilium, external surface between anterior and inferior gluteal lines
I: Femur, anterior border of greater trochanter

Actions

• Abducts the hip
• Internally rotates the hip
• Slightly flexes the hip

Innervation

• Superior gluteal nerve
• L4–S1

Functional Anatomy

Gluteus minimus lies deep and slightly anterior to gluteus medius. Together these muscles have the primary action of abducting the hip. Gluteus minimus is able to flex and internally rotate the hip because of its anterior origin on the ilium and insertion on the greater trochanter. It parallels the anterior deltoid in the shoulder joint.

When we stand, the hip is held in by the unified action of the gluteus minimus, gluteus medius, and quadratus lumborum (see Chapter 7). This action assists in proper alignment of the hip over the rest of the lower extremity. Weakness in these muscles allows the pelvis to shift laterally during standing, walking, or running. This presents as an inability to keep the pelvis centered over the knee and foot when standing on one leg. When walking, an inability to maintain sagittal movement results in a "waddling," frontal-oriented gait pattern.

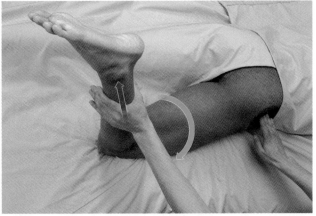

8-50

Piriformis • pir'i *form* is • Latin "**piri**" *pear* "**forma**" *shape*

Attachments
O: Sacrum, anterior surface
I: Femur, superior border of greater trochanter

Actions
- Externally rotates the hip
- Abducts the hip

Innervation
- Sacral plexus
- L4–S2

Functional Anatomy

Piriformis is the most superior of the six deep hip external rotators. These six muscles parallel the rotator cuff in the shoulder by stabilizing the hip joint at the greater trochanter. The other deep external rotators of the hip are the superior and inferior gemellus, obturator internus and externus, and the quadratus femoris.

The piriformis is unique in that it is strongly associated with the sciatic nerve. In some people, the nerve runs deep to piriformis, whereas in others the nerve weaves through the muscle, and still others have a split nerve with part running deep to piriformis and part superficial. Tightness in the deep six external rotators, and specifically the piriformis, can compress the nerve, causing pain, weakness, and altered sensation in the lower extremity.

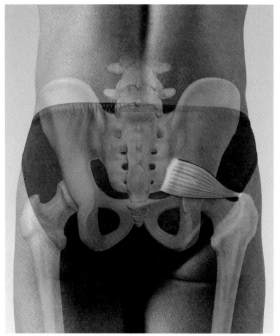

8-51

Palpating Piriformis

Positioning: client prone.

1. Standing at the client's side facing the hip, locate the lateral edge of the sacrum with your fingertips.
2. Slide your fingertips laterally and distally toward the greater trochanter. *(Caution: the sciatic nerve lies near the muscle belly of piriformis. To avoid compressing it, palpate following the oblique muscle fibers.)*
3. Palpate and follow the muscles fibers as they converge and insert on the superior surface of the greater trochanter.
4. Client gently resists external rotation of the hip to ensure proper location.

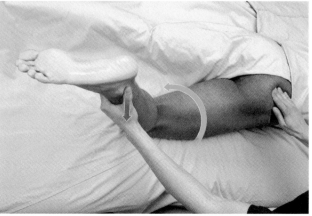

8-52

Superior Gemellus • *su per'e or je mel'us* • Latin "**superior**" *higher* "**geminus**" *twin*

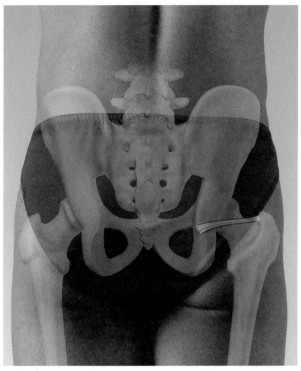

8-53

Palpating Superior Gemellus

Positioning: client prone.

1. Standing at the client's side facing the hip, locate the ischial spine with your fingertips.

2. Slide your fingertips laterally toward the greater trochanter.

3. Palpate and follow the muscles fibers as they converge and insert on the medial surface of the greater trochanter.

4. Client gently resists external rotation of the hip to ensure proper location.

Attachments

O: Ischium, external surface of spine
I: Femur, medial surface of greater trochanter

Actions

• Externally rotates the hip
• Adducts the hip

Innervation

• Sacral plexus
• L5–S2

Functional Anatomy

Superior gemellus lies just inferior to the piriformis and superior to obturator internus in the deep six external rotator group. The other deep external rotators of the hip are inferior gemellus, obturator internus and externus, and quadratus femoris. Just as the rotator cuff stabilizes the shoulder, these muscles stabilize the hip joint at the greater trochanter.

When the lower extremity is not planted, the deep six external rotators turn the femur out. During activities involving weight bearing on the lower extremity, these muscles prevent the femur from internally rotating, allowing the knee to dive inward. This posture is called *genu valgus* (or "knock-knees") and is shown in Figure 8-10. With the foot planted, the superior gemellus and piriformis will also tilt the pelvis laterally. This function occurs when the weight is shifted from one foot to the other, such as with walking or running. The lateral shift of the pelvis assists with trunk rotation and also helps initiate changes in movement directions such as cutting or pivoting.

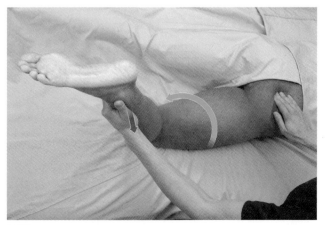

8-54

Inferior Gemellus   in *fer'e or jeme lus* • Latin "**inferior**" *lower* "**geminus**" *twin*

Attachments

O: Ischium, proximal part of tuberosity
I: Femur, medial surface of greater trochanter

Actions

• Externally rotates the hip
• Adducts the hip

Innervation

• Sacral plexus
• L5–S2

Functional Anatomy

Inferior gemellus lies just inferior to the obturator internus and superior to obturator externus in the deep six external rotator group. The other deep external rotators of the hip are the piriformis, superior gemellus, and quadratus femoris. The deep six muscles stabilize the hip joint at the greater trochanter.

The deep six external rotators turn the femur out when the lower extremity is not planted. When we bear weight on the lower extremity, these muscles prevent the femur from turning in and allowing the knee to dive inward. This "knock-kneed" posture is called *genu valgus* (see Figure 8-10).

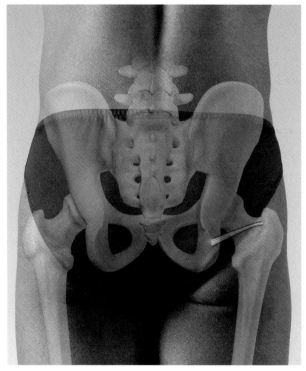

8-55

Palpating Inferior Gemellus

Positioning: client prone.

1. Standing at the client's side facing the hip, locate the proximal ischial tuberosity with your fingertips.

2. Slide your fingertips laterally toward the greater trochanter.

3. Palpate and follow the muscles fibers as they converge and insert on the medial surface of the greater trochanter.

4. Client gently resists external rotation of the hip to ensure proper location.

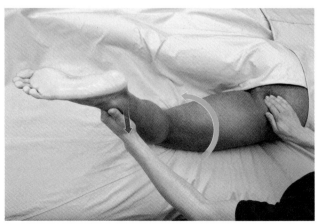

8-56

Obturator Internus ● *ob'tur a tor* in *ter'nus* • Latin "**obtur**" *close* "**internus**" *internal*

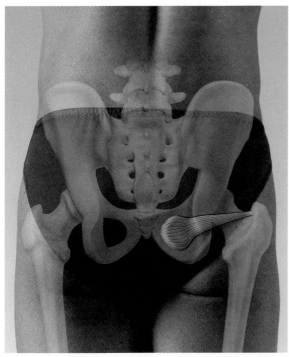

8-57

Palpating Obturator Internus

Positioning: client prone.

1. Standing at the client's side facing the hip, locate the inferior surface of the obturator foramen with your fingertips.
2. Slide your fingertips laterally toward the greater trochanter.
3. Palpate and follow the muscle fibers as they converge and insert on the medial surface of the greater trochanter.
4. Client gently resists external rotation of the hip to ensure proper location.

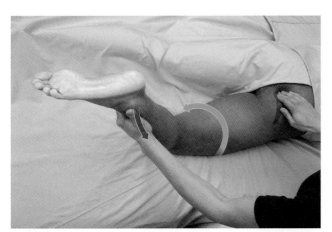

8-58

Attachments

O: Ischium, inferior surface of obturator foramen
I: Femur, medial surface of greater trochanter

Actions

• Externally rotates the hip
• Adducts the hip

Innervation

• Sacral plexus
• L5–S2

Functional Anatomy

Obturator internus lies just inferior to the gemellus superior and superior to gemellus inferior in the deep six external rotator group. The deep six muscles parallel the rotator cuff in the shoulder, they stabilize the hip joint at the greater trochanter.

The deep six external rotators turn the femur out when the lower extremity is not planted. When the lower extremity bears weight, these muscles oppose the *genu valgus* (or "knock-kneed") posture (see Figure 8-10).

Obturator Externus ● *ob'tur a tor ek ster'nus* • Latin **"obtur"** *close* **"externus"** *external*

Attachments

O: Pubis and ischium, superior and inferior rami
I: Femur, trochanteric fossa

Actions

* Externally rotates the hip
* Adducts the hip

Innervation

* Obturator nerve
* L3–L4

Functional Anatomy

Obturator externus lies anterior to quadratus femoris, posterior to pectineus, and just inferior to the gemellus inferior. One of the deep external rotators of the hip, it helps stabilize the hip joint at the greater trochanter.

The deep six external rotators turn the femur out when the lower extremity is not planted. When the lower extremity bears weight, these muscles keep the femur and knee from rotating into the *genu valgus* (or "knock-kneed") posture (see Figure 8-10).

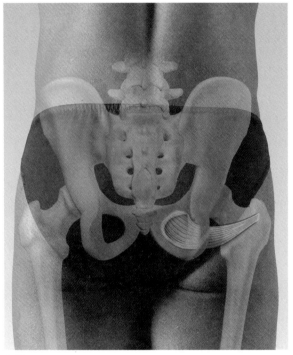

8-59

Palpating Obturator Externus

Positioning: client prone.

1. Standing at the client's side facing the hip, locate the proximal ischial tuberosity with your fingertips.

2. Slide your fingertips laterally and distally toward the greater trochanter.

3. Palpate and follow the muscle fibers as they converge and insert on the trochanteric fossa, just distal to gemellus inferior.

4. Client gently resists external rotation of the hip to ensure proper location.

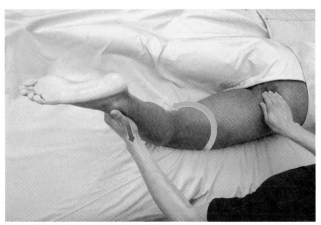

8-60

Quadratus Femoris 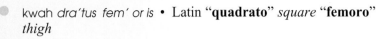 kwah *dra'tus fem' or is* • Latin "**quadrato**" *square* "**femoro**" *thigh*

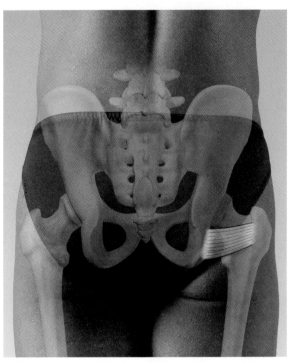

8-61

Palpating Quadratus Femoris

Positioning: client prone.

1. Standing at the client's side facing the hip, locate the proximal ischial tuberosity with your fingertips.

2. Slide your fingertips laterally and distally toward the greater trochanter.

3. Palpate and follow the muscle fibers as they converge and insert between the greater and lesser trochanters.

4. Client gently resists external rotation of the hip to ensure proper location.

Attachments

O: Ischium, lateral ischial tuberosity
I: Femur, crest between greater and lesser trochanters

Actions

• Externally rotates the hip
• Adducts the hip

Innervation

• Sacral plexus
• L4–S2

Functional Anatomy

Quadratus femoris lies posterior to the obturator externus, inferior to gemellus inferior, and superior to adductor magnus. The other deep external rotators of the hip are the piriformis, gemellus superior, and obturator internus. Together these muscles help maintain rotational alignment of the femoral head within the acetabulum.

The deep six external rotators turn the femur out when the lower extremity is not planted. When supporting bodyweight on the lower extremity, these muscles prevent the femur from turning in and allowing the knee to dive inward. This posture is called *genu valgus* or "knock-kneed" in more common terms.

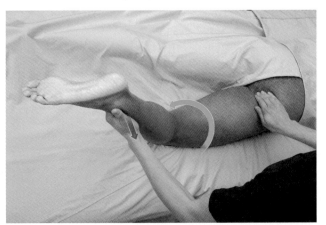

8-62

Biceps Femoris ● bi'seps fem'or is • Latin "**bi**" *two* "**ceps**" *head* "**femoro**" *thigh*

Attachments

O: Long head: ischial tuberosity
O: Short head: lateral lip of linea aspera
I: Fibula, head and lateral condyle of tibia

Actions

• Extends the hip
• Externally rotates the hip
• Flexes the knee
• Externally rotates the flexed knee

Innervation

• Sciatic nerve
• L5–S3

Functional Anatomy

Biceps femoris is the most lateral of the hamstring muscles. It is superficial on the posterior thigh, except where it dives under the gluteus maximus just distal to its origin on the ischial tuberosity. The hamstring group also includes the semimembranosis and semitendinosis. These muscles act as postural stabilizers more than the antagonist quadriceps muscles. They help the gluteus maximus and rectus abdominus maintain a posterior tilt on the pelvis. Like rectus femoris, biceps femoris is a two-joint muscle, crossing both the hip and the knee.

Biceps femoris, along with semimembranosis and semitendinosis, extends the hip and pulls the femur back when the lower extremity is not fixed. This action is used when we swing the leg back during walking and running. The hamstring muscles contract eccentrically to decelerate these movements. When the quadriceps group is excessively strong or the hamstrings are excessively tight, deceleration can end in injury to the hamstring muscles.

When the lower extremity is fixed, the hamstring muscles, along with the powerful gluteus maximus, straighten the body, pulling the pelvis back over the knee and foot. This "hip-hinging" function is critical during movements like standing, lifting, and pushing with the legs, such as with jumping.

The hamstrings also flex the knee and biceps femoris externally rotates it as well. Rotation at the knee is possible only when the knee is slightly flexed. Full extension locks the tibiofemoral joint and prevents rotation. Rotation on a flexed knee is practical when weight bearing to change the direction of movement in the lower body. This movement, commonly known as a plant and pivot, is critical in sports such as tennis, soccer, football, and basketball.

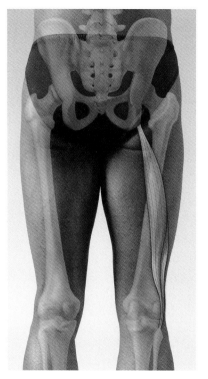

8-63

Palpating Biceps Femoris

Positioning: client prone with knee slightly flexed.

1. Standing at the client's side facing the thigh, locate the lateral proximal border of the popliteal fossa with your palm.
2. Slide your palm slightly proximally toward the ischial tuberosity.
3. Palpate and follow the muscle fibers as they dive under the gluteus maximus and attach to the ischial tuberosity.
4. Client gently resists flexion and external rotation of the knee to ensure proper location.

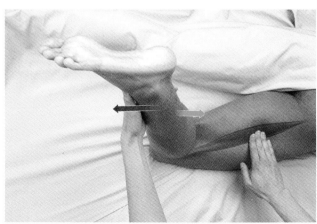

8-64

Semimembranosis

sem'e mem *bra no'sus* • Latin "**semi**" *half* "**membranosus**" *membranous*

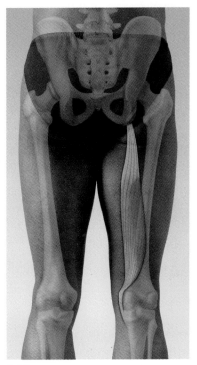

8-65

Palpating Semimembranosis

Positioning: client prone with knee slightly flexed.

1. Standing at the client's side facing the thigh, locate the medial proximal border of the popliteal fossa with your palm.

2. Slide your palm slightly proximally toward the ischial tuberosity.

3. Palpate and follow the muscle fibers posterior and medial to the gracilis up to midthigh.

4. Client gently resists flexion and internal rotation of the knee to ensure proper location.

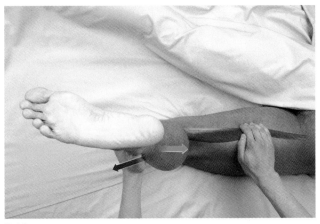

8-66

Attachments

O: Ischium, ischial tuberosity
I: Tibia, posteromedial portion of medial condyle

Actions

• Extends the hip
• Internally rotates the hip
• Flexes the knee
• Internally rotates the flexed knee

Innervation

Functional Anatomy

Semimembranosis is the most medial muscle in the hamstring group, lying between adductor magnus and semitendinosis. It is superficial on the posterior thigh, except where it dives under the gluteus maximus just distal to its origin on the ischial tuberosity. The hamstring muscles act as postural stabilizers more than the antagonist quadriceps muscles. They help the gluteus maximus and rectus abdominus maintain a posterior tilt on the pelvis. Like rectus femoris and biceps femoris, semimembranosis is a two-joint muscle, crossing both the hip and the knee.

Semimembranosis, along with biceps femoris and semitendinosis, extends the hip and pulls the femur back when the lower extremity is not fixed. We use this action to swing the leg back during walking and running. To decelerate these movements, the hamstring muscles contract eccentrically, and can be injured if they are tight or the quadriceps group is significantly stronger.

When the lower extremity is fixed, the hamstrings and gluteus maximus straighten the body, pulling the pelvis back over the knee and foot. This "hip-hinging" function is critical during movements like standing, lifting, and pushing with the legs, such as with jumping.

The hamstrings also flex the knee. Semimembranosis and semitendinosis have the additional action of internally rotating the knee, a movement that is possible only when the knee is slightly flexed. Full extension locks the tibiofemoral joint and prevents rotation. Rotation on a flexed knee is practical when weight bearing to change the direction of movement in the lower body. This plant and pivot movement is critical in sports such as tennis, soccer, football, and basketball.

Semitendinosis   ●   sem'e ten *di no'*sus   •   Latin "**semi**" *half* "**tendinosus**" *tendinous*

Attachments

O: Ischium, ischial tuberosity
I: Tibia, medial shaft via the pes anserine tendon

Actions

- Extends the hip
- Internally rotates the hip
- Flexes the knee
- Internally rotates the flexed knee

Innervation

- Sciatic nerve
- L4–S2

Functional Anatomy

Semitendinosis is part of the hamstring group. This slender muscle lies medial to biceps femoris and superficial to semi-membranosus. It is superficial on the posterior thigh, except where it dives under the gluteus maximus just distal to its origin on the ischial tuberosity. Semitendinosis forms the posterior third of the pes anserine group. The hamstring muscles stabilize posture and help the gluteus maximus and rectus abdominus maintain a posterior tilt on the pelvis. Like rectus femoris and biceps femoris, semimembranosis is a two-joint muscle, crossing both the hip and the knee.

    Semitendinosis, along with biceps femoris and semi-membranosis, extends the hip and pulls the femur back when the lower extremity is not fixed, as during walking and running. When we decelerate, the hamstring muscles contract eccentrically and can be injured if they are excessively tight or the quadriceps group is significantly stronger.

    When the lower extremity is fixed, the hamstring muscles, along with the powerful gluteus maximus, straighten the body, pulling the pelvis back over the knee and foot. This "hip-hinging" function is critical during movements like standing, lifting, and pushing with the legs, such as with jumping.

    The hamstrings also flex the knee, and both semitendinosis and semimembranosis internally rotate the knee. Rotation at the knee is possible only when the knee is slightly flexed, as full extension locks the tibiofemoral joint. Rotation on a flexed knee is necessary in the plant and pivot movement used in sports such as tennis, soccer, football, and basketball.

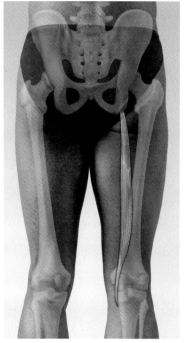

8-67

Palpating Semitendinosis

Positioning: client prone with knee slightly flexed.

1. Standing at the client's side facing the thigh, locate the medial proximal border of the popliteal fossa with your palm.
2. Slide your palm slightly proximally toward the ischial tuberosity.
3. Palpate and follow the muscle fibers proximally as they run parallel and medial to biceps femoris.
4. Client gently resists flexion and internal rotation of the knee to ensure proper location.

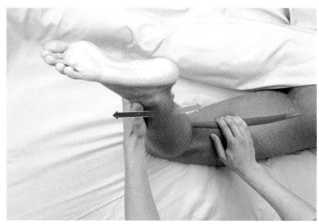

8-68

Popliteus   pop li *te'us* • **"poplit"** Latin *back of the knee*

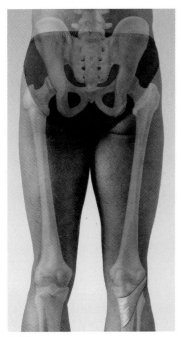

8-69

Palpating Popliteus

Positioning: client prone with knee slightly flexed.

1. Standing at the client's side facing the knee, locate the medial tibial condyle with your fingertips.

2. Curl your fingertips posteriorly onto the distal border of the popliteal fossa finding the posterior shaft of the tibia. *(Caution: the popliteal fossa contains the popliteal artery and vein, the tibial and common peroneal nerves, and lymph nodes. To avoid these structures, palpate the distal border of the fossa.)*

3. Palpate and follow the oblique fibers of popliteus toward the lateral femoral condyle.

4. Client gently resists internal rotation of the knee with a neutral foot to ensure proper location.

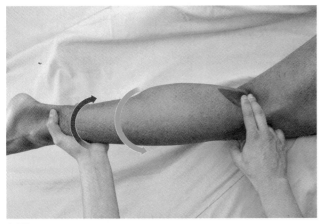

8-70

Attachments

O: Femur, lateral condyle
I: Tibia, proximal posterior surface

Actions

• Flexes the knee
• Internally rotates the knee

Innervation

Functional Anatomy

Popliteus lies at an angle across the back of the knee. It connects the lateral condyle of the femur and the posterior tibia, creating rotation at the tibiofemoral joint. If the foot is not fixed, the tibia will rotate medially on the femur. If it is fixed, the femur will rotate laterally on the tibia.

The main function of the popliteus muscle is to unlock the "screw-home" mechanism. This mechanism, which is possible because the medial femoral condyle is larger than the lateral, involves locking the tibiofemoral joint through rotation. As the knee extends, the tibia spins externally on the femur until it reaches full external rotation. This is the "locked" position. A simple way to observe this is to first sit in a chair facing forward. Straighten one knee fully, watching the position of your foot as you do so. As you reach full knee extension, your foot should turn out slightly. This happens when the tibia turns on the femur. You can also observe it by standing and gently locking (fully extending) and unlocking (slightly flexing or "softening") the knee.

When popliteus initiates internal rotation of the tibia and flexion of the knee, this subtle movement "unlocks" the knee and allows the hamstrings to continue flexion and/or rotation. Hyperextension of the knee can damage the popliteus muscle, creating pain and swelling in the back of the knee as well as dysfunction in the lower extremity.

◗ SYNERGISTS/ANTAGONISTS: HIP

Motion	Muscles Involved	Motion	Muscles Involved
Flexion 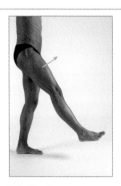 **Hip flexion.**	Psoas Iliacus Sartorius Tensor Fascia Latae Rectus Femoris Pectineus Adductor Brevis Adductor Longus Adductor Magnus (anterior fibers) Gluteus medius (anterior fibers) Gluteus minimus	Extension 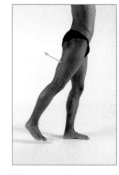 **Hip extension.**	Adductor Magnus (posterior fibers) Gluteus maximus Gluteus medius (posterior fibers) Biceps femoris (long head) Semimembranosis Semitendinosis
Abduction 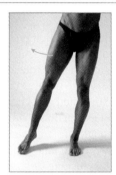 **Hip abduction.**	Sartorius Tensor Fascia Latae Piriformis Gluteus maximus (upper fibers) Gluteus medius Gluteus minimus	Adduction 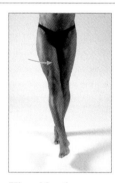 **Hip adduction.**	Pectineus Adductor Brevis Adductor Longus Gracilis Adductor Magnus Gluteus maximus (lower fibers) Gemellus Superior Gemellus Inferior Obturator Internus Obturator Externus Quadratus Femoris
Internal Rotation 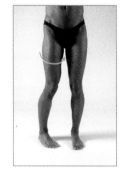 **Hip internal rotation.**	Tensor Fascia Latae Gluteus medius (anterior fibers) Gluteus minimus Semimembranosis Semitendinosis	External Rotation 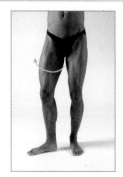 **Hip external rotation.**	Psoas Iliacus Sartorius Adductor Brevis Gluteus maximus Gluteus medius (posterior fibers) Piriformis Gemellus Superior Gemellus Inferior Obturator Internus Quadratus Femoris Biceps femoris (long head)

▶ SYNERGISTS/ANTAGONISTS: KNEE

Knee Motion	Muscles Involved	Knee Motion	Muscles Involved
Flexion	Sartorius	Extension	Rectus Femoris
	Gracilis		Vastus Lateralis
	Biceps femoris		Vastus Intermedius
	Semimembranosis		Vastus Medialis
	Semitendinosis		
	Popliteus		
	Gastrocnemius (see Chapter 9)		

Knee flexion.   **Knee extension.**

Knee Motion	Muscles Involved	Knee Motion	Muscles Involved
Internal Rotation	Sartorius	External Rotation	Gracilis
	Semimembranosis		Biceps femoris
	Semitendinosis		
	Popliteus		

Knee internal rotation.   **Knee external rotation.**

❱ PUTTING IT IN MOTION

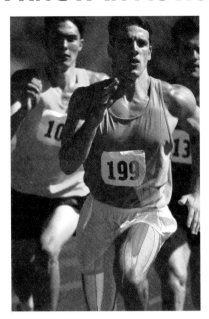

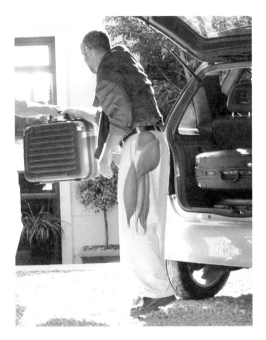

Running. Alternating opposite motions of the hips and knees drive the running motion. Powerful hip extensors and knee flexors bring one leg back as the other drives forward using the hip flexors and knee extensors. The body maintains its sagittal plane motion through the stabilizing efforts of the deep six external rotators as well as the adductors and smaller gluteal muscles.

Lifting. The hip and knee must work in concert with the trunk and upper body to lift objects from the ground. Powerful muscles like the gluteus maximus and quadriceps muscles drive the motion while stabilizers like gluteus medius and the adductor group maintain a steady body position.

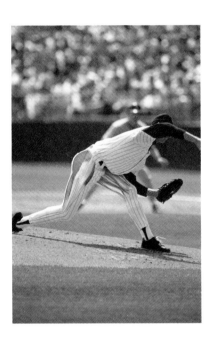

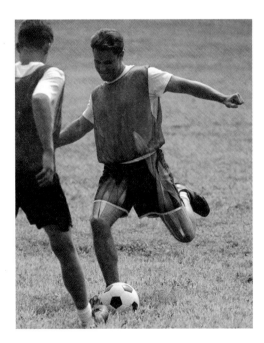

Throwing. As with running, throwing requires different movements on each side of the body. This movement is more complex because it takes place in multiple planes. The front or *lead* leg plants while the body rotates around it bringing the chest and arm forward. The quadriceps, hamstrings, and gluteals accept the body's weight while the rotators of the hip and knee pivots the body around the foot. The back or *trail* leg uses the adductors to control the motion before swinging through and accepting the body's weight for the follow through motion.

Kicking. Kicking is similar to throwing in that there is a planted lead leg and a swinging trail leg. Again, the body must pivot around the planted lead leg in order to position the body for powerful sagittal motion. In kicking, the trail leg does not contact the ground as it does with throwing. The hip flexors and knee extensors are maximally recruited to place greatest force at the foot for kicking. The gluteus maximus, hamstrings, and adductors must slow this motion once the ball has been contacted.

SUMMARY

- The pelvic girdle is made up of the ilium, ischium, pubis, sacrum, and coccyx. The ilium, ischium, and pubis converge at the acetabulum, forming the socket of the ball-and-socket coxal joint.
- The sacroiliac joints and pubic symphysis allow slight movement in the pelvic girdle.
- The head of the femur forms the ball of the ball-and-socket coxal joint and can move in all planes to produce flexion, extension, abduction, adduction, internal rotation, and external rotation at the hip.
- The knee consists of two joints: the tibiofemoral joint and the patellofemoral joint. Together, these joints allow flexion, extension, internal rotation, and external rotation at the knee. Movement of the patella maintains the leverage of the quadriceps muscles as the knee flexes and extends.
- As with the shoulder, the deeper, smaller muscles in the hip, such as the deep six external rotators, tend to stabilize the joints. The larger, more superficial muscles, such as the gluteals, create powerful movements.
- The inguinal region, deep posterior hip, and posterior knee contain several vulnerable structures, including lymph nodes and vessels, veins, arteries, and nerves. Avoid these during palpation.
- Balanced flexibility and strength in the muscles of the pelvis, hip, and thigh enhance posture and minimize injury such as patellar tracking problems, muscle strains, and ligament sprains.
- Coordinated movement of the muscles of the pelvis, thigh, and knee is required during walking and running as well as powerful movements such as lifting, throwing, and kicking.

FOR REVIEW

Multiple Choice

1. The bones that make up the coxal joint are:
   A. the ilium, sacrum, ischium, and pubis
   B. the sacrum, coccyx, coxae, and femur
   C. the ilium, ischium, pubis, and femur
   D. the sacrum, coccyx, and coxae

2. The bones that make up the pelvic girdle are:
   A. the ilium, sacrum, ischium, and pubis
   B. the sacrum, coccyx, coxae, and femur
   C. the ilium, ischium, pubis, and femur
   D. the sacrum, coccyx, and coxae

3. The coxal joint is a:
   A. hinge joint
   B. ball-and-socket joint
   C. modified hinge joint
   D. gliding joint

4. The tibiofemoral joint is a:
   A. hinge joint
   B. ball-and-socket joint
   C. modified hinge joint
   D. gliding joint

5. The pelvic muscle that bridges the spine and the hip is the:
   A. psoas
   B. sartorius
   C. biceps femoris
   D. piriformis

6. The muscle that is most closely associated with the sciatic nerve is the:
   A. psoas
   B. sartorius
   C. biceps femoris
   D. piriformis

7. The motion that all the gluteal muscles have in common is:
   A. hip extension
   B. hip internal rotation
   C. hip abduction
   D. hip adduction

8. The only quadriceps muscle that acts on the hip joint is the:
   A. vastus lateralis
   B. rectus femoris
   C. vastus medialis
   D. vastus intermedius

9. The hamstring muscle responsible for externally rotating the knee is:
   A. semimembranosis
   B. semitendinosis
   C. biceps femoris
   D. both A and B are correct

10. The three muscles that connect to the pes anserine tendon are the:
    A. adductor magnus, gracilis, semitendinosis
    B. biceps femoris, semitendinosis, semimembranosis
    C. sartorius, gracilis, semimembranosis
    D. sartorius, gracilis, semitendinosis

Matching

Different muscle attachments are listed below. Match the correct muscle with its attachment.

11. _____ Ilium, anterolateral lip of iliac crest

12. _____ Femur, middle one-third of medial lip of linea aspera

13. _____ Femur, intertrochanteric line and medial lip of linea aspera

14. _____ T12–L5 vertebrae, transverse processes, lateral bodies and corresponding intevertebral disks.

15. _____ Pubis, superior ramus

16. _____ Femur, trochanteric fossa

17. _____ Femur, gluteal tuberosity and lateral tibial condyle via the iliotibial band

18. _____ Ischium, proximal part of tuberosity

19. _____ Tibia, proximal posterior surface

20. _____ Tibia, posteromedial portion of medial condyle

A. Obturator externus

B. Semimembranosis

C. Gluteus maximus

D. Gemellus inferior

E. Tensor fascia latae

F. Pectineus

G. Popliteus

H. Adductor longus

I. Vastus medialis

J. Psoas

Different muscle actions are listed below. Match the correct muscle with its action. Answers may be used more than once.

21. _____ Gluteus medius

22. _____ Popliteus

23. _____ Iliacus

24. _____ Adductor Brevis

25. _____ Gracilis

26. _____ Biceps Femoris

27. _____ Vastus intermedius

28. _____ Semitendinosis

29. _____ Gluteus minimus

30. _____ Piriformis

A. Flexes the hip
B. Extends the hip
C. Abducts the hip
D. Adducts the hip
E. Internally rotates the hip
F. Externally rotates the hip
G. Flexes the knee
H. Extends the knee
I. Internally rotates the knee
J. Externally rotates the knee

Short Answer

31. Describe the general structure of the pelvic girdle and compare it to that of the shoulder girdle. Do the same for the coxal joint and glenohumeral joint.

32. Briefly describe the importance of a proper balance of strength between the muscles of the quadriceps relative to patellar tracking.

33. Briefly describe the joints and motions involved in planting and pivoting the lower extremity. What activities or sports require this type of movement?

Try This!

Activity: Find a partner and have him or her perform one of the skills identified in the *Putting It in Motion* segment. Identify the specific actions of the hip and knee that make up this skill. Write them down. Use the synergist list to identify which muscles work together to create this movement. Make sure you put the actions in the correct sequence. See if you can discover which muscles are stabilizing or steering the joint into position and which are responsible for powering the movement.

Switch partners and perform a different skill from *Putting It in Motion*. Repeat the steps above. Confirm your findings with the *Putting It in Motion* segment on the student CD included with your textbook. To further your understanding, practice this activity with skills not identified in *Putting It in Motion*.

SUGGESTED READINGS

Aminaka N, Gribble PA. Patellar taping, patellofemoral pain syndrome, lower extremity kinematics, and dynamic postural control. *J Athl Train.* 2008;43(1):21–28.

Cote KP, Brunet ME II, Gansneder BM, et al. Effects of pronated and supinated foot postures on static and dynamic posture stability. *J Athl Train.* 2005;40(1):41–46.

Devan MR, Pescatello LS, Faghri P, et al. A prospective study of overuse knee injuries among female athletes with muscle imbalances and structural abnormalities. *J Athl Train.* 2004;39(3):263–267.

Fairclough J, Hayashi K, Toumi H, et al. The functional anatomy of the iliotibial band during flexion and extension of the knee: implications for understanding iliotibial band syndrome. *J Anat.* 2006;208(3):309–316.

Hanson AM, Padua DA, Blackburn JT, et al. Muscle Activation During Side-Step Cutting Maneuvers in Male and Female Soccer Athletes. *J Athl Train.* 2008;43(2):133–143.

Moss RI, DeVita P, Dawson ML. A biomechanical analysis of patellofemoral stress syndrome. *J Athl Train.* 1992;7(1):64–66, 68–69.

Pettitt R, Dolski A. Corrective neuromuscular approach to the treatment of iliotibial band friction syndrome: a case report. *J Athl Train.* 2000;35(1):96–99.

Richards J, Thewlis D, Selfe J, et al. A biomechanical investigation of a single-limb squat: implications for lower extremity rehabilitation exercises. *J Athl Train.* 2008;43(5):477–482.

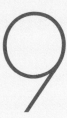

Leg, Ankle, and Foot

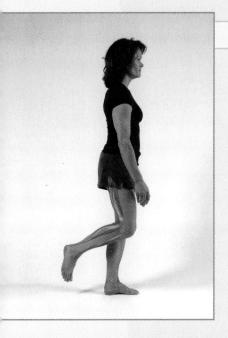

Learning Objectives

After working through this chapter you should be able to:

- Identify the main structures of the leg, ankle, and foot, including bones, joints, special structures, and deep and superficial muscles.
- Identify normal posture and postural deviations of the leg, ankle, and foot.
- Label and palpate the major surface landmarks of the leg, ankle, and foot.
- Draw, label, palpate, and fire the superficial and deep muscles of the leg, ankle, and foot.
- Locate the attachments and nerve supply of the muscles of the leg, ankle, and foot.
- Identify and demonstrate all actions of the muscles of the leg, ankle, and foot.
- Describe the events of human gait and identify the muscles involved in each phase.
- Demonstrate passive and resisted range of motion of the ankle and foot.
- Describe the unique functional anatomy and relationships between each muscle of the leg, ankle, and foot.
- Identify both the synergists and antagonists involved in each movement of the ankle and foot (e.g., plantarflexion, dorsiflexion).
- Identify muscles used in performing four coordinated movements of the ankle and foot: walking, running, skating, and blading.

▶ OVERVIEW OF THE REGION

The lower leg, ankle, and foot are structurally similar to the forearm, wrist, and hand. Both have parallel bones (radius and ulna in the forearm and tibia and fibula in the leg) connected by an interosseous membrane. Moving distally, the joints become more complex and then terminate in multi-jointed complexes—the hand and foot, respectively.

Whereas both the foot and hand are capable of multiple motions, the lower extremity tends to be more stable as it must bear the weight of the body. The lower leg allows minimal motion at its proximal and distal joints, stabilizing the lower extremity during propulsion activities such as walking, running, and jumping. The ankle hinges sagittally, pointedly driving the body forward. Finally, the foot is the most mobile structure, absorbing the shock of ground contact and adapting to various surfaces.

▶ SURFACE ANATOMY OF THE LEG, ANKLE, AND FOOT

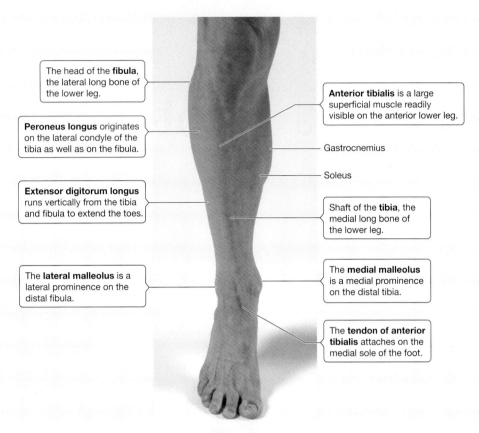

The head of the **fibula**, the lateral long bone of the lower leg.

Peroneus longus originates on the lateral condyle of the tibia as well as on the fibula.

Extensor digitorum longus runs vertically from the tibia and fibula to extend the toes.

The **lateral malleolus** is a lateral prominence on the distal fibula.

Anterior tibialis is a large superficial muscle readily visible on the anterior lower leg.

Gastrocnemius

Soleus

Shaft of the **tibia**, the medial long bone of the lower leg.

The **medial malleolus** is a medial prominence on the distal tibia.

The **tendon of anterior tibialis** attaches on the medial sole of the foot.

9-1A. Anterior view.

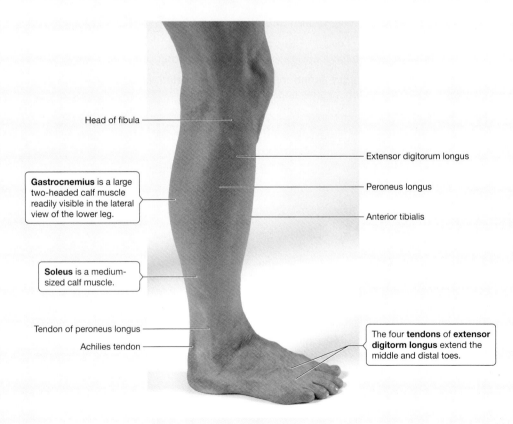

Head of fibula

Gastrocnemius is a large two-headed calf muscle readily visible in the lateral view of the lower leg.

Soleus is a medium-sized calf muscle.

Tendon of peroneus longus

Achilies tendon

Extensor digitorum longus

Peroneus longus

Anterior tibialis

The four **tendons** of **extensor digitorm longus** extend the middle and distal toes.

9-1B. Lateral view.

▶ SURFACE ANATOMY OF THE LEG, ANKLE, AND FOOT

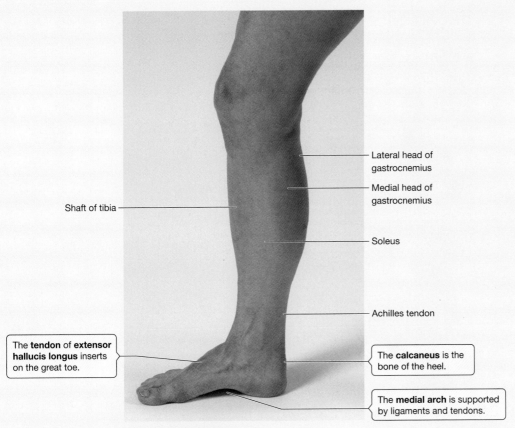

Shaft of tibia

Lateral head of gastrocnemius

Medial head of gastrocnemius

Soleus

Achilles tendon

The **tendon** of **extensor hallucis longus** inserts on the great toe.

The **calcaneus** is the bone of the heel.

The **medial arch** is supported by ligaments and tendons.

9-1C. Medial view.

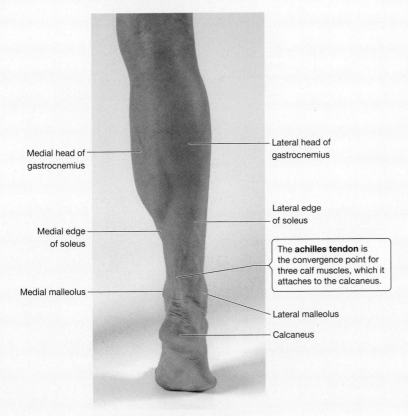

Medial head of gastrocnemius

Lateral head of gastrocnemius

Lateral edge of soleus

The **achilles tendon** is the convergence point for three calf muscles, which it attaches to the calcaneus.

Medial edge of soleus

Medial malleolus

Lateral malleolus

Calcaneus

9-1D. Posterior view.

▶ SKELETAL STRUCTURES OF LEG, ANKLE, AND FOOT

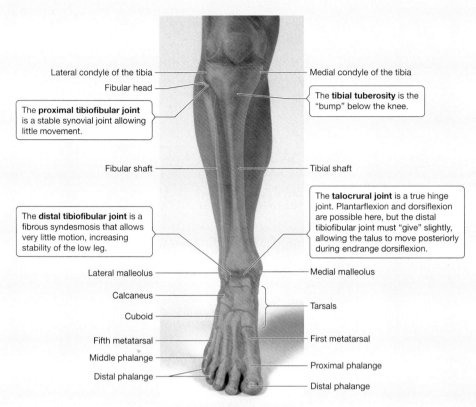

Lateral condyle of the tibia

Fibular head

The **proximal tibiofibular joint** is a stable synovial joint allowing little movement.

Fibular shaft

The **distal tibiofibular joint** is a fibrous syndesmosis that allows very little motion, increasing stability of the low leg.

Lateral malleolus

Calcaneus

Cuboid

Fifth metatarsal

Middle phalange

Distal phalange

Medial condyle of the tibia

The **tibial tuberosity** is the "bump" below the knee.

Tibial shaft

The **talocrural joint** is a true hinge joint. Plantarflexion and dorsiflexion are possible here, but the distal tibiofibular joint must "give" slightly, allowing the talus to move posteriorly during endrange dorsiflexion.

Medial malleolus

Tarsals

First metatarsal

Proximal phalange

Distal phalange

9-2A. Anterior view.

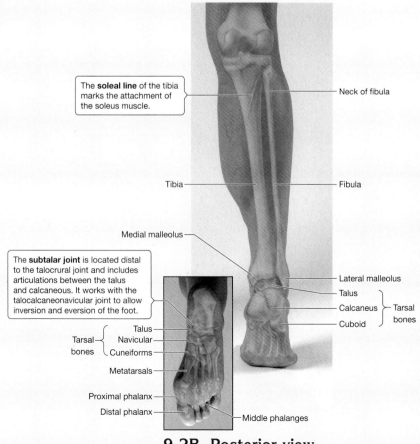

The **soleal line** of the tibia marks the attachment of the soleus muscle.

Neck of fibula

Tibia

Fibula

Medial malleolus

The **subtalar joint** is located distal to the talocrural joint and includes articulations between the talus and calcaneous. It works with the talocalcaneonavicular joint to allow inversion and eversion of the foot.

Lateral malleolus

Talus

Calcaneus ⎫
           ⎬ Tarsal
Cuboid   ⎭ bones

Tarsal ⎧ Talus
bones ⎨ Navicular
       ⎩ Cuneiforms

Metatarsals

Proximal phalanx

Distal phalanx

Middle phalanges

9-2B. Posterior view.

▶ SKELETAL STRUCTURES OF LEG, ANKLE, AND FOOT

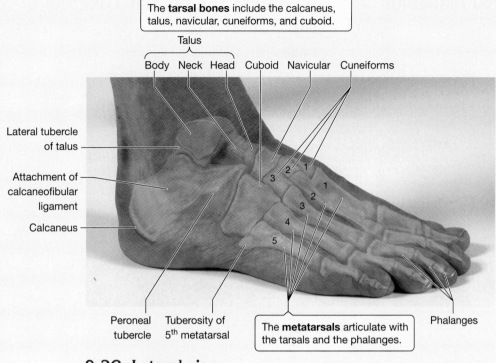

The **tarsal bones** include the calcaneus, talus, navicular, cuneiforms, and cuboid.

Talus

Body   Neck   Head   Cuboid   Navicular   Cuneiforms

Lateral tubercle of talus

Attachment of calcaneofibular ligament

Calcaneus

Peroneal tubercle

Tuberosity of 5th metatarsal

The **metatarsals** articulate with the tarsals and the phalanges.

Phalanges

9-2C. Lateral view.

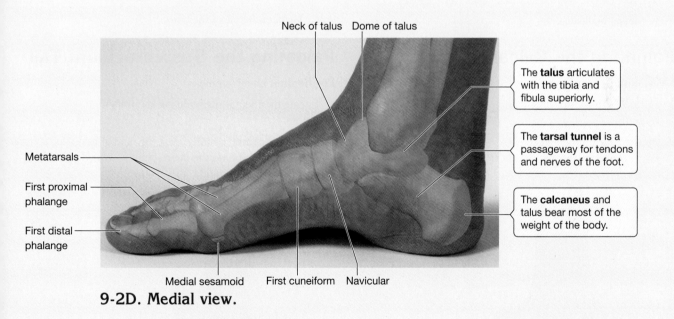

Neck of talus   Dome of talus

The **talus** articulates with the tibia and fibula superiorly.

The **tarsal tunnel** is a passageway for tendons and nerves of the foot.

The **calcaneus** and talus bear most of the weight of the body.

Metatarsals

First proximal phalange

First distal phalange

Medial sesamoid   First cuneiform   Navicular

9-2D. Medial view.

▶ BONY LANDMARKS OF SKELETAL STRUCTURES

Palpating the Medial Malleolus

Positioning: client supine.

1. Locate the medial ankle with your fingertips.
2. Explore the large protrusion at the distal end of the tibia, called the medial malleolus.

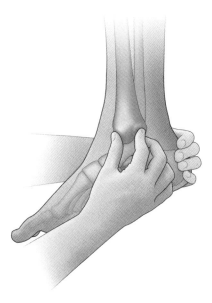

9-3A. **Medial malleolus.**

Palpating the Calcaneus

Positioning: client supine.

1. Locate the posterior heel with your thumb and fingertips.
2. Pincer your thumb and fingers together, palpating the large, round calcaneus.

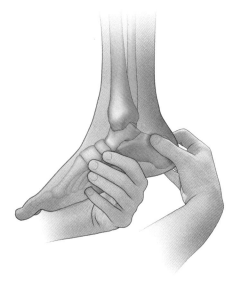

9-3B. **Calcaneus.**

Palpating the Medial Tubercle of the Talus

Positioning: client supine.

1. Locate the medial calcaneus with your thumb.
2. Slide your thumb anteriorly and slightly proximally toward the medial malleolus onto the small, rounded medial tubercle of the talus.

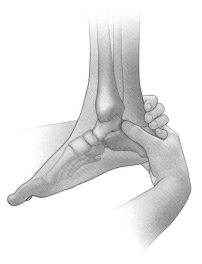

9-3C. **Medial tubercle of the talus.**

Palpating the Sustentaculum Tali

Positioning: client supine.

1. Locate the medial malleolus of the tibia with your thumb.
2. Slide your thumb distally, past the medial tubercle of the talus and onto the deep, blunt protrusion of the sustentaculum tali.

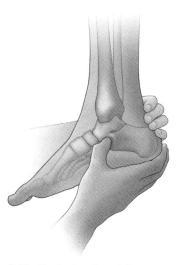

9-3D. **Sustentaculum tali.**

Palpating the Navicular

Positioning: client supine.

1. Locate the medial malleolus of the tibia with your thumb.
2. Slide your thumb distally and anteriorly toward the medial arch and onto the rounded medial protrusion of the navicular.

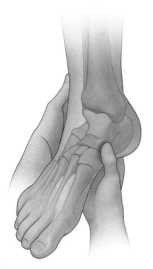

9-3E. Navicular.

Palpating the Cuneiforms

Positioning: client supine.

1. Locate the navicular with your thumb.
2. Slide your thumb distally and laterally onto the dorsal surface of the foot, palpating the flat, dorsal surfaces of the cuneiforms.

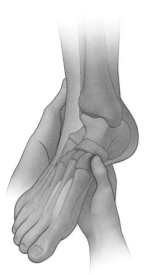

9-3F. Cuneiforms.

Palpating the Lateral Malleolus

Positioning: client supine.

1. Locate the lateral ankle with your thumb.
2. Explore the large protrusion at the distal end of the fibula, called the lateral malleolus.

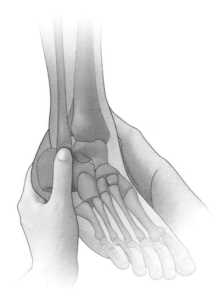

9-3G. Lateral malleolus.

Palpating the Talus

Positioning: client supine with ankle plantarflexed.

1. Locate the lateral malleolus with your thumb.
2. Slide your thumb medially and distally onto the deep, slightly rounded surface of the dome of the talus.

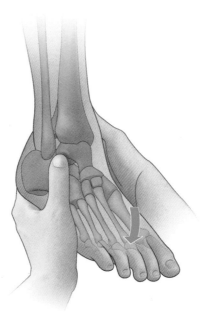

9-3H. Talus.

Palpating the Sinus Tarsi

Positioning: client supine.

1. Locate the lateral malleolus with your thumb.

2. Slide your thumb distally and slightly anteriorly, palpating the deep sinus tarsi that is deep and lateral to the dome of the talus.

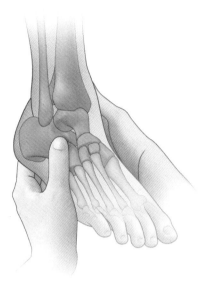

9-3I. **Sinus tarsi.**

Palpating the Cuboid

Positioning: client supine.

1. Locate the lateral calcaneus with your thumb.

2. Slide your thumb distally and anteriorly onto the flat dorsal surface of the cuboid.

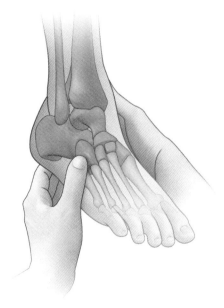

9-3J. **Cuboid.**

Palpating the Peroneal Tubercle

Positioning: client supine.

1. Locate the lateral malleolus with your thumb.

2. Slide your thumb distally onto the small protruding peroneal tubercle, located on the lateral surface of the calcaneus.

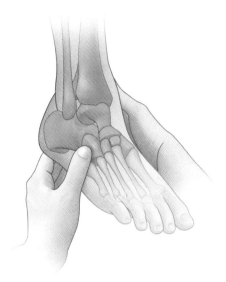

9-3K. **Peroneal tubercle.**

Palpating the Base of the Fifth Metatarsal

Positioning: client supine.

1. Locate the lateral edge of the foot, just below the 5th toe, with your thumb.

2. Slide your thumb proximally along the edge of the foot until you locate the sharp, lateral protrusion of the base of the 5th metatarsal.

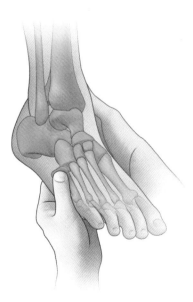

9-3L. **Base of the fifth metatarsal.**

Palpating the Medial Tubercle of the Calcaneus

Positioning: client supine.

1. Locate the plantar surface of the calcaneus with your thumb.

2. Slide your thumb distally and medially, palpating the deep medial tubercle of the calcaneus.

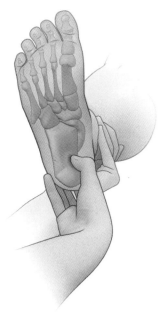

9-3M. **Medial Tubercle of the Calcaneus.**

Palpating the Sesamoids

Positioning: client supine with great toe extended.

1. Locate the distal end of the first metatarsal with your thumb.

2. Palpate the small, round sesamoid bones located side-by-side just proximal to the first metatarsophalangeal joint.

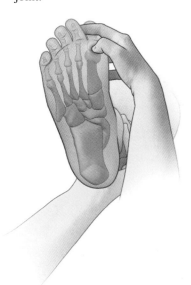

9-3N. **Sesamoids.**

Palpating the Metatarsal Heads

Positioning: client supine.

1. Locate the distal end of the first metatarsal with your thumb.

2. Slide your thumb laterally, palpating the heads of the second, third, fourth, and fifth metatarsals.

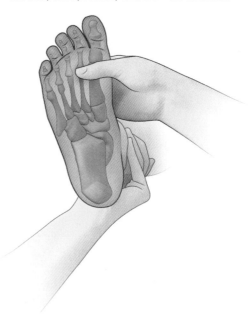

9-3O. **Metatarsal Heads.**

Palpating the Phalanges

Positioning: client supine.

1. Pincer grasp the toes between your thumb and fingertips.

2. Palpate the plantar and dorsal surface of the phalanges as well as the interphalangeal joints.

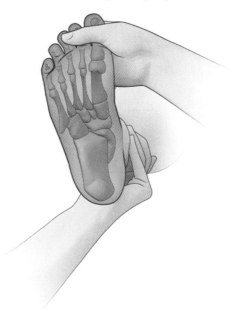

9-3P. **Phalanges.**

▶ MUSCLE ATTACHMENT SITES

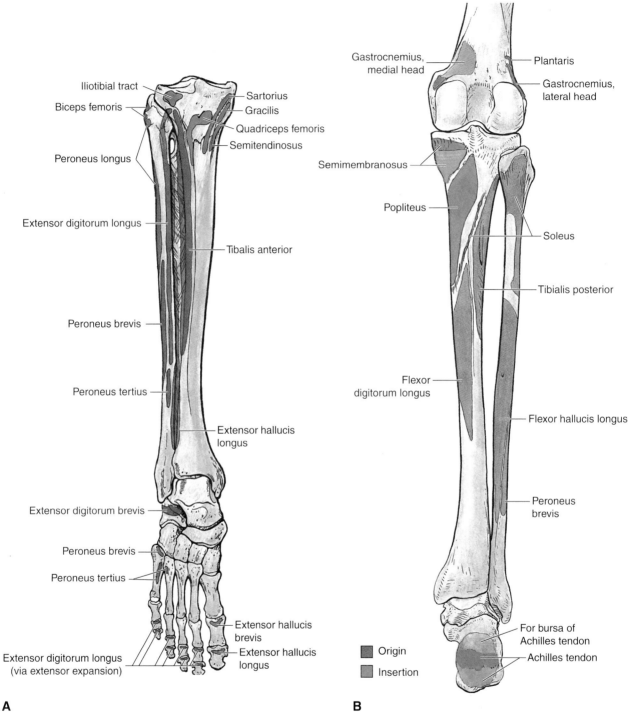

A   **B**

9-4 A. Muscle attachments of the lower leg, ankle, and foot: anterior view. **B.** Muscle attachments of the lower leg, ankle, and foot: posterior view. *(continues)*

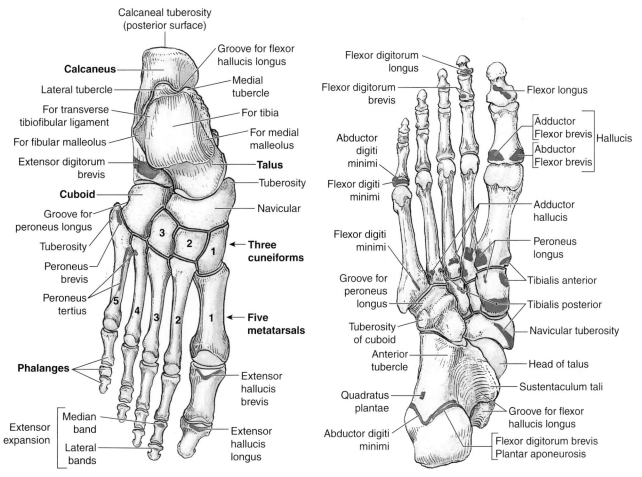

9-4 *(continued)* **C.** Muscle attachments of the foot: dorsal surface. **D.** Muscle attachments of the foot: plantar surface.

▶ LIGAMENTS OF THE LEG, ANKLE, AND FOOT

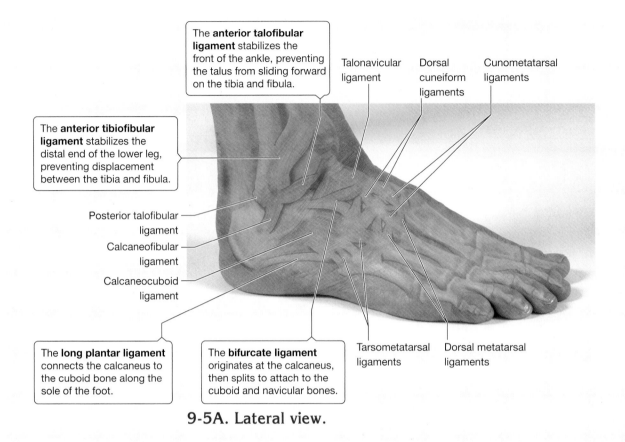

The **anterior talofibular ligament** stabilizes the front of the ankle, preventing the talus from sliding forward on the tibia and fibula.

The **anterior tibiofibular ligament** stabilizes the distal end of the lower leg, preventing displacement between the tibia and fibula.

Talonavicular ligament

Dorsal cuneiform ligaments

Cunometatarsal ligaments

Posterior talofibular ligament

Calcaneofibular ligament

Calcaneocuboid ligament

The **long plantar ligament** connects the calcaneus to the cuboid bone along the sole of the foot.

The **bifurcate ligament** originates at the calcaneus, then splits to attach to the cuboid and navicular bones.

Tarsometatarsal ligaments

Dorsal metatarsal ligaments

9-5A. Lateral view.

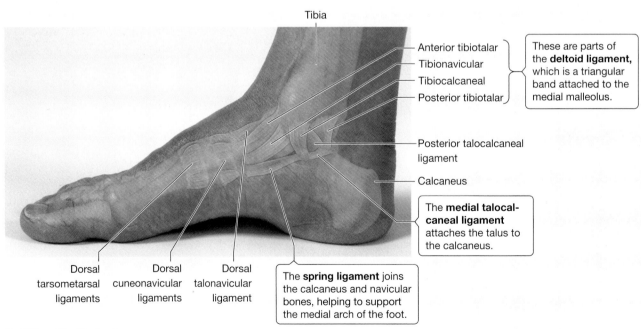

Tibia

Anterior tibiotalar
Tibionavicular
Tibiocalcaneal
Posterior tibiotalar

These are parts of the **deltoid ligament,** which is a triangular band attached to the medial malleolus.

Posterior talocalcaneal ligament

Calcaneus

The **medial talocalcaneal ligament** attaches the talus to the calcaneus.

Dorsal tarsometatarsal ligaments

Dorsal cuneonavicular ligaments

Dorsal talonavicular ligament

The **spring ligament** joins the calcaneus and navicular bones, helping to support the medial arch of the foot.

9-5B. Medial view.

◗ LIGAMENTS OF THE LEG, ANKLE, AND FOOT

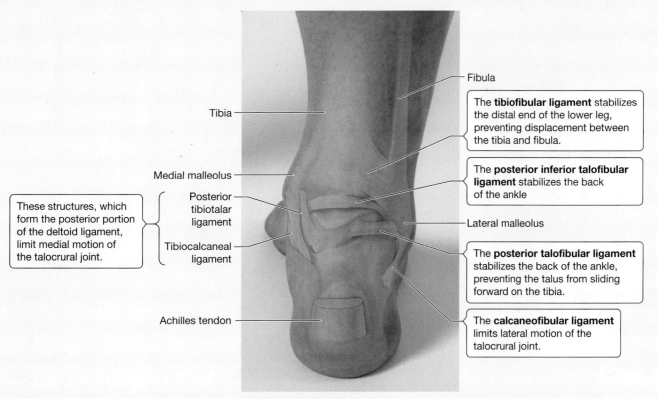

Tibia

Fibula

The **tibiofibular ligament** stabilizes the distal end of the lower leg, preventing displacement between the tibia and fibula.

Medial malleolus

The **posterior inferior talofibular ligament** stabilizes the back of the ankle

Posterior tibiotalar ligament

Lateral malleolus

These structures, which form the posterior portion of the deltoid ligament, limit medial motion of the talocrural joint.

Tibiocalcaneal ligament

The **posterior talofibular ligament** stabilizes the back of the ankle, preventing the talus from sliding forward on the tibia.

Achilles tendon

The **calcaneofibular ligament** limits lateral motion of the talocrural joint.

9-5C. Posterior view.

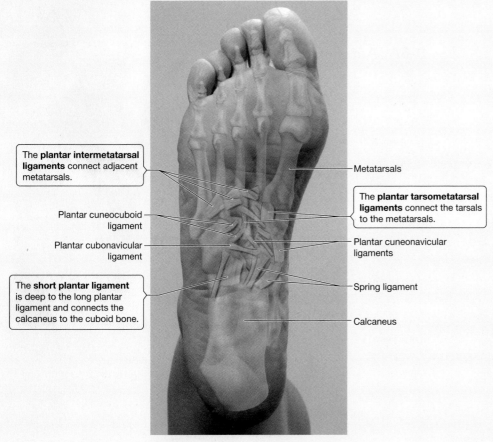

The **plantar intermetatarsal ligaments** connect adjacent metatarsals.

Metatarsals

The **plantar tarsometatarsal ligaments** connect the tarsals to the metatarsals.

Plantar cuneocuboid ligament

Plantar cubonavicular ligament

Plantar cuneonavicular ligaments

The **short plantar ligament** is deep to the long plantar ligament and connects the calcaneus to the cuboid bone.

Spring ligament

Calcaneus

9-5D. Inferior view.

▶ SUPERFICIAL MUSCLES OF THE LEG, ANKLE, AND FOOT

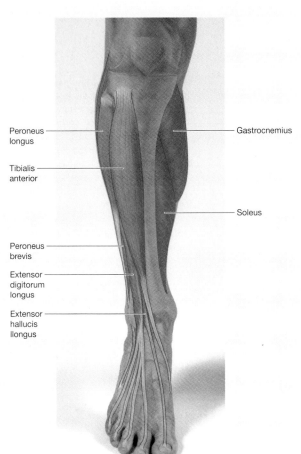

Peroneus longus

Tibialis anterior

Peroneus brevis

Extensor digitorum longus

Extensor hallucis llongus

Gastrocnemius

Soleus

9-6A. Anterior view.

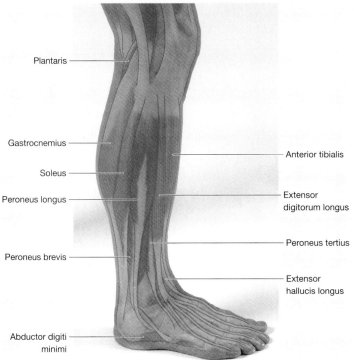

Plantaris

Gastrocnemius

Soleus

Peroneus longus

Peroneus brevis

Abductor digiti minimi

Anterior tibialis

Extensor digitorum longus

Peroneus tertius

Extensor hallucis longus

9-6B. Lateral view.

▶ SUPERFICIAL MUSCLES OF THE LEG, ANKLE, AND FOOT

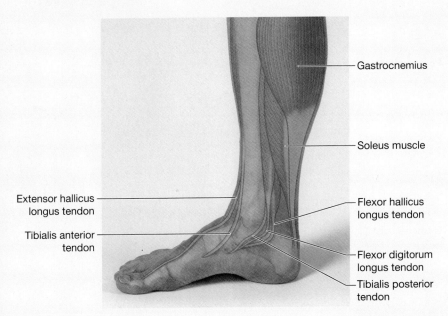

Gastrocnemius

Soleus muscle

Extensor hallicus longus tendon

Flexor hallicus longus tendon

Tibialis anterior tendon

Flexor digitorum longus tendon

Tibialis posterior tendon

9-6C. Medial view.

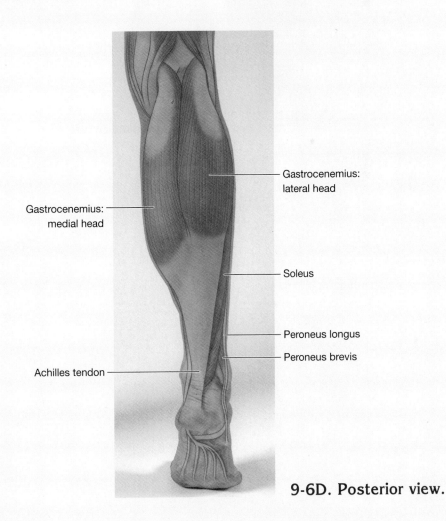

Gastrocenemius: lateral head

Gastrocenemius: medial head

Soleus

Peroneus longus

Peroneus brevis

Achilles tendon

9-6D. Posterior view.

▶ DEEP MUSCLES OF THE LEG, ANKLE, AND FOOT

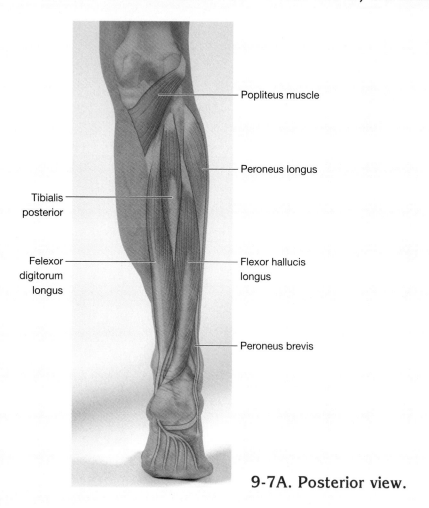

Popliteus muscle

Peroneus longus

Tibialis posterior

Felexor digitorum longus

Flexor hallucis longus

Peroneus brevis

9-7A. Posterior view.

▶ DEEP MUSCLES OF THE LEG, ANKLE, AND FOOT

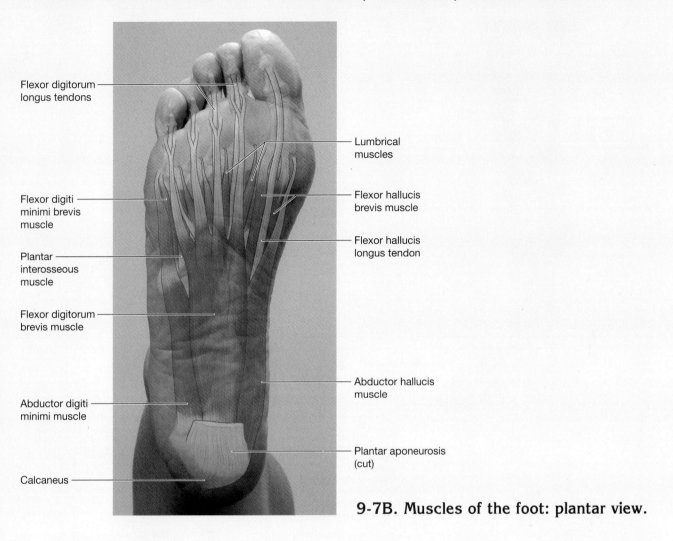

Flexor digitorum longus tendons

Lumbrical muscles

Flexor digiti minimi brevis muscle

Flexor hallucis brevis muscle

Plantar interosseous muscle

Flexor hallucis longus tendon

Flexor digitorum brevis muscle

Abductor hallucis muscle

Abductor digiti minimi muscle

Plantar aponeurosis (cut)

Calcaneus

9-7B. Muscles of the foot: plantar view.

▶ SPECIAL STRUCTURES OF THE LEG, ANKLE, AND FOOT

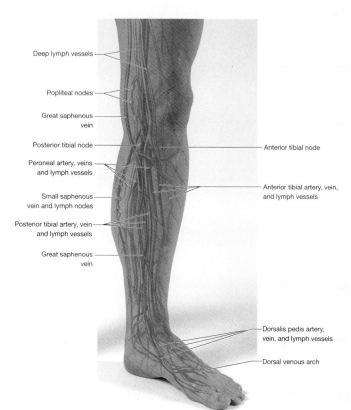

Deep lymph vessels

Popliteal nodes

Great saphenous vein

Posterior tibial node

Peroneal artery, veins and lymph vessels

Small saphenous vein and lymph nodes

Posterior tibial artery, vein and lymph vessels

Great saphenous vein

Anterior tibial node

Anterior tibial artery, vein, and lymph vessels

Dorsalis pedis artery, vein, and lymph vessels

Dorsal venous arch

9-8A. Blood vessels and lymphatics of the lower leg, ankle, and foot: anterior viw.

The **popliteal artery** is a continuation of the femoral artery of the thigh. Just inferior to the head of the fibula, it branches into the anterior and posterior tibial arteries.

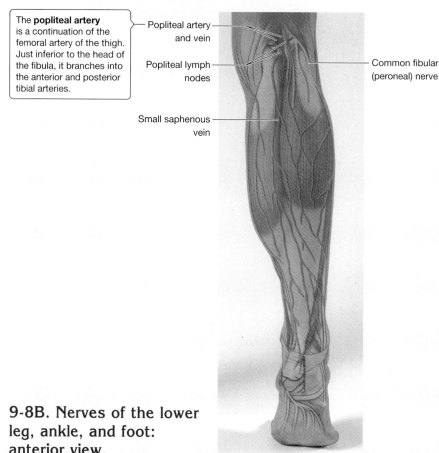

Popliteal artery and vein

Popliteal lymph nodes

Small saphenous vein

Common fibular (peroneal) nerve

9-8B. Nerves of the lower leg, ankle, and foot: anterior view.

▶ SPECIAL STRUCTURES OF THE LEG, ANKLE, AND FOOT

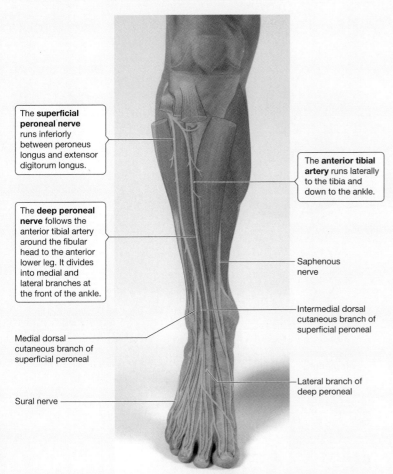

The **superficial peroneal nerve** runs inferiorly between peroneus longus and extensor digitorum longus.

The **deep peroneal nerve** follows the anterior tibial artery around the fibular head to the anterior lower leg. It divides into medial and lateral branches at the front of the ankle.

Medial dorsal cutaneous branch of superficial peroneal

Sural nerve

The **anterior tibial artery** runs laterally to the tibia and down to the ankle.

Saphenous nerve

Intermedial dorsal cutaneous branch of superficial peroneal

Lateral branch of deep peroneal

9-8C. Anterior view.

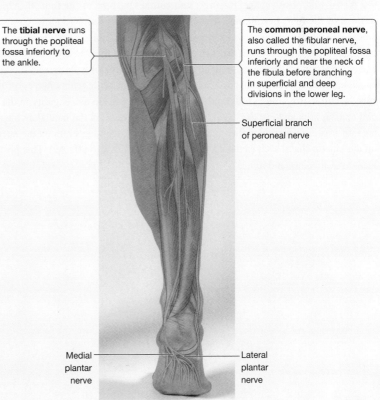

The **tibial nerve** runs through the popliteal fossa inferiorly to the ankle.

The **common peroneal nerve**, also called the fibular nerve, runs through the popliteal fossa inferiorly and near the neck of the fibula before branching in superficial and deep divisions in the lower leg.

Superficial branch of peroneal nerve

Medial plantar nerve

Lateral plantar nerve

9-8D. Posterior view.

▶ POSTURE OF THE ANKLE AND FOOT

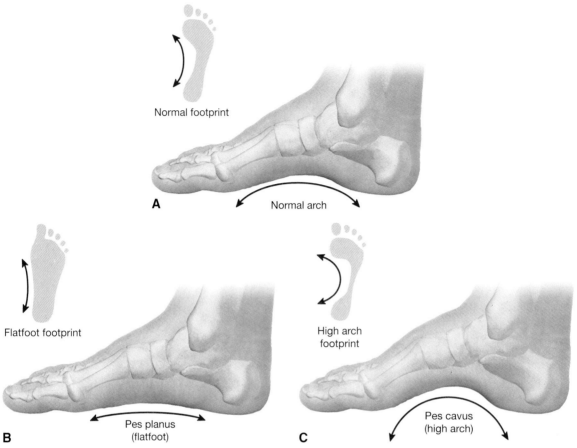

9-9 **A. Normal posture, architecture, and contact pattern of the foot. B. Abnormal posture, architecture, and contact pattern of the foot: pes planus.** A well-maintained medial arch requires passive tension from the joint capsules and ligaments as well as dynamic stabilization from the intrinsic muscles of the foot. A fallen arch, or *pes planus*, describes a decrease in the medial arch and excessive pronation in the foot. This posture creates decreased ability to transmit force and excessive strain on the medial structures of the foot. Structures further up the kinetic chain, such as the knee, hip, and spine, are also affected. This posture is often associated with genu valgus posture of the knee and hip. **C. Abnormal posture, architecture, and contact pattern of the foot: pes cavus.** Rigidity in the ankle and foot can lead to excessive medial arch. A high arch, or pes cavus, describes this increase in the medial arch and excessive supination in the foot. This posture creates decreased ability to absorb shock and excessive strain on the lateral structures of the foot. Structures further up the kinetic chain, such as the knee, hip, and spine, are also affected. This posture is often associated with genu varus posture of the knee and hip.

MOVEMENTS AVAILABLE: ANKLE

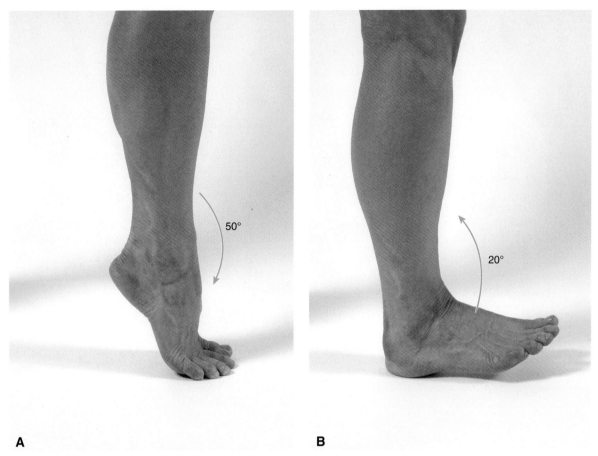

A   **B**

9-10 **A.** Ankle plantarflexion. **B.** Ankle dorsiflexion.

▶ MOVEMENTS AVAILABLE: FOOT

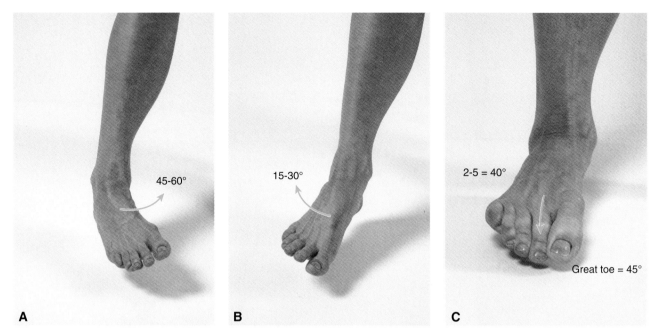

9-11 **A.** Foot inversion. **B.** Foot eversion. **C.** Toe flexion. *(continues)*

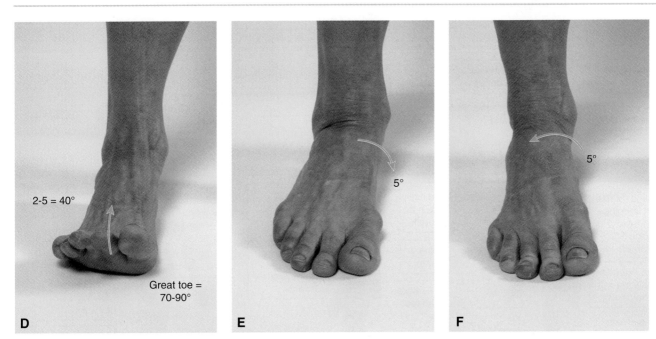

9-11 *(continued)* **D.** Toe extension. **E.** Foot pronation. **F.** Foot supination.

◗ GAIT

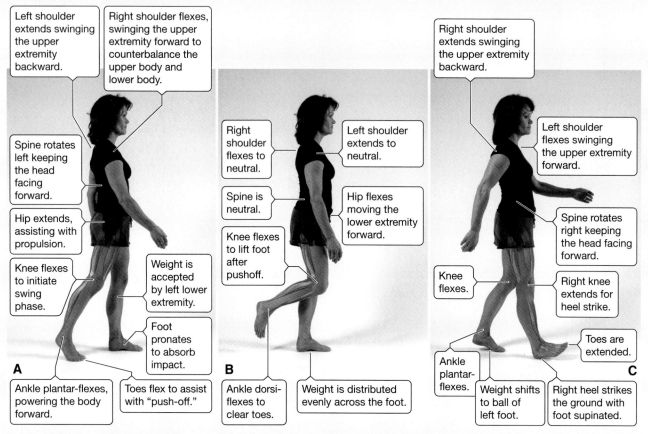

9-12. Gait. Human gait is very complex and requires movement in the lower extremity, pelvis, spine, and upper extremity. Weight is shifted between the right and left lower extremities as the spine rotates and arms swing to counterbalance the shifting weight. It is helpful to break the gait cycle into phases for evaluation: a *stance phase* where the weight of the body is accepted by the lower extremity and a *swing phase* where the non–weight bearing extremity is lifted and swung forward. These phases occur simultaneously with one extremity standing while the other swings. **A.** Stance phase: left. **B.** Swing phase: right. **C.** Double stance. *(continues)*

▶ GAIT

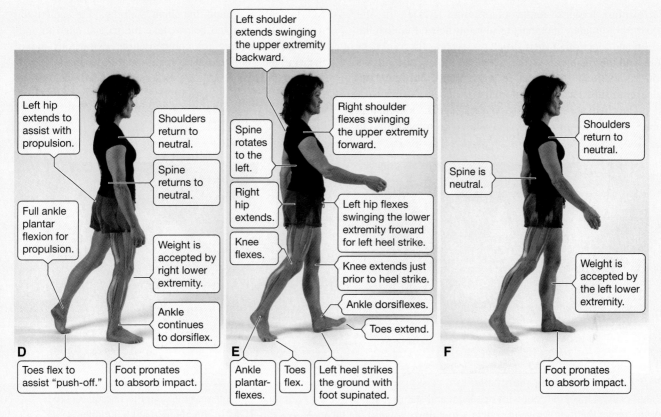

Left shoulder extends swinging the upper extremity backward.

Left hip extends to assist with propulsion.

Shoulders return to neutral.

Spine rotates to the left.

Right shoulder flexes swinging the upper extremity forward.

Spine returns to neutral.

Full ankle plantar flexion for propulsion.

Right hip extends.

Left hip flexes swinging the lower extremity froward for left heel strike.

Knee flexes.

Weight is accepted by right lower extremity.

Knee extends just prior to heel strike.

Ankle continues to dorsiflex.

Ankle dorsiflexes.

Toes extend.

Shoulders return to neutral.

Spine is neutral.

Weight is accepted by the left lower extremity.

D

E

F

Toes flex to assist "push-off."

Foot pronates to absorb impact.

Ankle plantar-flexes.

Toes flex.

Left heel strikes the ground with foot supinated.

Foot pronates to absorb impact.

9-12. Gait. *(continued)* **D.** Stance phase: right. **E.** Double stance. **F.** Stance phase: left.

▶ PASSIVE RANGE OF MOTION

Performing passive range of motion (ROM) in the talocrural, subtalar, and phalangeal joints helps establish the health and function of inert structures, such as the joint capsule, and the ligaments of the ankle and foot. It also allows you to evaluate the relative movements between the talocrural, subtalar, and distal joints.

The client should be lying on a massage or examination table. Ask the client to relax and allow you to perform the ROM exercises without the client "helping." For each of the movements illustrated below, take the foot through to endfeel while watching for compensation (extraneous movement) in the tibiofemoral or coxal joint. Procedures for performing passive ROM are described toward the end of Chapter 3.

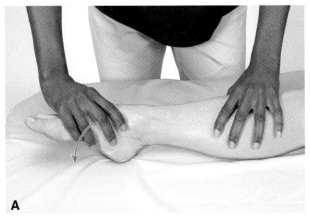
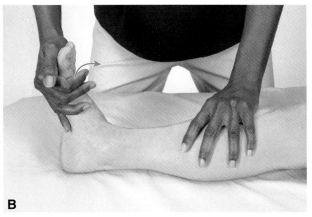

A

B

9-13 A. Passive ankle plantarflexion. The blue arrow indicates the direction of movement. Stand at the supine client's side. Grasp the foot with one hand and stabilize the lower leg with the other. Instruct the client to remain relaxed as you move the foot. Move the client's foot down toward the table. Assess the ROM of the anterior ankle ligaments, joint capsule, and muscles that dorsiflex the ankle the lower leg with the other. Instruct the client to remain relaxed as you move the foot. Move the client's foot up away from the table. Assess the ROM of the posterior ankle ligaments, joint capsule, and muscles that plantarflex the ankle. **B. Passive ankle dorsiflexion.** Stand at the supine client's side. Grasp the bottom of the foot with one hand and stabilize the lower leg with the other. Instruct the client to remain relaxed as you move the foot. Move the client's foot up away from the table. Assess the ROM of the posterior ankle ligaments, joint capsule, and muscles that plantarflex the ankle.

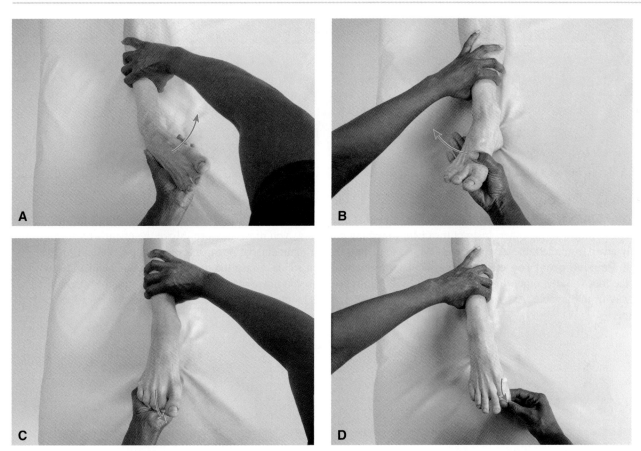

9-14 A. Passive foot inversion. Stand at the supine client's side. Grasp the foot with one hand and stabilize the lower leg with the other. Instruct the client to remain relaxed as you move the foot. Move the client's foot medially toward their other foot. Assess the ROM of the lateral ankle ligaments, joint capsule, and muscles that evert the foot.
B. Passive foot eversion. Stand at the supine client's side. Grasp the foot with one hand and stabilize the lower leg with the other. Instruct the client to remain relaxed as you move the foot. Move the client's foot laterally away from their other foot. Assess the ROM of the medial ankle ligaments, joint capsule, and muscles that invert the foot.
C. Passive toe flexion. Stand at the supine client's side. Grasp the toes with one hand and stabilize the foot with the other. Instruct the client to remain relaxed as you move the toes. Move the client's toes inferiorly toward the table. Assess the ROM of the dorsal digital ligaments, joint capsules, and muscles that extend the toes. **D. Passive great toe flexion.** Stand at the supine client's side. Grasp the great toe with one hand and stabilize the foot with the other. Instruct the client to remain relaxed as you move the toe. Move the client's toe inferiorly toward the table. Assess the ROM of the dorsal digital ligaments, joint capsules, and muscles that extend the great toe. *(continues)*

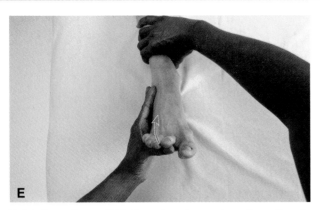

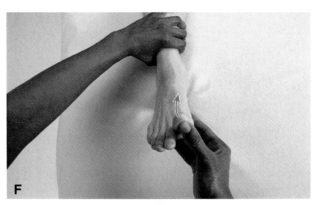

9-14 *(continued)* **E. Passive toe extension.** Stand at the supine client's side. Grasp the toes with one hand and stabilize the foot with the other. Instruct the client to remain relaxed as you move the toes. Move the client's toes superiorly away from the table. Assess the ROM of the plantar digital ligaments, joint capsules, and muscles that flex the toes. **F. Passive great toe extension.** Stand at the supine client's side. Grasp the great toe with one hand and stabilize the foot with the other. Instruct the client to remain relaxed as you move the toe. Move the client's toe superiorly away from the table. Assess the ROM of the plantar digital ligaments, joint capsules, and muscles that flex the great toe.

RESISTED RANGE OF MOTION

Performing resisted range of motion (ROM) helps establish the health and function of the dynamic stabilizers and prime movers in the ankle and foot. Evaluating functional strength and endurance helps you to identify balance and potential imbalance between the muscles that stabilize and steer the lower extremity. Procedures for performing and grading resisted ROM are outlined in Chapter 3.

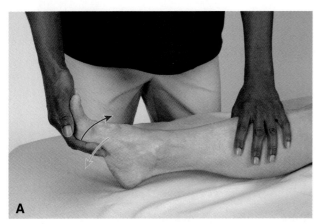 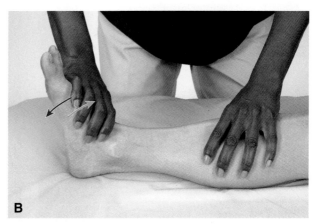

9-15 A. Resisted ankle plantarflexion. The green arrow indicates the direction of movement of the client and the red arrow indicates the direction of resistance from the practitioner. Stand facing your supine client. Place the palm of one hand on the bottom of the client's foot and the other on top of the lower leg to stabilize. Instruct the client to meet your resistance by pushing the foot down as you gently but firmly press the foot up. Assess the strength and endurance of the muscles that plantarflex the foot. B. Resisted ankle dorsiflexion. Stand facing your supine client. Place the palm of one hand on the top of the client's foot and the other on top of the lower leg to stabilize. Instruct the client to meet your resistance by pulling the foot up as you gently but firmly press the foot down. Assess the strength and endurance of the muscles that dorsiflex the foot.

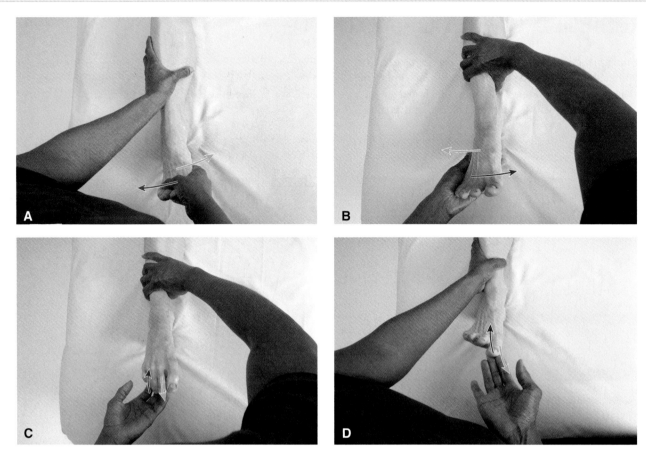

9-16 A. Resisted foot inversion. Stand facing your supine client. Place the palm of one hand on the inside of the client's foot and the other on top of the lower leg to stabilize. Instruct the client to meet your resistance by pulling the foot medially as you gently but firmly press the foot laterally. Assess the strength and endurance of the muscles that invert the foot. **B. Resisted foot eversion.** Stand facing your supine client. Place the palm of one hand on the outside of the client's foot and the other on top of the lower leg to stabilize. Instruct the client to meet your resistance by pushing the foot laterally as you gently but firmly press the foot medially. Assess the strength and endurance of the muscles that evert the foot. **C. Resisted toe flexion.** Stand facing your supine client. Place the fingertips of one hand on the bottom of the client's toes and the other on top of the lower leg to stabilize. Instruct the client to meet your resistance by pulling the toes down as you gently but firmly press the toes up. Assess the strength and endurance of the muscles that flex the toes. **D. Resisted great toe flexion.** Stand facing your supine client. Place the fingertips of one hand on the bottom of the client's great toe and the other on top of the lower leg to stabilize. Instruct the client to meet your resistance by pulling the toe down as you gently but firmly press the toe up. Assess the strength and endurance of the muscles that flex the great toe. *(continues)*

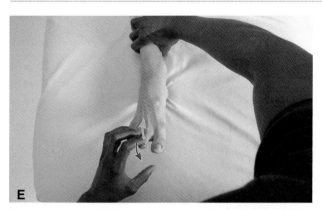

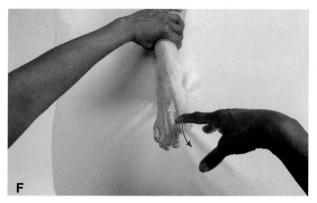

9-16 *(continued)* **E. Resisted toe extension.** Stand facing your supine client. Place the fingertips of one hand on the top of the client's toes and the other on top of the lower leg to stabilize. Instruct the client to meet your resistance by pulling the toes up as you gently but firmly press the toes down. Assess the strength and endurance of the muscles that extend the toes. **F. Resisted great toe extension.** Stand facing your supine client. Place the fingertips of one hand on the top of the client's great toe and the other on top of the lower leg to stabilize. Instruct the client to meet your resistance by pulling the toe up as you gently but firmly press the toe down. Assess the strength and endurance of the muscles that extend the great toe.

Tibialis Anterior
  tib e a'lis an *ter'e or* • Latin **"tibialis"** *of the tibia* **"anterior"** *front*

Attachments
O: Tibia, lateral condyle and proximal half and interosseous membrane

I: Medial cuneiform, plantar surface, and base of first metatarsal

Actions
- Dorsiflexes the ankle
- Inverts the foot

Innervation
- Deep peroneal nerve
- L4–S1

Functional Anatomy

Anterior tibialis is a large, superficial muscle on the front of the lower leg. Its function changes according to the position of the foot. If the foot is free, anterior tibialis raises the distal end of the foot up (dorsiflexion). This function keeps the toes from catching on the ground during the swing phase of gait. Maintaining this dorsiflexed position also allows the heel to strike the ground first, positioning for optimal shock absorption during the transition from heel strike to stance phase.

When the foot is fixed or planted, anterior tibialis pulls the lower leg over the foot (also called dorsiflexion). This function occurs during the stance phase of gait. Once heel strike has occurred, anterior tibialis continues to contract, pulling the center of gravity over and anterior to the foot. Overuse or weakness in this function creates irritation or tendonitis in this muscle. This is one of several causes of anterior lower leg pain, which is commonly called "shin splints."

Finally, anterior tibialis helps support the medial arch of the foot. Its tendon traverses the dorsal foot under the extensor retinaculum. Here it bends medially around the malleolus prior to attaching on the plantar surfaces of the medial cuneiform and base of the first metatarsal. This tendon angle gives anterior tibialis leverage to raise the center of the medial arch and limit or control pronation. It works synergistically with posterior tibialis to maintain the height of the arch and antagonistically with peroneus longus during pronation and supination of the foot.

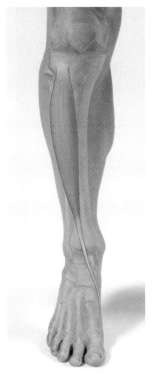

9-17

Palpating Tibialis Anterior

Positioning: client supine.

1. Standing at the client's feet, locate the lateral edge of the client's tibial shaft with the thumb of one hand.

2. Slide your thumb laterally onto the muscle belly of tibialis anterior.

3. Continue to palpate distally as the muscle converges to tendon toward the front of the ankle.

4. Client resists ankle dorsiflexion to ensure proper location.

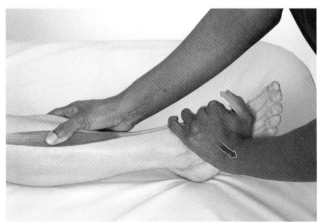

9-18

Extensor Digitorum Longus

eks ten′sor dij i to′rum long′gus • Latin
"**extensor**" *extender* "**digitorum**" *of the digits*
"**longus**" *long*

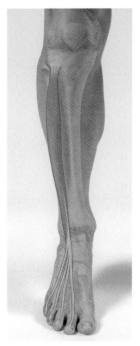

9-19

Palpating Extensor Digitorum Longus

Positioning: client supine.

1. Standing at the client's feet, locate the lateral edge of the tibia with the thumb of one hand.

2. Slide your thumb laterally past tibialis anterior and onto the muscle belly of extensor digitorum longus.

3. Continue to palpate distally as the muscle converges then branches to four tendons on the dorsal surface of the foot.

4. Client resists extension of toes 2–5 to ensure proper location.

Attachments

O: Tibia, lateral condyle, proximal anterior fibula, and interosseous membrane

I: Middle and distal phalanges 2–5, by four tendons to dorsal surfaces

Actions

• Extends the 2nd through 5th metatarsophalangeal and interphalangeal joints
• Dorsiflexes the ankle
• Everts the foot

Innervation

• Peroneal nerve
• L4–S1

Functional Anatomy

Extensor digitorum longus lies laterally to anterior tibialis. Its main function is to extend the four smaller toes. The muscle belly divides distally into four distinct tendons on the top of the foot before inserting on the middle and distal phalanges. Because it crosses all of the distal joints, it is able to extend the toes at the metacarpophalangeal and interphalangeal joints.

Extensor digitorum longus traverses the entire lower leg, giving it some leverage on the ankle. It assists tibialis anterior and extensor hallucis longus in dorsiflexing the ankle when the foot is free or fixed. Because it lies on the lateral side of the lower leg and foot, it is also able to assist the peroneals in everting the foot.

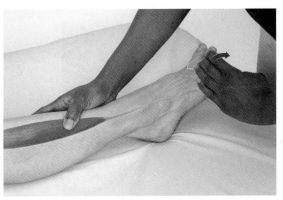

9-20

Extensor Hallucis Longus

eks ten'*sor* hal'*u* sis long'*gus* • Latin "**extensor**" *extender* "**hallux**" *great toe* "**longus**" *long*

Attachments

O: Fibula, middle of anterior surface and interosseous membrane
I: First distal phalanx, base on dorsal surface

Actions

* Extends first metarsophalangeal and interphalangeal joints
* Dorsiflexes the ankle
* Inverts the foot

Innervation

* Deep peroneal nerve
* L4–S1

Functional Anatomy

Extensor hallucis longus lies between anterior tibialis and extensor digitorum longus. It is deeper than the other two muscles, making it more difficult to palpate. Its main function is to extend the great toe. The muscle belly lies slightly laterally then converges to tendon under the extensor retinaculum. Here it must bend medially before inserting on the middle and distal phalanx of the great toe. Because it crosses all of the distal joints, it is able to extend the toe at the metacarpophalangeal and interphalangeal joints.

Extensor hallucis assists tibialis anterior and extensor digitorum longus in dorsiflexing the ankle when the foot is free or fixed. The bend in extensor hallucis longus at the extensor retinaculum provides leverage for inversion of the foot. Here it assists anterior tibialis, posterior tibialis, flexor digitorum longus, and flexor hallucis longus. The bend in the muscle also allows it to control pronation of the foot along with tibialis anterior and the deep posterior muscles.

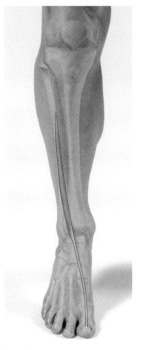

9-21

Palpating Extensor Hallucis Longus

Positioning: client supine.

1. Extensor hallucis longus lies deep between tibialis anterior and extensor digitorum longus. Standing at the client's feet, locate the distal musculotendinous junction of tibialis anterior with the thumb of one hand.

2. Slide your thumb slightly laterally onto the tendon of extensor hallucis longus.

3. Continue to palpate the tendon distally under the extensor retinaculum onto the dorsal surface of the big toe.

4. Client resists extension of the big toe to ensure proper location.

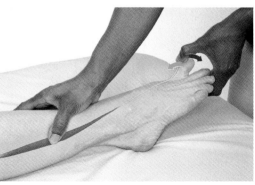

9-22

Peroneus Longus   *per o ne'yus lon'gus* • Greek **"perone"** *fibula* Latin **"longus"** *long*

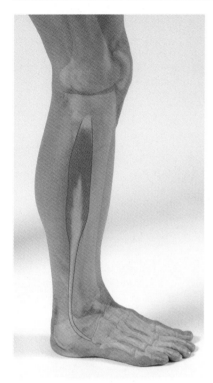

9-23

Palpating Peroneus Longus

Positioning: client supine.

1. Standing at the client's feet, locate the lateral surface of the head of the fibula with your thumb.

2. Palpate distally onto the muscle belly of peroneus longus.

3. Continue to palpate distally following the tendon as it converges with the other peroneals posterior to the lateral malleolus.

4. Client resists foot eversion to ensure proper location.

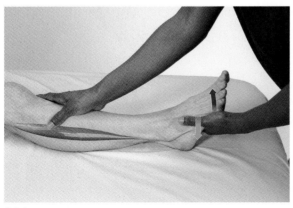

9-24

Attachments

O: Tibia, lateral condyle, head and lateral two-thirds of fibula
I: First metatarsal and medial cuneiform, lateral sides

Actions

• Plantarflexes the ankle
• Everts the foot

Innervation

• Superficial peroneal nerve
• L4–S1

Functional Anatomy

Peroneus longus is a long, pennate muscle located superficially on the lateral leg. Its tendon runs behind the lateral malleolus, extends across the bottom of the foot, and inserts near anterior tibialis. Together, peroneus longus and anterior tibialis form the "anatomical stirrup." These two continuous muscles are primary dynamic stabilizers of the transverse and medial arches of the foot. Both structures are integral in shock absorption at the foot and adaptation to uneven surfaces.

Peroneus longus works with peroneus brevis and peroneus tertius to evert the foot. This action is essential prior to planting the foot in order to achieve accurate position on the ground. It is also activated when moving the body laterally, in the frontal plane. Here the peroneus longus serves a similar function to anterior tibialis, pulling the center of gravity from medial to lateral over the foot. This type of side-stepping movement is common when walking over and around objects; for example, when hiking. It is also utilized in sports such as football, soccer, and basketball to initiate and control direction changes. Activities that require pushing from side to side, such as skiing and skating, rely on the peroneals to help power the movement.

Peroneus longus and peroneus brevis both insert on the plantar surface of the foot. Because of this, they contribute to plantarflexion of the ankle. Several large and small muscles work together to plantarflex the ankle during movements such as lifting, walking, running, and jumping.

Peroneus Brevis

per o ne'yus brev'is • Greek "**perone**" *fibula* Latin "**brevi**" *short*

Attachments

O: Fibula, distal two-thirds of lateral surface
I: Fifth metatarsal, lateral side of tuberosity at base

Actions

• Plantarflexes the ankle
• Everts the foot

Innervation

• Superficial peroneal nerve
• L4–S1

Functional Anatomy

Peroneus brevis is a short, pennate muscle located deep to the distal portion of peroneus longus on the lateral leg. Its tendon runs behind the lateral malleolus and inserts on the base of the fifth metatarsal. The tendons of peroneus longus and brevis are separated by the peroneal tubercle of the calcaneus. Peroneus brevis does not have the long tendon that peroneus longus has, giving it less leverage plantarflexing the foot.

Peroneus brevis primarily works with peroneus longus and peroneus tertius to evert the foot. This action is essential prior to planting the foot in order to achieve accurate position on the ground. It is also activated when moving the body laterally, in the frontal plane. Here the peroneals serve a similar function to anterior tibialis, pulling the center of gravity from medial to lateral over the foot. This type of side-stepping movement is common when walking over and around objects and in sports such as football, soccer, and basketball. The peroneals also help power activities, such as skiing and skating, that require pushing from side to side.

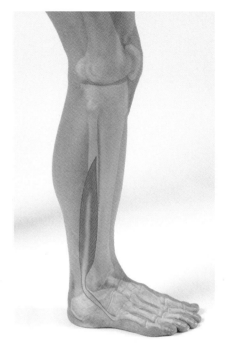

9-25

Palpating Peroneus Brevis

Positioning: client supine.

1. Peroneus brevis is deep to peroneus longus, making it difficult to distinguish. Standing at the client's feet, locate the posterior edge of the lateral malleolus with your thumb.

2. Slide your thumb posteriorly locating the tendons of peroneus brevis and peroneus longus.

3. Differentiate the tendon of peroneus brevis as the more anterior of the two and follow it to the tubercle of the fifth metarsal.

4. Client resists foot eversion to ensure proper location.

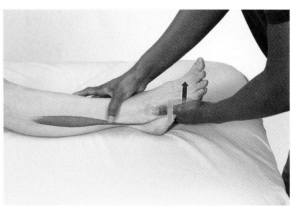

9-26

Peroneus Tertius • per *o ne'us ter'shus* • Greek "**perone**" *fibula* Latin "**terti**" *third*

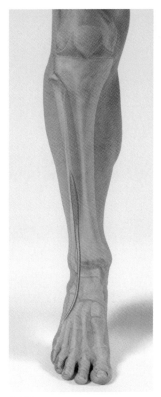

9-27

Palpating Peroneus Tertius

Positioning: client supine.

1. Standing at the client's feet, locate the medial edge of the lateral malleolus with your thumb.

2. Slide your thumb medially and superiorly onto the fibers of peroneus tertius.

3. Continue to palpate distally following the tendon under the extensor retinaculum onto the dorsal surface of the base of the fifth metatarsal.

4. Client resists foot eversion to ensure proper location.

Attachments

O: Fibula, distal one-third of anterior surface and interosseous membrane
I: Fifth metatarsal, dorsal surface of base

Actions

• Dorsiflexes the ankle
• Everts the foot

Innervation

• Deep peroneal nerve
• L4–S1

Functional Anatomy

Peroneus tertius is a short, pennate muscle located deep and anterior to peroneus longus and brevis. Its muscle belly lies between peroneus longus and extensor digitorum longus. The tendon of peroneus tertius runs in front of the lateral malleolus and inserts on the top of the base of the fifth metatarsal. This dorsal insertion makes it the only peroneal muscle that dorsiflexes the ankle.

Peroneus tertius primarily works with peroneus longus and peroneus brevis to evert the foot. This action is essential prior to planting the foot in order to achieve accurate position on the ground. It is also activated when moving the body laterally, in the frontal plane. Together, the peroneals pull the center of gravity from medial to lateral over the foot, achieving a type of side-stepping movement used in hiking, football, soccer, and basketball to initiate and control direction changes. The peroneals also help power activities that require pushing from side-to-side, such as skiing and skating.

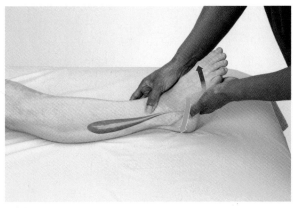

9-28

Gastrocnemius ● gas trok *ne'me us* • Greek "**gaster**" *belly* "**cnemi**" *leg*

Attachments

O: Medial head: femur, posterior medial condyle
O: Lateral head: femur, posterior lateral condyle
I: Calcaneous, posterior surface via the Achilles tendon

Actions

* Plantarflexes the ankle
* Flexes the knee

Innervation

* Tibial nerve
* S1–S2

Functional Anatomy

Gastrocnemius is the largest and most superficial of the three *triceps surae* (triceps 5 *three heads* and surae 5 *calf*) muscles. The plantaris and soleus are also part of this group, which converges into the achilles tendon and inserts on the posterior surface of the calcaneous.

Gastrocnemius is a very powerful two-headed muscle that dominates the back of the leg. Its two heads are easily located and followed inferiorly to the achilles tendon. Gastrocnemius contains mainly fast-twitch fibers, which are recruited rapidly but fatigue quickly. This fiber distribution is indicative of its role in generating explosive power during lifting, sprinting, and jumping.

Soleus is a synergist to gastrocnemius for plantarflexion. Which of these two muscles is most active during this movement is mainly driven by the position of the knee. If the knee is extending or extended (as when rising from a squatting or seated position or jumping), the gastrocnemius is more active. If the knee is flexed (as with relaxed walking or static standing), the soleus is more active.

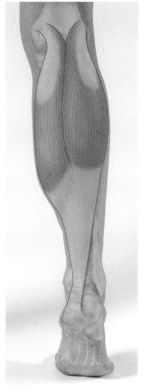

9-29

Palpating Gastrocnemius

Positioning: client prone.

1. Standing next to the client's lower leg, locate the bulk of muscle just distal to the popliteal fossa with your palm.

2. Slide your hand medially and laterally to differentiate the two large heads of gastrocnemius.

3. Continue to palpate distally as the gastrocnemius converges into the achilles tendon.

4. Client resists ankle plantarflexion to ensure proper location.

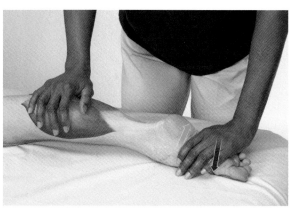

9-30

Soleus ● *so'le us* • Latin "**solum**" *bottom*

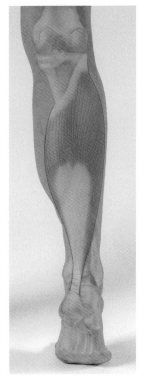

9-31

Palpating Soleus

Positioning: client prone with knee slightly flexed.

1. Standing next to the client's lower leg, locate the medial and lateral heads of gastrocnemius with your palm.

2. Slide your hand distally then grasp medial and lateral to gastrocnemius onto the edges of soleus.

3. Continue to palpate distally as soleus converges into the achilles tendon.

4. Client resists ankle plantarflexion to ensure proper location.

Attachments
O: Tibia, soleal line and posterior surface, posterior head and proximal surface of fibula
I: Calcaneous, posterior surface via the Achilles tendon

Actions
• Plantarflexes the ankle

Innervation
• Tibial nerve
• L5–S2

Functional Anatomy

Soleus is middle in size and location of the three *triceps surae* (triceps = *three heads* and surae = *calf*) muscles, which converge into the achilles tendon and insert on the posterior surface of the calcaneous. The plantaris and gastrocnemius are also part of this group.

Although a large muscle, soleus is composed of more slow-twitch than fast-twitch fibers. This fiber distribution is indicative of soleus' function as a fatigue-resistant postural muscle. Whereas gastrocnemius is recruited for explosive, powerful movements such as lifting, sprinting, and jumping, soleus drives less intense activities such as standing, walking, and jogging. Which muscle is most active is mainly driven by the position of the knee. If the knee is extending or extended (as when rising from a squatting or seated position or jumping), the gastrocnemius is more active. If the knee is flexed (as with relaxed walking or static standing), the soleus is more active.

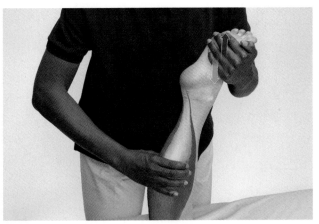

9-32

Plantaris • plan tar'is • Latin "**planta**" *sole of the foot*

Attachments

O: Femur, distal part of lateral supracondylar line
I: Calcaneous, posterior surface via the Achilles tendon

Actions

• Plantarflexes the ankle
• Flexes the knee

Innervation

• Tibial nerve
• L4–S1

Functional Anatomy

Plantaris is the deepest and smallest of the three *triceps surae* muscles. The triceps surae group is three calf muscles that converge into the achilles tendon (also called the calcaneus tendon) and insert on the posterior surface of the calcaneous. Soleus and gastrocnemius are also part of this group.

Plantaris is often compared to the palmaris longus found in the forearm because of its small muscle belly and long tendon. It is a direct synergist to gastrocnemius, but lacks the power of the larger muscle. Its small belly lies very near the medial head of gastrocnemius, and is often indistinguishable. The long tendon of plantaris is located deep in the posterior leg between the gastrocnemius and soleus. The function of plantaris is poorly understood, but it is believed to contribute to ankle plantarflexion and knee flexion during walking and running.

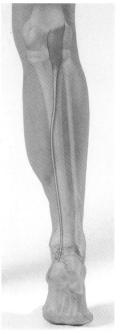

9-33

Palpating Plantaris

Positioning: client prone.

1. Standing next to the client's lower leg, locate the posterior surface of fibular head with your thumb.

2. Slide your thumb medially and distally between the two heads of gastrocnemius and onto the small belly of plantaris.

3. Continue to palpate plantaris before it dives between the heads of gastrocnemius. *(Caution: The popliteal fossa contains the popliteal artery and vein, the tibial nerve and common peroneal nerve, and lymph nodes. To avoid these structures, palpate the distal border of the fossa.)*

4. Client resists ankle plantarflexion to ensure proper location.

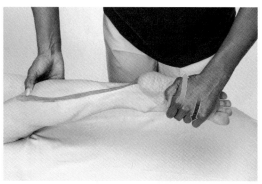

9-34

Tibialis Posterior   tib e a'lis po ster'e or • Latin "**tibialis**" *of the tibia* "**posterior**" *back*

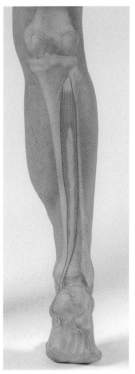

9-35

Palpating Tibialis Posterior

Positioning: client prone with flexed knee.

1. Standing next the client's lower leg, locate the medial edge of the tibia with your fingertips.

2. Slide your fingers posteriorly and hook around the edge of the tibia onto the fibers of posterior tibialis.

3. Continue to palpate the feathered fibers of posterior tibialis deep in the posterior leg between the tibia and fibula.

4. Client resists plantarflexion and inversion to ensure proper location.

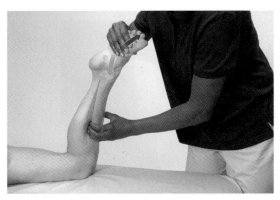

9-36

Attachments

O: Lateral, posterior tibia, proximal two-thirds of medial fibula, and interosseous membrane
I: Navicular tuberosity, cuneiforms 1–3, cuboid, and bases of metarsals 2–4

Actions

• Plantarflexes the ankle
• Inverts the foot

Innervation

• Tibial nerve
• L4–S1

Functional Anatomy

Posterior tibialis is the deepest muscle in the posterior leg. It is located deep to gastrocnemius and soleus, between flexor digitorum longus and flexor hallucis longus. Its tendon takes a sharp angle through a space between the posterior medial malleolus and calcaneus, called the tarsal tunnel, and onto the bottom of the foot. There, it inserts like a spiderweb onto eight separate bones. The other muscles of the tarsal tunnel include the flexor digitorum longus and flexor hallucis longus. (Hint: To remember this group, think of **T**om *tibialis posterior*, **D**ick *flexor digitorum longus*, and **H**arry *flexor hallucis longus*. You can also replace the "and" with **N** to remind yourself that the *posterior tibial nerve* also runs through the tunnel.)

Tibialis posterior runs medially and inserts on the bottom of the foot. This insertion enables it to invert the foot and plantarflex the ankle. More importantly, its broad insertion helps maintain the mechanical architecture of the medial arch and control pronation of the foot. Its influence on the arch is arguably greater than that of tibialis anterior, and some kinesiologists consider it to be the medial half of the "anatomical stirrup."

Tibialis posterior is most active during weight-bearing activities such as walking, running, and jumping. Maintaining proper strength and endurance in this and the other arch-supporting muscles is necessary to prevent a type of "shin splints" resulting from tendonitis of posterior tibialis. Such tendonitis is common, particularly in individuals with *pes planus* or an overpronated foot, which puts excessive strain on the muscle as it fires to maintain the medial arch.

Flexor Digitorum Longus

fleks′or dij i *to′rum* lon′*gus* • Latin "**flexor**" *bender* "**digitorum**" *of the digits* "**longus**" *long*

Attachments

O: Tibia, middle of posterior surface
I: Distal phalanges 2–5, by four tendons to base of plantar surfaces

Actions

- Flexes the second through fifth metatarsophalangeal and interphalangeal joints
- Plantarflexes the ankle
- Inverts the foot

Innervation

- Tibial nerve
- L5–S1

Functional Anatomy

Flexor digitorum longus lies deep to gastrocnemius and soleus and medial to posterior tibialis. It traverses the tarsal tunnel, along with posterior tibialis and flexor hallucis longus. These three muscles invert the foot and plantarflex the ankle. Flexor digitorum longus also flexes the smaller toes at the metacarpophalangeal and interphalangeal joints.

Flexor digitorum longus is one of several muscles that dynamically stabilize the medial arch of the foot. It is activated during weight-bearing activities such as walking, running, and jumping, and controls pronation of the foot. It also works with the foot's intrinsic muscles to make balance adjustments and conform the foot to whatever surface it contacts.

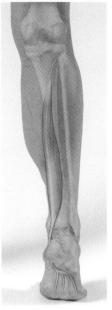

9-37

Palpating Flexor Digitorum Longus

Positioning: client prone.

1. Standing at the client's feet, locate the medial malleolus with your thumb.
2. Slide your thumb posteriorly and superiorly into the space between the tibial shaft and achilles tendon and onto flexor digitorum longus. *(Caution: The tibial artery and nerve also run posterior to the medial malleolus. Be sure to reposition your thumb if the client reports numbness or tingling, or you feel a pulse.)*
3. Continue to palpate proximally deep to the medial edge of soleus following flexor digitorum longus.
4. Client resists flexion of toes 2–5 to ensure proper location.

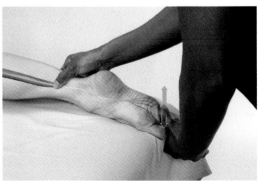

9-38

Flexor Hallucis Longus

fleks′ or hal′u sis long′gus • Latin "**flexor**" *bender* "**hallux**" *great toe* "**longus**" *long*

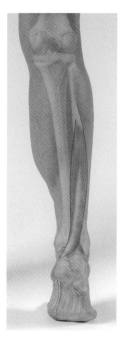

9-39

Palpating Flexor Hallucis Longus

Positioning: client prone.

1. Standing at the client's feet, locate the medial malleolus with your thumb.

2. Slide your thumb posteriorly and superiorly into the space between the malleolus and achilles tendon and onto the three tendons located there. *(Caution: The tibial artery and nerve also run posterior to the medial malleolus. Be sure to reposition your thumb if the client reports numbness or tingling, or you feel a pulse.)*

3. Continue to palpate the most posterior tendon, which is flexor hallucis longus.

4. Client resists flexion of the great toe to ensure proper location.

Attachments

O: Fibula, distal posterior surface and interosseous membrane

I: First distal phalanx, base on plantar surface

Actions

- Flexes the first metatarsophalangeal and interphalangeal joint
- Plantarflexes the ankle
- Inverts the foot

Innervation

- Tibial nerve
- L5–S2

Functional Anatomy

Flexor hallucis longus lies deep to gastrocnemius and soleus and lateral to posterior tibialis. Along with posterior tibialis and flexor digitorum longus, it traverses the tarsal tunnel to invert the foot and plantarflex the ankle. Flexor hallucis longus also flexes the great toe at the metacarpophalangeal and interphalangeal joint.

Flexor hallucis longus is one of several muscles that dynamically stabilize the medial arch of the foot. It controls pronation of the foot during weight-bearing activities such as walking, running, and jumping. It also works with the foot's intrinsic muscles to make balance adjustments and conform the foot to whatever surface it contacts.

Flexor hallucis longus is a primary muscle for "push off" during gait and propulsion of the body. The center of gravity shifts from the heel, across the foot, and onto the big toe at the end of the stance phase of gait. Forces generated by the hip, thigh, knee, and lower leg move through the foot and big toe, propelling the body forward. Flexor hallucis longus plays a significant role in directing those forces.

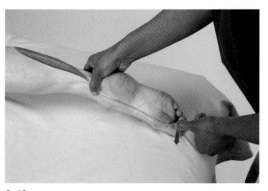

9-40

▶ TABLE 9-1. INTRINSIC MUSCLES OF THE FOOT

Muscle	Location	Action	Function
Extensor digitorum brevis	O: Lateral and dorsal calcaneus I: Dorsal aponeurosis of toes 2–4	Extends toes	Lifts toes 2–4 during gait. Assists with dorsiflexion
Extensor hallucis brevis	O: Dorsal calcaneus I: Base of first distal phalanx	Extends great toe	Lifts great toe during gait. Assists with dorsiflexion
Dorsal interossei	O: Adjacent sides of metatarsals I: Bases of proximal phalanges and dorsal digital expansions	Abducts toes	Adjust foot and toe position for balance.
Plantar interossei	O: Bases and medial sides of metatarsals 3–5 I: Medials sides of base of proximal phalanges 3–5	Adducts toes 3–5	Adjust foot and toe position for balance.

▶ TABLE 9-1. INTRINSIC MUSCLES OF THE FOOT *(continued)*

Muscle	Location	Action	Function
Lumbricals	O: Tendons of flexor digitorum longus I: Medially on the dorsal digital expansions of toes 2–5	Flexes the proximal phalanges	Adjust foot and toe position for balance.
Opponens digiti minimi	O: Dorsal surface of tubercle of 5th metatarsal I: Base of 5th proximal phalanx	Abducts fifth toe	Assists in supination of the foot.
Flexor digiti minimi	O: Base of 5th metatarsal and peroneus longus tendon sheath I: Proximal phalanx of 5th toes	Flexes small toe	Adjusts toe position for balance.
Adductor hallucis	O: Base of 2nd–4th metatarsals and peroneus longus tendon sheath (oblique head) O: Metatarsophalangeal ligaments 3–5 (transverse head) I: Base of first proximal phalanx and lateral sesamoid bone	Adducts great toe	Adjusts great toe position for balance and propulsion.

(continues)

▶ TABLE 9-1. INTRINSIC MUSCLES OF THE FOOT *(continued)*

Muscle	Location	Action	Function
Flexor hallucis brevis	O: Plantar surface of cuboid, lateral cuneiform, and tendon of tibialis posterior I: Sesamoid bones and medial and lateral sides of base of first proximal phalanx	Flexes great toe	Assists with balance and propulsion.
Abductor digiti minimi	O: Medial and lateral tuberosity of calcaneus and plantar aponeurosis I: Lateral side of 5th proximal phalanx	Abducts small toe	Adjusts toe position for balance.
Flexor digitorum brevis	O: Medial part of calcaneal tuberosity and plantar aponeurosis I: By individual tendons to the middle phalanges of toes 2–5	Flexes toes 2–5 at the proximal interphalangeal joint	Adjusts foot and toe position for balance.
Abductor hallucis	O: Medial part of calcaneal tuberosity I: Base of first proximal phalanx and medial sesamoid	Abducts great toe	Adjusts great toe position for balance and propulsion.

▶ SYNERGISTS/ANTAGONISTS: ANKLE AND FOOT

Motion		Muscles Involved	Motion		Muscles Involved
Plantarflexion	Ankle plantarflexion.	Gastrocnemius Soleus Plantaris Peroneus longus Peroneus brevis Tibialis posterior Flexor digitorum longus Flexor hallucis longus	Dorsiflexion	Ankle dorsiflexion.	Tibialis anterior Extensor digitorum longus Extensor hallucis longus Peroneus tertius
Inversion	Foot inversion.	Tibialis anterior Extensor hallucis longus Tibialis posterior Flexor digitorum longus Flexor hallucis longus	Eversion	Foot eversion.	Extensor digitorum longus Peroneus longus Peroneus brevis
Toe Flexion	Toe flexion.	Flexor digitorum longus (2–5) Flexor hallucis longus (1)	Toe Extension	Toe extension.	Extensor digitorum longus (2–5) Extensor hallucis longus (1)

❱ PUTTING IT IN MOTION

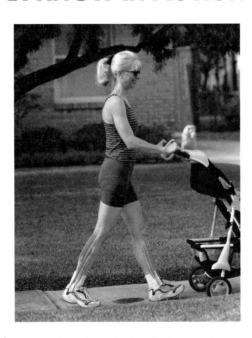

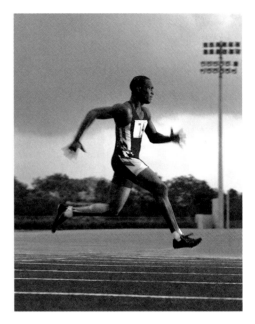

Walking. Coordinated weight-shifting from one leg to the other drives the walking pattern. The swinging leg moves through hip flexion, knee extension, ankle dorsiflexion, and toe extension. The stance leg drives the movement through hip extension, ankle plantarflexion, and toe flexion, especially with the big toe. Controlled pronation of the foot absorbs shock and accurately directs forces across the foot.

Running. Running requires greater force production than walking. The major difference between walking and running is the presence of a *flight phase*. There is a time in the running cycle when both feet are off the ground. This requires greater concentric forces to propel the body off the ground and eccentric forces to "catch" the body upon landing. The same muscles, hip extensors and ankle plantarflexors, drive the movement.

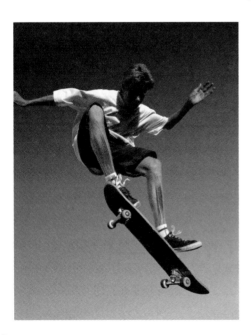

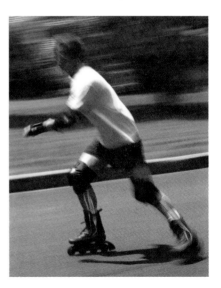

Skating. Skateboarding requires a variety of powerful and fine movements of the ankle and foot. The gastrocnemius and soleus create jumping motions necessary to propel the body and board into the air. The peroneals evert the foot and the anterior and posterior tibialis muscles invert the foot to guide the position of the board and control landings.

Blading. Rollerblading and skiing are frontal plane movements that rely heavily on the medial and lateral muscles of the lower leg. The peroneals drive the pushing motion (eversion) along with the hip abductors. The tibialis anterior, tibialis posterior, flexor digitorum longus, and flexor hallucis longus work with the intrinsic muscles of the foot to maintain foot position during this movement. The hip adductors are also heavily recruited during this side-to-side motion.

SUMMARY

- The tibia and fibula of the lower leg create the proximal and distal tibiofemoral joints. Both joints have very limited mobility, providing stability to the lower extremity.
- The ankle joint, or talocrural joint, allows only plantarflexion and dorsiflexion.
- The subtalar joint is more mobile and allows inversion and eversion of the foot.
- The foot is a complex network of bones, joints, and ligaments that allows several motions, including the surface-adapting and shock-absorbing motions pronation and supination.
- Several extrinsic muscles move the ankle and foot simultaneously while intrinsic muscles generate fine foot motions.
- Powerful movements of the ankle and foot are generated by large, superficial muscles, including the soleus and gastrocnemius.
- Gait is a complex movement pattern of the entire body, but is driven by the lower extremity.
- The muscles of the lower leg, ankle, and foot work together to create functional movements, such as walking, running, lifting, and skating.

FOR REVIEW

Multiple Choice

1. The bones that form the talocrural joint are:
   A. the femur, tibia, and fibula
   B. the tibia, fibula, and calcaneus
   C. the tibia, fibula, and talus
   D. the tibia, calcaneus, and talus

2. The bones that form the subtalar joint are:
   A. the tibia, fibula, and talus
   B. the talus and calcaneus
   C. the tibia and calcaneus
   D. the navicular and calcaneus

3. The movements allowed by the talocrural joint are:
   A. plantarflexion and dorsiflexion
   B. inversion and eversion
   C. pronation and supination
   D. all of the above

4. The movements allowed by the subtalar joint are:
   A. toe flexion and extension
   B. plantarflexion and dorsiflexion
   C. inversion and eversion
   D. both B and C are correct

5. A muscle that inserts on eight separate bones of the foot is:
   A. tibialis anterior
   B. tibialis posterior
   C. gastrocnemius
   D. flexor hallucis longus

6. Two muscles that cross the knee and the ankle are:
   A. gastrocnemius and soleus
   B. soleus and plantaris
   C. plantaris and gastrocnemius
   D. all of the above

7. A muscle that helps control pronation is:
   A. anterior tibialis
   B. posterior tibialis
   C. flexor digitorum longus
   D. all of the above

8. A posterior muscle that is considered "postural" is:
   A. gastrocnemius
   B. flexor digitorum longus
   C. soleus
   D. flexor hallucis longus

9. The muscles of the "triceps surae" are:
   A. plantaris, soleus, and gastrocnemius
   B. tibialis posterior, flexor digitorum longus, and flexor hallucis longus
   C. tibialis anterior, extensor digitorum longus, and extensor hallucis longus
   D. peroneus longus, brevis, and tertius

10. A muscle that pulls the lower leg over the foot during walking is:
    A. tibialis posterior
    B. soleus
    C. plantaris
    D. tibialis anterior

Matching

Different muscle attachments are listed below. Match the correct muscle with its attachment.

11. _____ Navicular tuberosity, cuneiforms 1–3, cuboid, and bases of metatarsals 2–4

12. _____ Tibia, lateral condyle, proximal anterior fibula, and interosseous membrane

13. _____ Tibia, soleal line and posterior surface, posterior head and proximal surface of fibula

14. _____ Distal phalanges 2–5, by four tendons to base of plantar surfaces

15. _____ Fibula, distal one-third of anterior surface and interosseous membrane

16. _____ Fibula, middle of anterior surface and interosseous membrane

17. _____ First metatarsal and medial cuneiform, lateral sides

18. _____ Medial cuneiform, plantar surface and base of first metatarsal

19. _____ Femur, distal part of lateral supracondylar line

20. _____ Fibula, distal posterior surface and interosseous membrane

A. Plantaris

B. Extensor hallucis longus

C. Tibialis posterior

D. Flexor hallucis longus

E. Peroneus longus

F. Tibialis anterior

G. Peroneus tertius

H. Soleus

I. Flexor digitorum longus

J. Extensor digitorum longus

Different muscle actions are listed below. Match the correct muscle with its action. Answers may be used more that once.

21. _____ Plantarflexion

22. _____ Dorsiflexion

23. _____ Inversion

24. _____ Eversion

25. _____ Toe flexion

26. _____ Great toe flexion

27. _____ Toe extension

28. _____ Great toe extension

A. Extensor digitorum longus

B. Peroneus brevis

C. Tibialis anterior

D. Flexor digitorum longus

E. Extensor hallucis longus

F. Soleus

G. Peroneus tertius

H. Flexor hallucis longus

I. Tibialis posterior

J. Peroneus longus

Short Answer

29. Describe the general structure of the lower leg, ankle, and foot and compare it to the forearm, wrist, and hand. Explain the differences.

30. Briefly describe the strength–balance relationship between the ankle plantarflexors and dorsiflexors. What is the purpose of this relationship?

31. Compare and contrast inversion and eversion and pronation and supination. How do these movements differ and what is their purpose?

Try This!

Activity: Find a partner and have him or her walk across the room or up and down a hall while you watch. Look at the movements of each lower extremity. Continue watching the hips, pelvis, and spine. Now look at their arm movement. Observe them from the front, back, and side. Take notes on what you are observing. What did you notice? Is the movement similar on the right and left? How is their range of motion? Do they move freely or stiffly? Can you identify the phases of their gait (swing phase and stance phase)? What muscles are making each part happen? What is happening at the foot, knee, hip, pelvis, spine, arms, and head?

Suggestions: Switch partners and repeat the activity. Share what you noticed with each other. Repeat the same process with running. It can be helpful to perform these activities on a treadmill if one is available.

SUGGESTED READINGS

Cote KP, Brunet ME II, Gansneder BM, et al. Effects of pronated and supinated foot postures on static and dynamic posture stability. *J Athl Train.* 2005;40(1):41–46.

Hanson AM, Padua DA, Blackburn JT, et al. Muscle activation during side-step cutting maneuvers in male and female soccer athletes. *J Athl Train.* 2008;43(2):133–143.

Hertel J. Functional anatomy, pathomechanics, and pathophysiology of lateral ankle instability. *J Athl Train.* 2002;37(4):364–375.

Hertel J, Gay MR, Denegar CR. Differences in postural control during single-leg stance among healthy individuals with different foot types. *J Athl Train.* 2002;37(2):129–132.

Richards J, Thewlis D, Selfe J, et al. A biomechanical investigation of a single-limb squat: implications for lower extremity rehabilitation exercises. *J Athl Train.* 2008;43(5):477–482.

Appendix
Answers to Chapter Review Questions

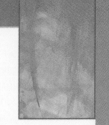

Chapter 1

1. D	15. B
2. C	16. F
3. B	17. I
4. B	18. D
5. C	19. G
6. C	20. C
7. A	21. B or E
8. D	22. A or D
9. D	23. C or F
10. B	24. B or E
11. E	25. B or E
12. A	26. C or F
13. H	27. B or E
14. J	28. A or D

29. Body standing upright, facing forward with feet together, arms at the sides, and palms facing forward.
30. Bones are firm and their shape remains constant upon palpation.
31. Muscles have a corrugated feel in a specific fiber direction and change shape as the body moves.
32. Regions:
    A. frontal
    B. sternal
    C. umbilical
    D. tibial
    E. crural
    F. antebrachial
    G. axillary
    H. mental

Chapter 2

1. B	11. F
2. C	12. C
3. A	13. H
4. D	14. D
5. C	15. A
6. B	16. J
7. A	17. G
8. C	18. I
9. B	19. B
10. C	20. E

21. *Functions of bone*
    A. Support and protection; serves as framework that supports all the soft tissues of the body and protects many critical organs.
    B. Movement; acts as rigid levers upon which muscles pull to produce movement.
    C. Hematopoiesis; blood-cell production occurs in the red bone marrow of bones.
    D. Storage of minerals and fats; phosphate and calcium form the "cement of bones and are stored for use in critical chemical functions." Fat is stored as yellow marrow in the center of mature long bones.

22. *Axial skeleton:* division of the skeleton comprised of the bones of the head and trunk, including the skull, mandible, hyoid, sternum, ribs, vertebrae, sacrum, and coccyx.
    Appendicular skeleton: division of the skeleton comprised of the bones of the shoulder girdle, upper limb, pelvic girdle, and lower limb. This includes the clavicle, scapula, humerus, radius, ulna, carpals, metacarpals, phalanges of the hand, ilium, ischium, pubis, femur, tibia, fibula, tarsals, metatarsals, and phalanges of the foot.

23. Bone shapes
    A. Long bone: longer than they are wide and have a shaft of diaphysis and ends called epiphyses
    B. Short bone: cube-shaped and composed mainly of spongy bone.
    C. Flat bone: thin, flattened, and tend to be curved. Location for hematopoiesis.
    D. Irregular bone: have unique shapes and do not fit into the other categories.
    E. Wormian bone: small, irregular bones that form areas of ossification outside of the usual cranial bone.

24. *Accessory motion:* movement of a joint's articulating surfaces relative to each other. Includes roll, spin, and glide.
    Physiological movements: gross movements of joints through the cardinal planes. Includes flexion, extension, abduction, adduction, and rotation.

25.

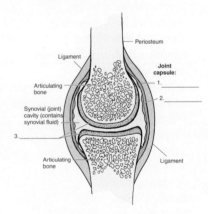

1. Osteocyte 2. Compact bone 3. Osteons 4. Periosteum 5. Volkmann canal 6. Haversian canal 7. Spongy bone

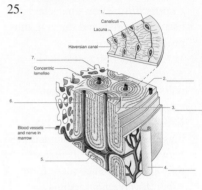

1. Fibrous capsule 2. Synovial membrane 3. Articular cartilage

Chapter 3

1. C	11. 1
2. D	12. 4
3. A	13. 2
4. A	14. 6
5. B	15. 3
6. D	16. 7
7. C	17. 10
8. B	18. 9
9. B	19. 5
10. D	20. 8

21. Motion, posture, protection, thermogenesis, vascular pump
22. *Extensibility:* allows muscle tissue to stretch without damage.
    Elasticity: allows muscle tissue to return to its original shape after lengthening or shortening.
    Excitability: muscle tissue can respond to electrical signals (from nerves).
    Conductivity: muscle tissue can propagate electrical signals (action potentials).
    Contractility: allows muscle tissue to shorten and thicken, thus producing force.
23. Force production factors
    Motor unit recruitment: more units recruited creates stronger contractions.
    Cross-sectional area: thicker muscles have greater interaction between myofilaments and are thus able to produce more force.
    Fiber arrangement: pennate muscles produce greater force than any other type.
    Muscle length: muscles generate maximal force when at resting length and this capacity diminishes if the muscle is shortened or stretched.
24. Intermediate fibers can produce energy aerobically or anaerobically, depending the type of training or activity that is most utilized by that muscle.
25. *Proprioception:* overall awareness of body position.
26. Muscle fiber
    A. Mitochondria
    B. Sarcomere
    C. Z line
    D. Sarcoplasmic reticulum
    E. Sarcolemma
    F. Transverse tubule
    G. Nucleus

Chapter 4

1. B		8. D	
2. D		9. B	
3. D		10. C	
4. A		11. C	
5. B		12. H	
6. A		13. E	
7. C		14. B	

15. A		23. E	
16. J		24. F	
17. I		25. C	
18. F		26. H	
19. G		27. G	
20. D		28. D	
21. J		29. A	
22. I		30. B	

31. *Scapulohumeral rhythm:* coordinated movement between the scapulothoracic and glenohumeral joints.
32. Both are ball-and-socket joints, but the glenohumeral joint has dramatically more mobility than the sternoclavicular joint.

Chapter 5

1. D		16. B	
2. A		17. F	
3. C		18. E	
4. C		19. A	
5. B		20. I	
6. C		21. F	
7. A		22. H	
8. D		23. C	
9. C		24. A	
10. B		25. I	
11. G		26. E	
12. J		27. G	
13. C		28. J	
14. D		29. D	
15. H		30. B	

31. The elbow flexes and extends due to movement of the hinging humeroulnar joint. The pivoting proximal and distal radioulnar joints allow pronation and supination of the forearm.
32. *Lateral epicondyle:* supinator, anconeus, extensor carpi radialis brevis, extensor carpi ulnaris, extensor digitorum, extensor digiti minimi
    Medial epicondyle: flexor carpi radialis, palmaris longus, flexor carpi ulnaris, flexor digitorum superficialis, pronator teres
33. The thumb is uniquely capable of *opposition* due to the presence of a saddle joint at the first carpometacarpal joint. This movement is not possible at any other joint of the hand.

Chapter 6

1. A		16. I	
2. C		17. J	
3. B		18. G	
4. D		19. F	
5. B		20. C	
6. A		21. A	
7. B		22. C or J	
8. C		23. G	
9. D		24. D	
10. D		25. I	
11. D		26. F	
12. H		27. H	
13. B		28. E	
14. E		29. B or F	
15. A		30. B or F	

31. The atlas and axis have different shapes and features than the rest of the cervical vertebrae. Together, they form a pivot joint that enhances the rotational movement of the head and neck.
32. The spinal cord traverses the vertebral foramen with spinal nerves threading through the lateral grooves between the transverse processes. The vertebral arteries and veins traverse the transverse foramen. Proper alignment between the skull and cervicalvertebrae is important for maintaining circulation and avoiding nerve compression in this region.
33. *Muscles that rotate head and neck to the same side:* longus colli, longus capitis, splenius capitis, splenius cervicis, rectus capitis posterior major, obliquus capitis inferior, rectus capitis anterior, levator scapula
    Muscles that rotate head and neck to the opposite side: sternocleidomastoid, scalenes, semispinalis, trapezius, rotatores, multifidi, semispinalis

Chapter 7

1. B		7. D	
2. C		8. A	
3. A		9. D	
4. D		10. B	
5. B		11. C	
6. C		12. J	

13. H 22. D
14. D 23. A
15. F 24. G
16. A 25. F
17. I 26. H
18. B 27. G
19. D 28. E
20. E 29. C
21. F 30. B

31. Both the thoracic and lumbar vertebrae have a body, transverse processes, a spinous process, and a vertebral foramen. The spinous processes of the thoracic vertebrae are flattened compared to the lumbar vertebrae. This is due to the kyphotic curve in the thoracic spine, which would be uncomfortable when lying supine and vulnerable to injury. The thoracic vertebrae also contain unique articulations for the ribs. The bodies of the lumbar vertebrae are much larger as they bare more of the body's weight than the vertebrae in thoracic spine.

32. The ribcage is made up anteriorly of the sternum while the ribs wrap from anterior to posterior, surrounding the internal organs. Posteriorly, the ribs attach to the thoracic vertebrae. True ribs attach directly to the sternum while false ribs attach via costocartilage and floating ribs have no anterior attachments. The costocartilage between the sternum and anterior ribs allows the ribcage to expand and contract as muscles pull on its surfaces, creating the movement of breathing.

33. Longissimus, spinalis, and quadratus lumbor are larger muscles that create movement. Semispinalis, rotatores, multifidi, interspinalis, and intertransversarii are small, deep muscles that stabilize the vertebrae. The diaphragm, serratus posterior superior, serratus posterior inferior, and levator costarum all contribute to inhalation for breathing.

Chapter 8

1. C   16. A
2. A   17. C
3. B   18. D
4. C   19. B
5. A   20. G
6. D   21. B
7. C   22. G
8. B   23. A
9. C   24. D
10. D 25. E
11. E 26. F
12. H 27. H
13. I 28. I
14. J 29. C
15. F 30. F

31. The pelvic girdle is formed by three fused bones: the ilium, ischium and pubis, and the sacrum. The pubic symphysis is a slightly moveable, cartilaginous joint and the two sacroiliac joints are very stable synovial joints. Slight movement is available at the pelvic girdle, which helps distribute forces in the lower extremities and absorb shock. Compared to the shoulder girdle, the pelvic girdle is much more stable and the bones are larger and more dense. This is due to the greater amount of bodyweight supported by the pelvic girdle.

    The coxal joint, like the glenohumeral joint, is a ball-and-socket synovial joint. It is triaxial, but has much less movement compared to the glenohumeral joint. This is due to the deeper socket formed by the acetabulum and strong ligaments that support the coxal joint.

32. The muscles of the quadriceps attach to the patella from the medial and lateral sides. If one of these muscles is stronger or less flexible than the others it will pull the patella towards its origin. This will alter the position of the patella in the femoral groove, causing dysfunction with the patellofemoral joint.

33. When the lower extremity plants and pivots, coordinated motions

between the subtalar, talocrural, tibiofemoral, and coxal joints must occur. Pivoting involves pronation or supination of the foot, rotation of the knee, and rotation of the hip. Sports such as tennis, racketball, basketball, volleyball, soccer, football, fielding and base running in baseball and softball, hockey, and lacross all require pivoting actions of the lower extremity.

Chapter 9

1. C   15. G
2. B   16. J
3. A   17. E
4. C   18. F
5. B   19. A
6. C   20. D
7. D   21. F
8. C   22. C
9. A   23. I
10. D 24. B,G,J
11. C   25. A
12. B   26. H
13. H 27. D
14. I   28. E

29. Both the forearm and low leg have two long bones joined by an interosseous membrane. The two joints of the forearm are able to rotate, while the low leg is more stable and has little or no movement in its proximal and distal articulations.

30. The plantarflexors are much stronger than the dorsiflexors. This is because the talocrural joint is a second class lever designed for forward propulsion.

31. Inversion and eversion occur at the subtalar joint while pronation and supination are complex movements of several ankle and foot joints. Pronation and supination occur when the foot is planted on the ground and these movements transmit forces along the length of the foot. Inversion and eversion are motions that position the foot when it is not planted on the ground.

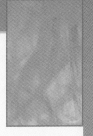

Abduction: joint movement occurring on the frontal plane around a sagittal axis that results in movement away from the midline.

Accessory motion: movement of a joint's articulating surfaces relative to each other.

Acetylcholine: neurotransmitter that crosses the synaptic cleft to propagate action potentials at the neuromuscular junction.

Action potential: change in cell membrane charge occurring in nerve, muscle, and other excitable tissue when excitation occurs.

Active range of motion: joint motion where a person moves a given body part through its possible motions independently, demonstrating their willingness and ability to voluntarily perform available motions at that joint.

Adduction: joint movement occurring on the frontal plane around a sagittal axis that results in movement towards the midline.

Adenosine triphosphate (ATP): compound that stores energy in cells.

Adipocytes: fat cells that store oil within their internal space.

Aerobic: utilizing oxygen for energy production. Also called *oxidative*.

Afferent fibers: sensory nerves that surround the intrafusal fibers of a muscle spindle and monitor the rate and magnitude of stretch within the muscle.

Afferent lymphatic vessel: structure that funnels lymph into a lymph node.

Agonist: muscle most involved in creating a movement.

Alpha motor neurons: motor nerves within a muscle spindle that prompt surrounding extrafusal fibers to contract and shorten the muscle, protecting it from harm.

Amphiarthrotic joint: joint surrounded by a pliable structure such as ligament or fibrocartilage.

Anaerobic: producing energy without oxygen.

Antagonist: muscle that performs the opposite action or actions to its agonist.

Anatomical terminology: universal system of communication to describe the human body regions and movements.

Anatomical position: reference body position characterized by the body erect and facing forward, feet parallel, arms extended at the sides, and palms facing forward.

Anatomy: the study of an organism's structures.

Anterior: regional term indicating toward the front.

Anterior pelvic tilt: postural deviation characterized by forward tipping of the pelvic girdle.

Appendicular skeleton: division of the skeleton comprised of the bones of the shoulder girdle, upper limb, pelvic girdle, and lower limb.

Approximation: limiting factor of joint movement being the body running into itself.

Aponeurosis: broad, flat tendon.

Arthrology: the study of joints.

Axial skeleton: division of skeleton comprised of the bones of the head and trunk, including the skull and associated bones, hyoid, sternum, ribs, vertebrae, sacrum, and coccyx.

Axis: part of a lever system that the lever itself turns around. Also called *fulcrum.*

Axon: lengthy extension of a nerve cell that receives impulses from the cell body and sends it down its length to a neighboring cell.

Ball-and-socket joint: synovial joint characterized by a spherical head on one bone fitting into a rounded cavity on another.

Biaxial: able to move in two planes of motion.

Bipennate: pennate muscle with fibers running obliquely along both sides of a central tendon.

Blood vessel: circulatory structure that is a pathway by which blood flows throughout the body.

Bone: type of supporting connective tissue made up of collagen fibers and minerals that form the skeleton.

Bony endfeel: limiting factor of joint movement being the contact of two bones.

Bony landmark: unique feature on a bone that identifies soft tissue attachments, articulating surfaces, channels, or other function.

Bursa: small, flattened sacs of synovial fluid that decrease friction between structures.

Bursitis: inflammation of a bursa resulting from trauma or excessive friction.

Calcium: mineral that is stored in bones, making up their cement along with phosphate. It is utilized in several chemical processes in the body, including maintaining the acid–base balance of the blood, transmitting nerve impulses, assisting in muscle contractions, maintaining blood pressure, and initiating blood clotting following injury.

Canaliculi: tiny canals that radiate from the central Haversian canals and bring microscopic blood vessels and nerve branches to outlying osteocytes.

Capsular endfeel: limiting factor of joint movement being the joint capsule.

Cardiac muscle: involuntary muscle that makes up the heart wall and creates the pulsing action necessary to circulate blood through the body.

Cartilage: a type of supporting connective tissue that varies in consistency and function by the proportion of proteins distributed through its matrix.

Cartilaginous joints: slightly moveable joints with cartilage separating the articular surfaces of adjacent bones.

Caudal: regional term indicating toward the feet.

Cell body: functional center of a neuron where the nucleus resides.

Cephalic: regional term indicating toward the head.

Chondroblasts: fibroblasts that secrete the proteins that make up the fibers in the extracellular matrix of cartilage.

Circular muscles: muscles with fiber arrangements surrounding an opening to form a sphincter.

Collagen fibers: long, straight strands of protein that give connective tissue tensile strength and flexibility.

Compact bone: dense portion of bone made up of concentric lamellar osteons and interstitial lamellae.

Concave: rounded inward.

Concentric contraction: isotonic muscle contraction where tension is generated, the muscle shortens, and joint angle decreases.

Condyle: rounded end of a bone that forms a joint.

Conductivity: ability to propagate electrical signals.

Connective tissue: one of the four basic types of tissue that is most abundance and found in most structures of human movement, including bone, ligament, tendon, and fascia.

Contractility: ability to shorten and thicken-thus producing force- in response to a specific stimulus.

Convex: rounded outward.

Convex–concave rule: rule that governs the direction of accessory motions roll and glide and states that the shape of the joint surface will determine movement: glide will occur in the same direction as rolling when a concave surface is moving on a fixed convex surface and gliding and rolling will occur in opposite directions if a convex surface is moving on a fixed concave surface.

Crest: long, narrow soft-tissue attachment site on a bone.

Cross-bridges: connections between myosin heads and active receptor sites on the actin filament during muscle contraction.

Deep: regional term indicating further from the surface of the body.

Deep fascia: network of dense connective tissue that forms a network around the muscles and their internal structures.

Deform: change shape.

Dendrite: short branches of a nerve cell that transmit impulses to the cell body.

Dense connective tissue: connective tissue containing many collagen fibers and little ground substance.

Depressions: basins and channels in bone that house muscles, tendons, nerves, and vessels.

Dermis: mostly dense connective tissue layer found deep to the epidermis and containing hair follicles, glands, nerves, blood vessels, and tiny muscles.

Diaphysis: shaft of a long bone made up of compact bone with yellow bone marrow filling the center.

Diarthrotic joint: joint characterized by large joint cavity.

Direct synergist: muscle that has all of its actions in common with its agonist.

Dislocation: displacement of normal bone formation at a joint.

Distal: regional term indicating away from the trunk.

Dynamic stabilizer: structures that limit or control movement by contracting and stretching.

Eccentric contraction: isotonic muscle contraction where tension is generated, the muscle lengthens, and the joint angle increases.

Edema: abnormal accumulation of fluid in the body's tissues.

Efferent lymphatic vessel: structure that funnels lymph out of a lymph node.

Elastic fibers: component of connective tissue that contains elastin and gives tissue resiliency, allowing it to return to its original shape.

Elastic cartilage: self-supporting cartilage with the highest proportion of elastic fibers found in the nose and ears.

Elasticity: ability to return to original shape after lengthening or shortening.

Elastin: protein found in elastic fibers that gives tissues a branched, wavy appearance and allow them to return to their original shape following stretching or deformation.

Ellipsoid joint: synovial joint characterized by oval-shaped joint surfaces that resemble flattened circles or ellipses.

Empty endfeel: abnormal endfeel characterized by abnormal motion allowed where a ligament or joint capsule should prevent it. Also called *loose endfeel.*

Endfeel: the perceived quality of movement at the end of a joint's available range of motion, determined using passive range of motion.

Endomysium: sheath of connective tissue that surrounds individual muscle cells.

Epicondyle: projection on a long bone near the articular end, above the condyle.

Epidermis: layer or epithelial tissue on the surface of the skin containing keratin, melanin, and immune cells.

Epimysium: sheath of connective tissue that surrounds bundles of muscle fascicles.

Epiphyseal plate: region where the epiphysis of a long bone meets the diaphysis. Also called a *growth plate.*

Epiphysis: bumpy end of a long bone that is composed of spongy bone surrounded by a thin layer of compact bone.

Epithelial tissue: one of the four basic types of tissue that covers the body's internal and external surfaces. It protects, absorbs, filters, and secretes substances in the body and regenerates easily.

Excitability: able to respond to a stimulus by producing electrical signals. Also called *irritability*.

Extensibility: ability to stretch without sustaining damage.

Extension: joint movement occurring on the sagittal plane around a frontal axis that results in an increase in joint angle.

External rotation: joint movement of the appendicular skeleton on the transverse plane around a longitudinal axis that turns away from the midline. Also known as *lateral rotation*.

Extracellular matrix: connective tissue component made up of various fibers suspended in ground substance.

Extrafusal fibers: muscle fibers within a muscle spindle that contract and shorten in response to stimulation by the alpha motor neurons.

Facet: flat projection of bone that forms a joint.

Fascia: thin membrane of loose or dense connective tissue that covers the structures of the body, protecting them and binding them into a structural unit.

Fascicle: bundle of muscle fibers surrounded by perimysium.

Fiber direction: alignment of muscle tissue that determines the direction of pull when the tissue contracts.

Fibroblast: cells that produce and secrete the proteins that make up the fibers in the extracellular matrix of connective tissue.

Fibrous capsule: outer portion of a synovial joint capsule that provides stability and protection for the joint.

Fibrous cartilage: cartilage made of a dense network of collagen fibers that cushions and enhances joint continuity found in the vertebral disks and meniscus of the knee.

Fibrous joints: stable union between bones with minimal joint cavity and collagen-dense connective tissue holding the bones tightly together.

First-class lever: mechanical system characterized by a central axis with the force on one side and the resistance on the other.

Fissure: a cleft somewhat like an enlarged crack or slit in a bone.

Flaccidity: decreased muscle tone.

Flat bones: type of bone that is thin, formed by ossification of a fibrous network, and includes the sternum, ilium, and several cranial bones. The spongy bone at the center of these is where hematopoiesis occurs.

Flexion: joint movement occurring on the sagittal plane around a frontal axis that results in a decrease in joint angle.

Flight phase: phase of running gait when neither foot is in contact with the ground.

Fluid connective tissue: connective tissue that contains plasma in the extracellular matrix.

Foramen: a small to large, usually circular opening in a bone.

Force: source of mechanical energy in a lever system that initiates motion.

Frontal axis: imaginary line that intersects the sagittal plane at a right angle around which flexion and extension occurs.

Frontal plane: plane of movement that divides the body vertically into anterior and posterior halves.

Fulcrum: part of a lever system that the lever itself turns around. Also called *axis*.

Fusiform muscles: muscles with fiber arrangements having a thick central belly and tapered ends.

Gait: manner of walking or running.

Gamma motor neurons: motor nerves that adjust the tension of muscle spindles to maintain their length-monitoring function.

Genu valgus: postural deviation characterized by lateral deviation of the leg in relationship to the thigh.

Genu varum: postural deviation characterized by medial deviation of the leg in relationship to the thigh.

Glandular epithelium: tissue that produces and delivers substances to the external or internal surfaces of the body or directly into the bloodstream.

Glide: accessory motion that occurs when a point on one bony surface comes in contact with a series of points on another.

Gliding joint: synovial joint characterized by flat articulating surfaces that allow small, planar movements.

Glycolysis: anaerobic energy production where glucose is converted to lactic acid.

Golgi tendon organ: proprioceptor woven into the connective tissue present in tendons that monitors changes in muscle tension generated by stretching or muscle contraction.

Gomphosis: specific fibrous joints at which teeth fit into sockets in the jaw.

Ground substance: unique fluid component of connective tissue that suspends the extracellular matrix and exists as either watery liquid or firm solid.

Growth plate: *see epiphyseal plate*

Guarding: sudden, involuntary muscle contraction characterized by jerky or shaky movements. Also called *muscle spasm*.

Heel strike: foot contact of lead foot on the ground during gait.

Haversian canals: longitudinal canals that allow blood vessels and nerves to traverse compact bone.

Head: large, round projection at the end of a long bone that forms a joint.

Hematopoiesis: process of blood cell formation that occurs in red bone marrow.

Hinge joint: synovial joint characterized by a cylindrical prominence on one bone that fits into a corresponding depression on another.

Hyaline cartilage: smooth, rubbery cartilage that helps reduce friction and is found in the voice box, between the ribs and sternum, and the articulating surfaces of bones.

Hypertonicity: excessive muscle tone.

Hypodermis: loose connective tissue layer found deep to the dermis of skin containing adipose cells that that cushion and protect underlying structures. See *superficial fascia*.

Inferior: regional term indicating toward the bottom.

Intermediate fibers: muscle fibers that have characteristics of both slow twitch and fast twitch fibers.

Internal rotation: joint movement of the appendicular skeleton on the transverse plane around a longitudinal axis that turns towards the midline. Also known as *medial rotation*.

Interstitial space: space between tissue cells.

Interosseous membrane: broad sheet of dense connective tissue that is thinner than ligaments and connects bones along the length of their shafts.

Intrafusal fibers: specialized muscle fibers within a muscle spindle that are surrounded by a coil of sensory nerve endings that monitor the rate and magnitude of stretch within the muscle.

Inverse myotatic reflex: relaxation of a muscle and contraction of its antagonist in response to excessive muscle tension, due to stimulation of the Golgi tendon organ.

Involuntary: not under conscious control.

Irregular bones: uniquely shaped bones, including the vertebrae and facial bones.

Irritability: able to respond to a stimulus by producing electrical signals. Also called *excitability*.

Isometric contraction: muscle contraction where tension is generated, but muscle length and joint angle do not change.

Isotonic contraction: muscle contraction where tension is generated and the muscle length and joint angle changes.

Joint: place of union between bones.

Joint capsule: network of dense connective tissue that wraps around an entire joint.

Joint cavity: space between articulating surfaces of bones.

Joint play: the amount of slack or "give" in the joint capsule and ligaments that surround a joint.

Keratin: tough, protective protein found in the epidermis of skin.

Kinesiology: the study of human movement.

Kyphosis: posterior curvature of the spine.

Lacunae: tiny cavities within the bone matrix that house osteocytes.

Lamellae: concentric circles of lacunae wrapped around central Haversian canals.

Lateral: regional term indicating away from the midline.

Left rotation: joint movement of the spine on the transverse plane around a longitudinal axis that turns the spine to the left.

Lever: rigid device that transmits or modifies forces to create movement.

Leverage: amount of force increase produced by a mechanical system. Also called *mechanical advantage*.

Ligament: fibrous structure made of dense connective tissue that connects bones to each other.

Line: long, narrow soft tissue attachment site on a bone.

Long bones: type of bone that is longer than it is wide and characterized by a distinct shaft and bumpy ends.

Longitudinal axis: imaginary line that intersects the transverse plane at a right angle around which rotation occurs.

Loose connective tissue: connective tissue that contains high levels of ground substance and few fibers.

Loose endfeel: abnormal endfeel characterized by abnormal motion allowed where a ligament or joint capsule should prevent it. Also called *empty endfeel*.

Lordosis: anterior curvature of the spine.

Lymph: excess fluid in the body's tissues.

Lymph node: tiny organ that cleanses lymph of foreign particles, viruses, and bacteria.

Macrophages: immune cells that respond to injury or infection.

Meatus: a tiny passageway in bone.

Mechanical advantage: amount of force increase produced by a lever. Also called *leverage*.

Mechanoreceptor: specialized nerve ending that deforms in response to pressure and assists with proprioception.

Medial: regional term indicating toward the midline.

Medullary cavity: central cavity of a long bone diaphysis that contains bone marrow.

Melanin: pigment protein found in the epidermis of skin.

Mitochondrion: principle energy source of a cell, which produces adenosine triphosphate (ATP).

Motor nerve: action-oriented nerves that carry out responses determined by the brain.

Motor neuron: neurons responsible for initiating motion.

Motor unit: a motor neuron and all of the muscle fibers it controls.

Multipennate: pennate muscle with fibers running on both sides of multiple tendons.

Muscle belly: portion of a muscle between its tendons.

Muscle spasm: sudden, involuntary muscle contraction characterized by jerky or shaky movements. Also called *guarding*.

Muscle spindle: proprioceptor distributed throughout skeletal muscle tissue that monitors changes in tissue length.

Muscle tissue: one of four basic types of tissue that contains contractile protein structures called myofibrils that allow this type of tissue to contract and generate movement.

Muscle tone: tension generated from continual motor unit activation.

Musculotendinous junction: location where the epimysium of a muscle begins to converge and form a tendon.

Myofibrils: specialized contractile proteins that make skeletal muscle tissue appear striated.

Myology: the study of muscles.

Myosin: protein that forms the thick filaments in muscle.

Myotatic reflex: contraction of muscles in response to a rapid stretching force, due to stimulation of the muscle spindle.

Nerve: part of the nervous system that controls and communicates with the rest of the body.

Nervous tissue: one of four basic types of tissue that is able to be stimulated, conduct a stimulus, and respond to stimulation.

Neuromuscular junction: connection between the axon of a nerve cell and a muscle cell.

Neuron: nerve cell.

Neurotransmitter: specialized chemical that crosses the synaptic cleft and stimulates or inhibits adjacent cells.

Nucleus: portion of a cell that contains its functional information and controls its operations.

Openings: holes and channels in bone that allow passage of nerves, vessels, muscles, and tendons. They also create air-filled cavities called *sinuses.*

Osseous tissue: see *bone*

Ossification: process where hyaline cartilage is replaced by bone tissue produced by osteoblasts.

Osteoarthritis: chronic inflammation of joint resulting from damage to the hyaline cartilage.

Osteoblasts: fibroblasts that secrete the proteins that make up the fibers in the extracellular matrix of bone.

Osteoclast: bone cells that break down old bone.

Osteocyte: bone cell.

Osteology: the study of bones.

Osteon: functional unit of bone comprised of the lamellae and Haversian canals. Also called a *Haversian system.*

Osteoporosis: pathology that results from depletion of bone minerals such as calcium and phosphate characterized by porous bone with decreased density.

Pacinian corpuscle: mechanoreceptor located within skin, connective tissue around muscles, and tendons that detect the initial application of vibration or deep pressure to monitor direction and speed of body movement.

Panniculus: flat, continuous sheet of muscle.

Passive range of motion: joint motion that occurs when the client is resting and the therapist moves a joint through its possible motions, used to determine joint endfeel.

Pennate: feather-shaped.

Perimysium: connective tissue sheath that surrounds muscle fascicles.

Periosteum: dense connective tissue that surrounds bone, nourishing and protecting it.

Pes cavus: postural deviation of the foot and ankle characterized by excessive medial arch and foot supination.

Pes planus: postural deviation of the foot and ankle characterized by decreased medial arch and excessive foot pronation.

Phosphate: mineral that is stored in bones, making up their cement along with calcium.

Physiological movements: gross movements of joints through the cardinal planes.

Physiology: the study of an organism's function.

Pivot joint: synovial joint characterized by a cylindrical segment of bone that fits into a corresponding cavity of another.

Posterior: regional term indicating toward the back.

Posterior pelvic tilt: postural deviation characterized by backward tipping of the pelvic girdle.

Power stroke: ratcheting action that occurs as myosin heads, bound to actin, pull the sarcomere together.

Process: prominence where soft tissue connects to the bone.

Projection: a bump found on a bone that helps form joints.

Prone: position lying face down.

Proprioception: overall awareness of body position.

Proximal: regional term indicating toward the trunk.

Quadriceps angle (Q-angle): angle formed by the line of traction of the quadriceps tendon on the patella and the line of traction of the patellar tendon on the tibial tubercle.

Ramus: bridgelike projection of bone.

Range of motion: the extent of movement possible at a joint.

Reciprocal inhibition: relaxation of a muscle on one side of a joint to accommodate contraction of muscles on the other side of that joint, due to stimulation of the muscle spindles and Golgi tendon organs.

Red bone marrow: loose connective tissue found in the interior cavity of certain types of bones where blood cells are made.

Reflexes: protective mechanisms that occur without thought.

Relative synergist: muscle that has only one or a few of its actions in common with its agonist.

Resistance: source of mechanical energy in a lever system exerted in opposition to force.

Resisted range of motion: joint motion that occurs when the client meets the resistance of the practitioner in attempting to produce movement of a joint, used to determine the health and function of contracting muscles and their corresponding tendons.

Reticular fibers: thin proteins found within connective tissue that resist force in multiple directions, helping to hold structures together.

Ridge: long, narrow soft tissue attachment site on a bone.

Right lymphatic duct: one of two terminal lymph vessels. It resides on the right side of the neck and empties into the right brachiocephalic vein in the chest.

Right rotation: joint movement of the spine on the transverse plane around a longitudinal axis that turns the spine to the right.

Roll: accessory joint motion that occurs when a series of points on one bony surface come in contact with a corresponding series of points on another.

Ruffini corpuscle: mechanoreceptor located throughout joint capsules that detect distortion and monitor joint position.

431

Saddle joint: synovial joint characterized by two bony surfaces that are concave in one direction and convex in the other.

Sagittal axis: imaginary line that intersects the frontal plane at a right angle around which abduction and adduction occurs.

Sagittal plane: plane of movement that divides the body vertically into right and left halves.

Sarcolemma: cell membrane of a muscle fiber that regulates chemical transport into and out of the fiber.

Sarcomere: functional unit of a muscle fiber, which includes structures from one Z line to the next.

Sarcoplasm: cytoplasm of a muscle cell.

Sarcoplasmic reticulum: network of fluid-filled chambers that covers each myofibril and stores calcium ions that help trigger muscle contractions.

Scoliosis: postural deviation characterized by lateral deviation and sometimes rotation of the spine.

Scapulohumeral rhythm: coordinated movement between the scapulothoracic and glenohumeral joints.

Screw-home mechanism: locking of the tibiofemoral joint through external rotation of the tibia.

Second-class lever: mechanical system characterized by a force on one end, the axis on the other end, and the resistance between the two.

Sensory epithelium: tissue containing specialized cells that are able to perceive and conduct specific stimuli.

Sesamoid bone: bone that is encased in tendon and functions to improve the leverage and strength of muscles that it contacts.

Sensory nerve: type of nerve that monitors the internal and external environment and relays this data to the brain.

Short bones: cube-shaped bones composed mainly of spongy bone that allow fine, gliding movements.

Skeletal muscle: voluntary muscle that creates movements at joints.

Skin: continuous structure that covers the body, protecting it from outside invaders and radiation, helps regulate internal temperature, excretes certain waste products, and facilitates interaction with the outside environment.

Sliding filament theory: explanation of how contractile proteins within the thick and thin filaments of the myofibrils bind and release to produce shortening in the sarcomere and result in muscle contractions.

Slow-twitch fiber: muscle fiber that uses aerobic energy production and is slow to contract and resistant to fatigue.

Smooth muscle: involuntary muscle that aid in digestion, urinary excretion, reproduction, circulation, and breathing.

Spin: accessory motion that occurs when one surface rotates clockwise or counterclockwise around a stationary longitudinal axis.

Spine: short, sharp, thornlike process of bone.

Spongy bone: a three-dimensional latticework of porous bony tissue filled with red bone marrow.

Spongy endfeel: abnormal endfeel characterized by a squishy or boggy endfeel.

Springy block: abnormal endfeel characterized by a rubbery or bouncy stoppage that occurs prior to end range.

Springy endfeel: limiting factor of joint movement being the stretching of muscles or tendons.

Stance phase: phase of gait characterized by weight being fully supported by the lower extremity.

Static stabilizer: structure that limits movement by resisting stretch.

Striation: visible alternating dark and light fibers within cardiac and skeletal muscle tissue.

Subserous fascia: dense connective tissue that separates the deep fascia from the membranes that line the thoracic and abdominal cavities.

Summation: process of recruiting more and more motor units to increase force production.

Superficial: regional term indicating closer to the surface.

Superficial fascia: loose connective tissue that lies directly under the dermis of this skin and stores fat and water and creates a passageway for nerves and vessels.

Superior: regional term indicating toward the top.

Supine: position of lying face up.

Supportive connective tissue: strong, solid connective tissue that contains calcium salts deposited in its ground substance.

Surface epithelium: tissue that contains sheetlike layers of cells located on the internal or external body surfaces functioning as a barrier or secretor.

Sutures: continuous periosteal connections between bones.

Swing phase: phase of gait characterized by leg lifting and moving forward to position for heel strike.

Symphysis: fibrocartilaginous union between the bones forming a joint.

Synapse: functional membrane to membrane contact between one nerve cell and another nerve cell, muscle cell, gland, or sensory receptor cell.

Synaptic cleft: space between the axon terminal and the postsynaptic membrane.

Synarthrotic joint: joints where articulating surfaces are very close together.

Syndesmosis: fibrous joints held together with cord or sheet of connective tissue.

Synergist: muscle that assists with the function of its agonist by stabilizing, steering, or contributing to a particular joint movement.

Synostosis: osseous union between the bones forming a joint.

Synovial fluid: lubricant found in bursae and synovial joints that decreases friction and creates gliding movements between structures.

Synovial joint: most mobile type of joint characterized by having a joint capsule, large joint cavity, and synovial fluid.

Synovial membrane: inner portion of a synovial joint capsule that produces synovial fluid.

Tendon: convergence of the dense connective tissue of myofascia that connects muscle to bone.

Thermogenesis: heat production in the body.

Thick filament: one of the contractile elements in muscular fibers composed to the protein myosin.

Thin filament: one of the contractile elements in muscular fibers composed of the protein actin.

Third-class lever: mechanical system characterized by a resistance on one end, the axis on the other end, and the force between the two.

Thixotropy: the ability of ground substance to become more liquid as movement and temperature of tissue increases.

Thoracic duct: largest lymphatic vessel in the body and one of two terminal vessels that empty into the brachiocephalic vein.

Tissue: a group of cells that share a similar structure and function.

Toe-off: pushing off of foot of trail leg for propulsion during gait.

Trabeculae: osseous struts that form and reform according to lines of stress and work like braces.

Transverse plane: plane of movement that divides the body horizontally into superior and inferior halves.

Transverse tubules: network of tubules that run at right angles to sarcomeres and transmit nerve impulses from the sarcolemma to the cell interior.

Triangular muscles: muscles with fiber arrangements that start at a broad base then converge to a single point.

Triaxial: able to move in all three planes of motion (sagittal, frontal, and transverse).

Trochanter: rounded attachment site on a bone.

Tropomyosin: protein that covers binding sites on actin molecules during rest.

Troponin: protein that keeps tropomyosin in place over actin's binding sites during rest, and moves it out of the way to allow muscle contraction.

Tubercle: rounded attachment site on a bone.

Tuberosity: rounded attachment site on a bone.

Uniaxial: able to move in a single plane of motion.

Unipennate: pennate muscle with fibers running obliquely from one side of a central tendon.

Vestibular apparatus: structures within the inner ear that interpret stimuli regarding head position and movement.

Volkmann's canals: channels that run perpendicular to the Haversian canals in compact bone and complete the pathway from the surface of the bone to its interior. Also called *perforating canals*.

Voluntary: under conscious control.

Wolff's Law: principle that describes the adaptations of bone as a result of stresses placed upon them, such as compression from gravity and tension from muscles and ligaments.

Wormian bone: small, irregular bone found along the sutures of the cranium.

Agur AMR, Dalley AF. *Grant's Atlas of Anatomy.* 11th Ed. Philadelphia: Lippincott, Williams & Wilkins; 2005.

American College of Sports Medicine. *ACSM's Resources for the Personal Trainer.* 2nd Ed. Thompson WR, Baldwin KE, Pire NI, et al., eds. Philadelphia: Lippincott, Williams & Wilkins; 2007.

Aminaka N, Gribble PA. Patellar taping, patellofemoral pain syndrome, lower extremity kinematics, and dynamic postural control. *J Athl Train.* 2008;43(1):21–28.

Archer P. *Therapeutic Massage in Athletics.* Philadelphia: Lippincott, Williams & Wilkins; 2007.

Behnke RS. *Kinetic Anatomy.* 2nd Ed. Champaign: Human Kinetics; 2006.

Benjamin MH, Toumi JR, Ralphs G, et al. Where tendons and ligaments meet bone: attachment sits ('entheses') in relation to exercise and/or mechanical load. *J Anat.* 2006;208(4):471–490.

Bernasconi SM, Tordi NR, Parratee FM, et al. Effects of two devices on the surface electromyography responses of eleven shoulder muscles during azarian in gymnastics. *J Strength Cond R.* 2006;20(1): 53–57.

Biel A. *Trail Guide to the Body.* 3rd Ed. Boulder: Books of Discovery; 2005.

Bongers PM. The cost of shoulder pain at work: variation in work tasks and good job opportunities are essential for prevention. *BMJ.* 2001;322(7278):64–65.

Boyde A. The real response of bone to exercise. *J Anat.* 2003;203(2):173–189.

Braun MB, Simonson S. *Introduction to Massage Therapy.* Philadelphia: Lippincott, Williams & Wilkins; 2005.

Brumitt J, Meira E. Scapula stabilization rehab exercise prescription. *Strength Cond J.* 2006;28(3):62–65.

Chandler J, Brown LE. *Conditioning for Strength and Human Performance.* Philadelphia: Lippincott, Williams & Wilkins; 2008.

Chek P. Corrective postural training and the massage therapist. *Massage Therapy Journal.* 1995;34(3):83.

Clarkson H. *Joint Motion and Function: A Research-Based Practical Guide.* Baltimore: Lippincott, Williams & Wilkins; 2005

Clay JH, Pounds DM. *Basic Clinical Massage Therapy: Integrating Anatomy and Treatment.* 2nd Ed. Philadelphia: Lippincott, Williams & Wilkins; 2008.

Cogley RM, Archambault TA, Fiberger JF, et al. Comparison of muscle activation using various hand positions during the push-up exercise. *J Strength Cond R.* 2005;19(3):628–633.

Cohen BJ. *Memmler's The Structure and Function of the Human Body.* 8th Ed. Philadelphia: Lippincott, Williams & Wilkins; 2005.

Cote KP, Brunet II ME, Gansneder BM, et al. Effects of pronated and supinated foot postures on static and dynamic posture stability. *J Athl Train.* 2005; 40(1):41–46.

Davies GJ, Zillmer DA. Functional progression of a patient through a rehabilitation program. *Orthop Phys Ther Clin N Am.* 2000;9: 103–118.

Devan MR, Pescatello LS, Faghri P, et al. A prospective study of overuse knee injuries among female athletes with muscle imbalances and structural abnormalities. *J Athl Train.* 2004;39(3):263–267.

Drysdale CL, Earl JE, Hertel J. Surface electromyographic activity of the abdominal muscles during pelvic-tilt and abdominal hollowing exercises. *J Athl Train.* 2004;39(1):32–36.

Eroschenko VP. *diFiores' Atlas of Histology with Functional Correlations.* 10th Ed. Philadelphia: Lippincott, Williams & Wilkins; 2005.

Fairclough J, Hayashi K, Toumi H, et al. The functional anatomy of the iliotibial band during flexion and extension of the knee: implications for understanding iliotibial band syndrome. *J Anat.* 2006;208(3): 309–316.

Falla D, Jull G, Russell T, et al. Effect of neck exercise on sitting posture in patients with chronic neck pain. *Phys Ther.* 2007;87:408–417.

Floyd RT. *Manual of Structural Kinesiology.* 16th Ed. Boston: McGraw-Hill; 2007.

Frost HM. From Wolff's law to the Utah paradigm: insights about bone physiology and its clinical applications. *Anat Rec.* 2001;262(4):398–419.

Grezios AZ, Gissis IT, Sotiropoulos AA, et al. Muscle-contraction properties in overarm throwing movements. *J Strength Cond R.* 2006;20(1):117–123.

Hanson AM, Padua DA, Blackburn JT, et al. Muscle Activation During Side-Step Cutting Maneuvers in Male and Female Soccer Athletes. *J Athl Train.* 2008;43(2):133–143.

Hendrickson T. *Massage for Orthopedic Conditions.* Baltimore: Lippincott, Williams & Wilkins; 2003.

Hertel J, Gay MR, Denegar CR. Differences in postural control during single-leg stance among healthy individuals with different foot types. *J Athl Train.* 2002; 37(2):129–132.

Hertel J. Functional anatomy, patho-mechanics, and pathophysiology of lateral ankle instability. *J Athl Train.* 2002;37(4):364–375.

Hoppenfeld S. *Physical Examination of the Spine & Extremities.* Norwalk: Appleton & Lange; 1976.

Jeran JJ, Chetlin RD. Training the shoulder complex in baseball pitchers: a sport-specific approach. *Strength Cond J.* 2005;27(4): 14–31.

Juhan D. *Job's Body.* 3rd Ed. Barrytown, NY: Station Hill; 2003.

Kendall FP, et al. *Muscles: Testing and Function with Posture and Pain.* 5th Ed. Baltimore: Lippincott, Williams & Wilkins; 2005.

Knudson DV, Morrison CS. *Qualitative Analysis of Human Movement.* 2nd Ed. Champaign: Human Kinetics; 2002.

Konrad P, Schmitz K, Denner A. Neuromuscular Evaluation of Trunk-Training Exercises. *J Athl Train.* 2001;36(2):109–118.

Lee TC, Staines A, Taylor D. Bone adaptation to load: microdamage as stimulus for bone remodeling. *J Anat.* 2002;201(6):437–446.

Magee DJ. *Orthopedic Physical Assessment.* 2nd Ed. Philadelphia: Saunders; 1992.

Mansell J, Tierney RT, Sitler MR, et al. Resistance training and head-neck segment dynamic stabilization in male and female collegiate soccer players. *J Athl Train.* 2005; 40(4):310–319.

Marieb EN. *Essentials of Human Anatomy & Physiology.* 8th Ed. San Francisco: Pearson; 2006.

McArdle WD, Katch FI, Katch VL. *Essentials of Exercise Physiology.* 2nd Ed. Baltimore: Lippincott, Williams & Wilkins; 2000.

McMullen J, Uhl TL. A kinetic chain approach for shoulder rehabilitation. *J Athl Train.* 2000;35(3):329–337.

Mills SE. *Histology for Pathologists.* 3rd Ed. Philadelphia: Lippincott, Williams & Wilkins; 2007.

Moore KL, Dalley AF II. *Clinically Oriented Anatomy. 4th Ed.* Baltimore: Lippincott, Williams & Wilkins; 1999.

Moss RI, DeVita P, Dawson ML. A biomechanical analysis of patellofemoral stress syndrome." *J Athl Train. 1992;*27(1):64–66, 68–69.

Muscolino J. The effects of postural distortion. *Massage Therapy Journal.* 2006;45(2):167.

Muscolino JE. *Kinesiology: The Skeletal System and Muscle Function.* St. Louis: Mosby; 2006.

Muscolino JE. *The Muscular System Manual: The Skeletal Muscles of the Human Body: 2nd Ed.* St. Louis: Elsevier; 2006.

Myers JB, Pasquale MR, Laudner KG, et al. On-the-field resistance-tubing exercises for throwers: an electromyographic analysis. *J Athl Train.* 2005;40(1):15–22.

Myers TW. *Anatomy Trains: Myofascial Meridians for Manual and Movement Therapists.* New York: Churchill Livingstone; 2001.

National Academy of Sports Medicine. *NASM Essentials of Personal Fitness Training.* 3rd Ed. Clark MA, Lucett SC, Corn RJ, eds. Philadelphia: Lippincott, Williams & Wilkins, 2008.

National Strength and Conditioning Association. *Essentials of Strength Training and Conditioning.* 2nd Ed. Baechle TR, Earle R, eds. Champaign: Human Kinetics; 2000.

National Strength and Conditioning Association. *NSCA's Essentials of Personal Training.* Earle RW, Baechle TR, eds. Champaign: Human Kinetics; 2004.

Netter FH. *Atlas of Human Anatomy.* 2nd Ed. East Hanover: Novartis; 1997.

Oatis CA. *Kinesiology: The Mechanics and Pathomechanics of Human Movement.* Baltimore: Lippincott, Williams & Wilkins; 2004.

Passero PL, Wyman BS, Bell JW, et al. Temporomandibular joint dysfunction syndrome: a clinical report. *Phys Ther.* 1985;65: 1203–1207.

Pettitt R, Dolski A. Corrective neuro-muscular approach to the treatment of iliotibial band friction syndrome: a case report. *J Athl Train.* 2000; 35(1):96–99.

Premkumar K. *The Massage Connection: Anatomy and Physiology.* 2nd Ed. Philadelphia: Lippincott, Williams & Wilkins; 2004.

Prentice WE. *Techniques in Musculo-skeletal Rehabilitation.* New York: McGraw-Hill; 2001.

Richards J, Thewlis D, Selfe J, et al. A biomechanical investigation of a single-limb squat: implications for lower extremity rehabilitation exercises. *J Athl Train.* 2008;43(5): 477–482.

Riemann BL, Lephart SM. The senso-rimotor system, part II: the role of proprioception in motor control and functional joint stability. *J Athl Train.* 2002;37(1):80–84.

Ronai P. Exercise modification and strategies to enhance shoulder function. *Strength Cond J.* 2005;27(4): 36–45.

Ruff C, Holt B, Trinkaus E. Who's afraid of the big bad Wolff? "Wolff's law" and bone functional adaptation. *Am J Phys Anthropol.* 2006;129(4):484–498.

Scannell JP, McGill SM. Lumbar posture-should it and can it, be modified? A study of passive tissue stiffness and lumbar position during activities of daily living. *Phys Ther.* 2003;83:907–917.

Scheumann DW. *The Balanced Body: A Guide to Deep Tissue and Neuromuscular Therapy.* 3rd Ed. Baltimore: Lippincott, Williams & Wilkins; 2007.

Stedman TL. *Stedman's Medical Dictionary for the Health Professions and Nursing: Illustrated.* 5th Ed. Philadelphia: Lippincott, Williams & Wilkins; 2005.

Terry GC, Chopp TM. Functional anatomy of the shoulder. *J Athl Train.* 2000;35(3):248–255.

Tortora GJ, Grabowski SR. *Principles of Anatomy and Physiology*. 8th Ed. New York: Harper Collins; 1996.

Tyson A. Identifying and treating rotator cuff imbalances. *Strenth Cond J*. 2006;28(2):92–95.

Tyson A. Rehab exercise prescription sequencing for shoulder external rotators. *Strength Cond J*. 2005;27(6): 39–41.

Tyson A. The importance of the posterior capsule of the shoulder in overhead athletes. *Strength Cond J*. 2005;27(4):60–62.

Udermann BE, Mayer JM, Graves JE, et al. Quantitative Assessment of Lumbar Paraspinal Muscle Endurance. *J Athl Train*. 2003;38(3):259–262.

Voight ML, Thompson BC. The role of the scapula in the rehabilitation of shoulder injuries. *J Athl Train*. 2000;35(3):364–372.

Wackerhage H, Rennie MJ. How nutrition and exercise maintain the human musculoskeletal mass. *J Anat*. 2006;208(4):417–431.

Weineck J. *Functional Anatomy in Sports*. 2nd Ed. DeKornfield TJ, Trans. St. Louis: Mosby-Year Book; 1990.

Wilmore JH, Costill DL. *Physiology of Sport and Exercise*. 3rd Ed. Champaign: Human Kinetics; 2004.

Zimmerman GR. Carpal tunnel syndrome. *J Athl Train*. 1994;29(1): 22–24, 26–28, 30.

Index

(continued above)

442

443